Neurology and Neurobiology

EDITORS

Victoria Chan-Palay
University Hospital, Zurich

Sanford L. Palay
The Harvard Medical School

ADVISORY BOARD

Albert J. Aguayo
McGill University

Günter Baumgartner
University Hospital, Zurich

Masao Ito
Tokyo University

Tong H. Joh
Cornell University Medical
College, New York

Bruce McEwen
Rockefeller University

William D. Willis, Jr.
The University of Texas,
Galveston

ADVANCES IN NEURAL REGENERATION RESEARCH

ADVANCES IN NEURAL REGENERATION RESEARCH

Proceedings of the Third International Neural Regeneration Symposium, Held at the Asilomar Conference Center, Pacific Grove, California, December 3-7, 1989

Editor

Fredrick J. Seil

Office of Regeneration Research Programs
V.A. Medical Center
Portland, Oregon

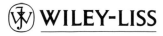

WILEY-LISS

A JOHN WILEY & SONS, INC., PUBLICATION
NEW YORK • CHICHESTER • BRISBANE • TORONTO • SINGAPORE

Address all Inquiries to the Publisher
Wiley-Liss, Inc., 41 East 11th Street, New York, NY 10003

The publication of this volume was facilitated by the authors and editors who submitted the text in a form suitable for direct reproduction without subsequent editing or proofreading by the publisher.

Library of Congress Cataloging-in-Publication Data

International Symposium on Neural Regeneration (3rd : 1989 : Pacific Grove, Calif.)
    Advances in neural regeneration research : proceedings of the Third International Neural Regeneration Symposium, held at the Asilomar Conference Center, Pacific Grove, California, December 3-7, 1989 / editor, Fredrick J. Seil.
        p.   cm. -- (Neurology and neurobiology ; v. 60)
    Includes bibliographical references.
    Includes index.
    ISBN 0-471-56849-X
    1. Nerves--Regeneration--Congresses.   I. Seil, Fredrick J.
II. Title.   III. Series.
    [DNLM: 1. Nerve Regeneration--congresses.   W1 NE337B v. 60 / WL 102 I6193a]
QP363.5.I58   1989
616.8--dc20
DNLM/DLC
for Library of Congress   90-12704
                                                              CIP

Contents

Contributors

J. Atkinson, Department of Neurosurgery, The Robert S. Dow Neurological Sciences Institute, Good Samaritan Hospital and Medical Center, Portland, OR 97210 **[329]**

Rita J. Balice-Gordon, Department of Anatomy and Neurobiology, Washington University School of Medicine, St. Louis, MO 63110 **[33]**

Utpal Banerjee, Department of Biology and Molecular Biology Institute, University of California Los Angeles, Los Angeles, CA 90024 **[309]**

Michael S. Beattie, Department of Anatomy and Surgery and the Neuroscience Program, Ohio State University, Columbus, OH 43210 **[57]**

Hilary P. Benton, MRC Molecular Neurobiology Unit, MRC Centre, Cambridge CB2 2QH, England **[277]**

Robert R. Bernhardt, Department of Biology and Institute of Gerontology, University of Michigan, Ann Arbor, MI 48109-1048 **[5]**

Jacqueline C. Bresnahan, Department of Anatomy and the Neuroscience Program, Ohio State University, Columbus, OH 43210 **[57]**

Jeremy P. Brockes, Ludwig Institute for Cancer Research, London W1P 8BT, England **[253]**

Michael Brown, Department of Physiology, University of Oxford, Oxford OX1 3PT, England **[125]**

P.B. Brown, Department of Physiology, West Virginia University Health Sciences Center, Morgantown, WV 26506 **[329]**

David Burke, Department of Neurology, The Prince Henry Hospital and School of Medicine, University of New South Wales, Sydney 2036, Australia **[379]**

Ajay B. Chitnis, Department of Biology and Institute of Gerontology, University of Michigan, Ann Arbor, MI 48109-1048 **[5]**

The numbers in brackets are the opening page numbers of the contributors' articles.

Brian Y. Cooper, Department of Neuroscience and Center for Neurobiological Sciences, University of Florida College of Medicine, Gainesville, FL 32610 **[355]**

Carl W. Cotman, Department of Psychobiology, University of California, Irvine, CA 92717 **[1]**

Samuel David, Centre for Research in Neuroscience, McGill University, and The Montreal General Hospital Research Institute, Montreal, Quebec, Canada H3G 1A4 **[185]**

Milan R. Dimitrijevic, Division of Restorative Neurology and Human Neurobiology, Baylor College of Medicine, Houston, TX 77030 **[391]**

Eduardo Eidelberg, Division of Neurosurgery, Audie L. Murphy Memorial Veteran's Hospital, and the University of Texas Health Sciences Center at San Antonio, San Antonio, TX 78284 **[369]**

Sergey Fedoroff, Department of Anatomy, University of Saskatchewan, Saskatoon, Saskatchewan S7N 0W0 **[161]**

S. Goderie, Division of Neurosurgery and Program in Neuroscience, Albany Medical College, Albany, NY 12208 **[199]**

Harry G. Goshgarian, Department of Anatomy and Cell Biology, Wayne State University School of Medicine, Detroit, MI 48201 **[341]**

Manuel B. Graeber, Max-Planck-Institute for Psychiatry, 8033 Martinsried, Federal Republic of Germany; present address: Center for Neurological Diseases, Brigham and Women's Hospital and Harvard Medical School, Boston, MA 02115 **[215]**

Anthony Graham, Lab of Eukaryotic Molecular Genetics, National Institute for Medical Research, London NW7 1AA, England **[291]**

Theo Hagg, Department of Biology, University of California San Diego School of Medicine, La Jolla, CA 92093 **[87]**

Michael R. Hanley, MRC Molecular Neurobiology Unit, MRC Centre, Cambridge CB2 2QH, England **[277]**

Bastian Hengerer, Department of Neurochemistry, Max-Planck-Institute for Psychiatry, 8033 Martinsried, Federal Republic of Germany **[125]**

Rolf Heumann, Department of Neurochemistry, Max-Planck-Institute for Psychiatry, 8033 Martinsried, Federal Republic of Germany **[125]**

H. Hirata, Department of Neurosurgery, The Robert S. Dow Neurological Sciences Institute, Good Samaritan Hospital and Medical Center, Portland, OR 97210; present address: Department of Anesthesiology, Yale University School of Medicine, New Haven, CT 06510 **[329]**

Paul Hunt, Lab of Eukaryotic Molecular Genetics, National Institute for Medical Research, London NW7 1AA, England **[291]**

H. Kettenmann, Institut für Neurobiologie, Universität Heidelberg,
Federal Republic of Germany [199]

H.K. Kimelberg, Division of Neurosurgery and Program in Neuroscience,
Albany Medical College, Albany, NY
12208 [199]

Georg W. Kreutzberg, Max-Planck-
Institute for Psychiatry, 8033 Martinsried, Federal Republic of Germany
[215]

Robb Krumlauf, Lab of Eukaryotic
Molecular Genetics, National Institute
for Medical Research, London NW7
1AA, England [291]

Albert T. Kulics, Department of
Physiology and Neurobiology, Northeastern Ohio University College of
Medicine, Rootstown, OH 44272
[355]

John Y. Kuwada, Department of
Biology and Institute of Gerontology,
University of Michigan, Ann Arbor,
MI 48109-1048 [5]

Story C. Landis, Department of
Neurosciences, Case Western Reserve
University School of Medicine,
Cleveland, OH 44106 [17]

M. Gail Leedy, Department of Anatomy, Ohio State University, Columbus, OH 43210 [57]

Jeff W. Lichtman, Department of
Anatomy and Neurobiology, Washing-
ton University School of Medicine,
St. Louis, MO 63110 [33]

Dan Lindholm, Department of Neur-
ochemistry, Max-Planck-Institute for
Psychiatry, 8033 Martinsried, Federal
Republic of Germany [125]

Mark A. Lissens, Division of Restor-
ative Neurology and Human Neurobi-
ology, Baylor College of Medicine,
Houston, TX 77030; present address:
Department of Physical Medicine and
Rehabilitation, University Hospitals
Leuven, Leuven, Belgium [391]

Francis J. Liuzzi, Department of
Anatomy and Neurobiology and Neur-
osurgery, Eastern Virginia Medical
School, Norfolk, VA 23501 [225]

Marston Manthorpe, Department of
Biology, University of California San
Diego School of Medicine, La Jolla,
CA 92093 [87]

H. Peter Matthiessen, Department of
Neurology, Molecular Neurobiology
Laboratory, University of Düsseldorf,
D-4000 Düsseldorf, Federal Republic
of Germany [147]

W. Barry McKay, Division of Restorative Neurology and Human Neurobiology, Baylor College of
Medicine, Houston, TX 77030 [391]

Ronald L. Meyer, Department of
Developmental and Cell Biology,
Developmental Biology Center, University of California, Irvine, CA
92717 [43]

Robert H. Miller, Center for Neuroscience, Case Western Reserve University School of Medicine, Cleveland, OH 44106 **[171]**

David Muir, Department of Biology, University of California San Diego School of Medicine, La Jolla, CA 92093 **[87]**

H.W. Müller, Department of Neurology, Molecular Neurobiology Laboratory, University of Düsseldorf, D-4000 Düsseldorf, Federal Republic of Germany **[147]**

Junichi Nabekura, Department of Anatomy and Neurobiology, Washington University School of Medicine, St. Louis, MO 63110 **[33]**

Monica M. Oblinger, Department of Cell Biology and Anatomy, The Chicago Medical School, North Chicago, IL 60064 **[257]**

E. O'Connor, Division of Neurosurgery and Program in Neuroscience, Albany Medical College, Albany, NY 12208 **[199]**

Hitoshi Okamoto, Department of Biology and Institute of Gerontology, University of Michigan, Ann Arbor, MI 48109-1048 **[5]**

Dörte Otto, Department of Anatomy and Cell Biology, University of Marburg, 6-3550 Marburg, Federal Republic of Germany **[115]**

S. Pang, Institute of Biophysics, Academica Sinica, Beijing, China **[199]**

Nancy Papalopulu, Lab of Eukaryotic Molecular Genetics, National Institute for Medical Research, London NW7 1AA, England **[291]**

Inder Perkash, Department of Surgery, Stanford University, and Spinal Cord Injury Service, VA Medical Center, Palo Alto, CA 94304 **[325]**

Hugh Perry, Department of Experimental Psychology, Oxford University, Oxford OX1 3PT, England **[125]**

Linda L. Phillips, Department of Neurosurgery, University of Virginia Health Sciences Center, Charlottesville, VA 22908 **[71]**

L.M. Pubols, Department of Neurosurgery, Robert S. Dow Neurological Sciences Institute, Good Samaritan Hospital and Medical Center, Portland, OR 97210 **[329]**

Mark M. Rich, Department of Anatomy and Neurobiology, Washington University School of Medicine, St. Louis, MO 63110 **[33]**

J. Murdoch Ritchie, Department of Pharmacology, Yale University School of Medicine, New Haven, CT 06510 **[237]**

Ronald D. Rogge, Department of Biology and Molecular Biology Institute, University of California Los Angeles, Los Angeles, CA 90024 **[309]**

Corinne Schmalenbach, Department of Neurology, Molecular Neurobiology Laboratory, University of Düsseldorf, D-4000 Düsseldorf, Federal Republic of Germany **[147]**

Fredrick J. Seil, Office of Regeneration Research Programs, V.A. Medical Center, Portland, OR 97201 [**xvii**]

D.A. Simone, Department of Neurosurgery, The Robert S. Dow Neurological Sciences Institute, Good Samaritan Hospital and Medical Center, Portland, OR 97210 [**329**]

George M. Smith, Center for Neuroscience, Case Western Reserve University School of Medicine, Cleveland, OH 44106 [**171**]

Oswald Steward, Department of Neuroscience, University of Virginia Health Sciences Center, Charlottesville, VA 22908 [**71**]

Enrique R. Torre, Department of Neuroscience and Neurological Surgery, University of Virginia Health Sciences Center, Charlottesville, VA 22908 [**71**]

Patricia A. Trimmer, Departments of Neuroscience and Neurological Surgery, University of Virginia Health Sciences Center, Charlottesville, VA 22908 [**71**]

Klaus Unsicker, Department of Anatomy and Cell Biology, University of Marburg, 6-3550 Marburg, Federal Republic of Germany [**115**]

Peter van Mier, Department of Anatomy and Neurobiology, Washington University School of Medicine, St. Louis, MO 63110 [**33**]

Silvio Varon, Department of Biology, University of California San Diego School of Medicine, La Jolla, CA 92093 [**87**]

Charles J. Vierck, Jr., Department of Neuroscience and Center for Neurobiological Sciences, University of Florida College of Medicine, Gainesville, FL 32610 [**355**]

Patricia Ann Walicke, Department of Neuroscience, University of California San Diego, La Jolla, CA 92093 [**103**]

Barry L. Whitsel, Department of Physiology, University of North Carolina School of Medicine, Chapel Hill, NC 27514 [**355**]

David Wilkinson, Lab of Eukaryotic Molecular Genetics, National Institute for Medical Research, London NW7 1AA, England [**291**]

Johnson Wong, Department of Cell Biology and Anatomy, The Chicago Medical School, North Chicago, IL 60064 [**257**]

Preface

Advances in neural regeneration research have occurred at a pace so rapid and over so many fronts that designing a program for the third symposium in a series of alternate-year symposia on neural regeneration was not a difficult task. What was difficult was restricting the scope of the symposium to five major topic areas. The five categories selected represent basic science and clinical areas of notable progress, and include (1) axonal growth and synaptic plasticity, (2) neural growth promoters and inhibitors, (3) spontaneous recovery of function after spinal cord injury, (4) astrocyte reactions in injury and regeneration, and (5) molecular mechanisms relevant to regeneration.

The chapters in this volume represent the invited papers presented at the Third International Symposium on Neural Regeneration held December 3–7, 1989, at the Asilomar Conference Center, Pacific Grove, California. The first chapter in each section is an introductory overview of the topic by the individual who chaired that session during the symposium. The remaining chapters review developments in specific areas under the major topic headings. The coverage of each of these areas is comprehensive and current, providing the reader with an up-to-date assessment of the status of the field.

What could, regrettably, not be included in this volume because of space constraints are the abstracts of over 60 posters displayed at the symposium. Needless to say, these posters contributed greatly to the interest, excitement, and success of the conference, and thanks are due to the poster exhibitors for their contributions. Also to be thanked for their contributions to the symposium are those speakers with a special role in the conference, namely the keynote speaker, Dr. Eric Shooter; the featured speakers, Drs. Barry Arnason, Stanley Kater, and Geoffrey Raisman; and the summary speaker, Dr. Georg Kreutzberg.

I am especially indebted to the Program Committee for their efforts in planning the symposium. This committee consisted of members of the VA Office of Regeneration Research Programs Advisory Board, including Drs.

Kevin Barron, Bruce Carlson, Lawrence Eng, Irvine McQuarrie, Inder Perkash, Paul Reier, David Stocum, Betty Uzman, and Stephen Waxman, and Dr. Mary Ellen Michel of the National Institute of Neurological Disorders and Stroke.

Finally, I would like to acknowledge those sponsoring organizations that made the symposium possible. They are the U.S. Department of Veterans Affairs (Medical Research Service), the Paralyzed Veterans of America (Spinal Cord Research Foundation), the National Institutes of Health (National Institute of Neurological Disorders and Stroke), and the American Paralysis Association (Carter-Wallace Foundation). The continuing support and promotion of neural regeneration research by these organizations is greatly appreciated.

Fredrick J. Seil

Advances in Neural Regeneration
Research, pages 1–4
© 1990 Wiley-Liss, Inc.

AXONAL GROWTH AND SYNAPTIC PLASTICITY

Carl W. Cotman

Department of Psychobiology, University

of California, Irvine, California 92717

The functional capacity of the central nervous system (CNS) depends on the state of its circuitries. These must be properly developed, maintained, and modified throughout life and even restored, insofar as possible, after injury. This section will focus on current topics related to issues in the development and plasticity of neuronal circuits. To understand the potential mechanisms facilitating the repair of the nervous system, one must understand how it grows early in life. Recent data shows, in fact, that some of the same mechanisms used in development are reactivated in the adult CNS after injury. Accordingly, contributions in this section deal with central issues in development as well as in regeneration and axon sprouting.

In essence, neurons early in life must locate their targets, survive, and differentiate as functional units, as a team of input cells and their target cells. The establishment and regeneration of the proper circuitry depends on the behavior of the growth cone at one level and, at the next level, on successful synapse formation and neuronal differentiation. John Kuwada and coworkers discuss work on zebra fish embryo, an elegant preparation for the study of pathfinding mechanisms that direct growth cones to their targets. This preparation has the advantage of being transparent, so fiber growth can be followed *in situ*. Such approaches combined with genetic mutations promise to reveal new basic mechanisms.

Target cells in both the peripheral and CNS play a critical role in setting the number of neurons which survive during development. Target cells also produce a factor(s) which influences, in part, the phenotype of the surviving neurons as described in the chapter by Story Landis. The initially noradrenergic character of the sympathetic neurons innervating the sweat glands is suppressed as these cells acquire subsequent cholinergic and peptidergic functions. The data on the development of phenotype in the sympathetic neurons innervating the sweat gland shows how this system makes a particular decision. The data may also provide clues on how other systems proceed to establish their neurotransmitter characteristics.

In the injured CNS., if neuronal loss is prevented, the optimal reestablishment of neural circuitry depends on the successful regeneration of damaged fibers and successful synapse formation. Recently, several strategies have become available that promote CNS fiber regeneration, e.g., peripheral nerve segments, transplants, artificial bridges, etc. A critical and largely unexplored area is the reestablishment of synaptic connections between axotomized neurons and their targets. Jeff Lichtman and coworkers describe their progress in monitoring this process in the living neuromuscular junction. They have succeeded in studying the kinetics and properties of synapse elimination and have shown that ACh receptors are lost prior to terminal retraction. This raises some intriguing questions on the mechanisms underlying this target-mediated selectivity.

Synapse rearrangement in the course of regeneration has been characterized in several systems. Perhaps the most detailed data is available on regeneration of the goldfish optic nerve after nerve crush. As Ron Meyer describes in his chapter, optic fibers invade the anterior region of the tectum by about 30 days, at which time there is rough topographical order. Over the next month or so, retinotopy improves markedly. It appears that activity plays a key role in the time course of this sorting process, but not the number of connections. NMDA receptor-mediated activity appears to participate in this retinotropic refinement of connections in the goldfish as well as in synaptic plasticity in other developing systems.

Progress on regeneration depends on the capacity to make functional synapses. In this regard, studies on axon sprouting have the potential to provide valuable information on the mechanisms in the mature brain. Sprouting is also interesting as a mechanism in its own right: It may participate, in select cases, in functional recovery. Alternatively, it may compete with regenerating fibers, particularly when sprouted fibers are phenotypically indistinguishable from those regenerating. Jacqueline Bresnahan and coworkers describe their studies on the effect of spinal cord injury on the somatic motor neurons mediating reproductive function and sexual behavior. The goal is to determine if changes in reflex behavior depend on synaptic input and how this might be regulated. Testosterone appears to act as a type of trophic factor in controlling the synaptic input to motor neurons in select nuclei involved in sexual responsiveness.

In recent years, axon sprouting and reactive synaptogenesis have been studied in greatest detail in the hippocampus. Oswald Steward and coworkers describe the various responses elicited in the genes of cytoskeletal proteins potentially involved in reactive growth. The induction or lack thereof illustrates that selectivity is the rule. An unexpected finding is the discovery of glial acidic fibrillary protein induction in zones outside those directly denervated. This contrasts with previous data on the induction of the protein. It suggests that all proteins are not expressed in proportion to their message levels in brain after injury. Other related studies show that a fetal form of several cytoskeletal proteins is induced (Geddes et al., 1990). The signals resulting in such responsiveness are currently unknown. Axonal sprouting and reactive synaptogenesis in some systems may be an ongoing process which can be released or stimulated by injury and which, in select cases, can participate in functional recovery (Cotman et al., 1981; Cotman and Anderson, 1989). The exact role must be evaluated in each case.

A goal of studies on animal models is to better understand the human brain. Recently, Carl Cotman and coworkers have begun to study the hippocampus in the normal aged brain and that of patients with Alzheimer's disease (AD). In AD subjects, neurons in the entorhinal cortex degenerate creating a natural lesion similar to the entorhinal lesion in the rodent brain. It appears as if axon sprouting and many of the accompanying events identified in the rodent brain also occur in the human brain. An exception is the formation of senile plaques, an apparent unfortunate end point of misdirected plasticity mechanisms (Geddes et al., 1986). As studies on animal models progress, it is important to identify similarities and differences as they occur in the course of injury to the human CNS.

REFERENCES

Geddes JW, Wong J, Choi BH, Kim RC, Cotman CW, Miller FD (1990). Increased expression of an embryonic, growth-associated mRNA in Alzheimer's disease. Neurosci Lett 109: 54-61.

Cotman CW, Nieto-Sampedro M, Harris E (1981). Synapse replacement in the nervous system of adult vertebrates. Physiol Rev 61: 684-784.

Cotman CW, Anderson KJ (1989). Neural plasticity and regeneration. In Siegel GJ (ed): "Basic Neurochemistry: Molecular, Cellular, and Medical Aspects, 4th ed.," New York: Raven Press.

Geddes JW, Anderson KJ, Cotman CW (1986). Senile plaques as aberrant sprout stimulating structures. Exper Neurol 94: 767-776.

**Advances in Neural Regeneration
Research, pages 5–16
© 1990 Wiley-Liss, Inc.**

GROWTH CONE GUIDANCE IN A SIMPLE VERTEBRATE NERVOUS SYSTEM

John Y. Kuwada, Hitoshi Okamoto, Robert R.
Bernhardt, and Ajay B. Chitnis
Department of Biology and Institute of
Gerontology, University of Michigan, Ann Arbor,
MI 48109-1048

INTRODUCTION

A number of different extrinsic cues have been shown
to influence the rate and direction of extension by growth
cones in a variety of animals. These include local cues
in the immediate environment of growth cones as well as
long-distance cues; attractive and inhibitory cues; and
cues specific for certain growth cones in addition to
nonspecific cues. Our understanding of these cues has
benefited from the analysis of pathfinding by identifiable
growth cones in relatively simple nervous systems. One
promising system is that of fish embryos where one can
experimentally investigate pathfinding by growth cones of
known identities at the single cell level.

Pathfinding by identified growth cones can be studied
in normal, experimentally manipulated, and mutant fish
embryos. Since the early fish embryo is transparent,
neurons which are 5 to 15 μm in diameter can be readily
visualized in living embryos. These neurons can be
labeled by backfilling them via their axons or by
intracellular injections with a variety of dyes and by
monoclonal antibodies which recognize epitopes on all or
subsets of neurons. These techniques have been utilized
to study growth cone guidance mechanism in the spinal cord
and brain of zebrafish embryos and the fin motor system of
Japanese medaka fish embryos.

PATHFINDING IN THE EMBRYONIC SPINAL CORD

The early (18-20 hr) cord of zebrafish embryos consists of neuroepithelial cells, floor plate cells, and approximately 18 neurons per hemisegment (Bernhardt et al., submitted). By this time 8 to 11 of these early neurons have projected growth cones and fall into 6

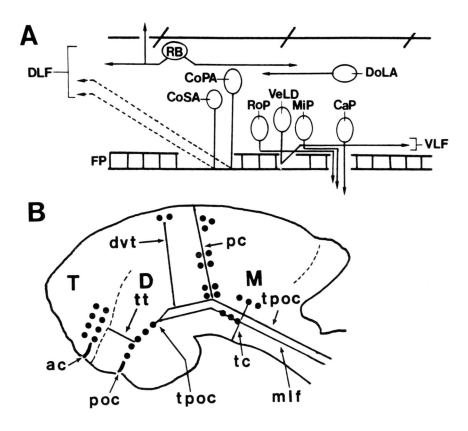

Figure 1. A schematic summarizing the neuronal classes and major axonal tracts in the A. spinal cord and B. brain of zebrafish embryos. In this and all other figures, unless otherwise noted, anterior is left, dorsal is up, the segment borders are indicated by diagonal lines, arrows at the ends of axons indicate that the axons extend further, and contralateral axons are indicated by dashed lines. T, telencephalon; D, diencephalon; M, mesencephalon.

classes of identified neurons (Fig. 1A). These are 3
primary motor neurons (RoP, MiP and CaP; Myers et al.,
1986), approximately 3 mechanosensory Rohon-Beard (RB)
neurons, 1 primary commissural interneuron (CoPA), 0-2
secondary commissural interneurons (CoSA), 0-1 dorsal
longitudinal (DoLA) interneuron, and 1 ventral
longitudinal interneuron (VeLD) (Bernhardt et al.,
submitted). Additionally, there are approximately 20
floor plate (FP) cells, which make up the ventral floor of
the cord and are arranged as a row of cells approximately
3 cells wide (Kuwada et al., in press; Fig. 2C,D) in each
segment. The floor plate cells are amongst the earliest
cells to become distinguishable in the cord and are
evident several hr prior to the first spinal growth cones.
These cells are presumably nonneuronal, extend no
processes, and differ from the other neuroepithelial cells
in shape. Additionally, the middle row of floor plate
cells is antigenically different from other neuroepithelial cells (Charles Kimmel, personal communication).

All the early spinal neurons project growth cones
which extend along precise, cell-specific pathways to
reach their termination sites in the CNS (Kuwada et al.,
submitted). These identified growth cones appear to
bypass some axons but follow others suggesting that they
can distinguish among the different axons they encounter.
Furthermore, analysis of the local environment of
identified growth cones rules out that simple, nonspecific
constraints such as mechanical barriers are responsible
for directionality of axon outgrowth. Most interestingly
the growth cones of the CoPA and VeLD neurons exhibit
cell-specific behaviors in the immediate vicinity of the
floor plate cells (Kuwada et al., in press).

The CoPA neuron projects a single growth cone from the
ventral pole of the cell body at 16-17 hr of development
(Fig. 2A, 3A). After emerging from the soma, the growth
cone extends ventrally along the superficial surface of
the cord between the endfeet of neuroepithelial cells and
the lateral cell bodies of neurons. In doing so it
bypasses the ipsilateral dorsal longitudinal fasciculus
(DLF) consisting of RB and DoLA axons and the ipsilateral
ventral longitudinal fasciculus (VLF) consisting of VeLD
axons. CoPA growth cones extend between the floor plate
cells and the basal lamina to cross the ventral midline.
While in apparent contact with the floor plate cells CoPA

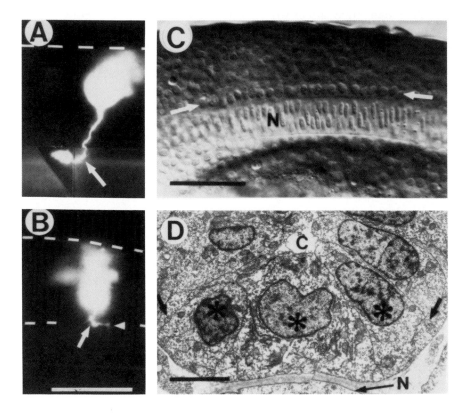

Figure 2. The CoPA and VeLD growth cones exhibit cell-
specific behaviors at the floor plate. A. Lucifer Yellow
filled CoPA neuron with a growth cone just past the
ventral midline from a 19 hr embryo. This is a
photomontage which displays the soma and the contralateral
growth cone, which are at different focal planes,
simultaneously. Arrow, point where the axon crosses the
ventral midline. B. VeLD growth cone which has just
turned posterior at the ventral floor of the cord in a 16
hr embryo. Arrowhead and arrow, leading edge and distal
part of the growth cone, respectively. Scale for A and B,
50 μm. C. Floor plate cells (arrows) from a **live** 17 hr
embryo. Scale, 50 μm. D. EM micrograph of the floor plate
cells (asterisks) in cross-section from a 20 hr embryo.
Arrows point to 2 axonal profiles, which may represent
VeLD axons, in contact with the lateral floor plate cells.
C, central canal; N, notochord; scale, 5 μm.

growth cones turn anterior. The CoPA growth cone then ascends along a rostrodorsal pathway and bypasses the contralateral VLF. When the growth cone reaches the contralateral DLF, it turns onto it and ascends toward the brain.

The VeLD neuron like the CoPA neuron projects a single growth cone from the ventral pole of its cell body (Fig. 2B, 3B). This growth cone extends towards the floor plate but does not cross the midline; rather it turns posterior along the floor plate cells in the ipsilateral cord. The VeLD growth cone extends along a caudodorsal pathway to reach the VLF and descends in the VLF.

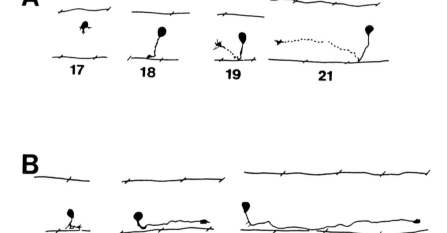

Figure 3. Development of CoPA and VeLD neurons. Camera lucida drawings of Lucifer Yellow-filled neurons at various stages (hr) in development. A. CoPA neuron. Scale, 50 μm. B. VeLD neurons. Scale, 50 μm.

These observations suggest that the floor plate may have multiple, cell-specific effects on identified spinal growth cones in the zebrafish embryo. More specifically our work has generated several interesting, testable hypotheses. 1) Floor plate cells attract some growth cones (CoPA and VeLD) to extend towards the ventral midline but not others. 2) Floor plate cells induce the CoPA growth cones to cross the midline and make cell-specific turns. 3) Floor plate cells inhibit the VeLD growth cone from crossing the midline and instead induce it to turn posterior. 4) Interactions with the floor plate cells may be necessary for commissural growth cones to turn onto the appropriate longitudinal pathway. These hypotheses can be tested by 1) laser ablation of floor plate cells, 2) transplantation of floor plate cells to ectopic sites, and 3) examination of Cyclops mutants in which the floor plate fails to develop (Charles Kimmel, personal communication). The results of such experiments are especially interesting in light of the finding that the floor plate can attract the growth cones of commissural neurons in the spinal cord of rat embryos (Dodd and Jessell, 1988; Tessier-Lavigne et al., 1988).

PATHFINDING IN THE EMBRYONIC BRAIN

The brain of early zebrafish embryos is also simple, and at 28 hr of development the forebrain and midbrain contains 8 main axonal tracts, which are arranged as a set of longitudinal tracts connected by commissures: anterior commissure (AC), telencephalic tract (TT), postoptic commissure (POC), tract of the postoptic commissure (TPOC), dorso-ventral diencephalic tract (DVT), posterior commissure (PC), median longitudinal fasciculus (MLF), and ventral tegmental commissure (TC) (Fig 1B; Chitnis and Kuwada, in press). Each tract is established by identified clusters of approximately 2 to 12 neurons found in discrete regions of the brain. These identified clusters of neurons project axons in a defined direction appropriate for the cluster and have axons with stereotyped trajectories suggesting that their growth cones follow cell-specific routes. For example, the three earliest tracts form at 17 hr when neurons in the ventral diencephalon and anterior tegmentum project axons posteriorly to establish the TPOC and the MLF, respectively; and telencephalic neurons project axons toward the ventral diencephalon to establish the TT.

Pathfinding by neurons whose growth cones extend into already established tracts also follow cell-specific routes. For example, neurons of the nucleus of the posterior commissure (nuc PC), which is located in the dorsolateral diencephalon just anterior to the tectum, project ventrally directed growth cones. These growth cones arrive at a site in the anterior tegmentum where 4 tracts meet (Fig. 4). At this site they could in principle turn anteriorly or posteriorly into the TPOC, posteriorly into the MLF, or towards the ventral midline in a ventral tegmental commissure. Yet nuc PC growth

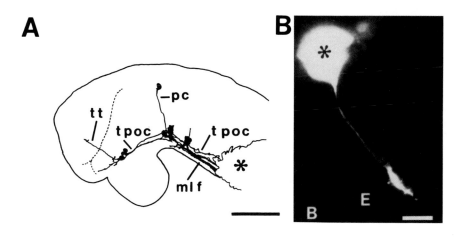

Figure 4. Nuc PC growth cones turn posterior onto the TPOC in the anterior tegmentum. A. A nuc PC neuron with an axon in the TPOC. Drawing of the TPOC bundles, MLF, and posterior commissure (open arrow) backlabeled with an application (asterisk) of the lipophilic dye, diI, in the hindbrain. The ventral TPOC bundle is contiguous with the MLF. Ventral tegmental commissure is not labeled by this application. Scale, 80 μm. B. LY-filled nuc PC neuron with its growth cone at the intersection of tracts in the anterior tegmentum. E, eye; scale, 20 μm.

cones always turn posteriorly into the TPOC. The pattern of pathfinding by these growth cones suggests the hypothesis that the growth cones of identified clusters of neurons establish the simple set of early tracts by selecting cluster-specific pathways in order to reach their targets in the brain. This hypothesis can be tested in the zebrafish brain by elimination of specific tracts like the TPOC and by transplanting identified clusters of neurons to ectopic sites.

PATHFINDING BY FIN MOTOR AXONS

The pectoral fin of Japanese medaka is a simple limb consisting of two muscles. The fin muscles are innervated by motor neurons found in the first 4 spinal segments. The two pools of motor neurons overlap extensively. Like axons in the brain and spinal cord of zebrafish embryos, fin motor axons extend along stereotyped pathways to reach the base of the fin bud in the medaka embryo (Fig. 5; Okamoto and Kuwada, unpublished data). Most interestingly these axons turn so as to form a plexus at the base of the fin bud: S1 axons posterior, S4 axons anterior, and S2 and S3 axons in both directions. Axons emerge from the plexus to innervate the extensor muscle first, then axons emerge to innervate the flexor muscle. Occasionally, a small bundle of S5 axons innervate the fin but at present it is not known if these axons are motor or sensory and why they only ocassionally innervate the fin.

In order to see if the fin bud normally influences outgrowth by fin motor neurons, fin motor axons were examined in mutant embryos missing a normal fin and in wildtype embryos in which fin buds were manipulated. The pl mutant lacks pectoral fins (Tomita, 1982): the fin buds begin to develop but arrest at an early stage when the apical ectodermal ridge has formed but before any other signs of limb differentiation. Despite the early arrest of fin bud development, the fin axons make their turns and fasciculate with each other to form a plexus, but fail to extend beyond the plexus into the abnormal fin bud. This suggests that if the fin bud does exert some influence on motor axon outgrowth, it does so early in fin bud development. Furthermore, development beyond the formation of the apical ectodermal ridge may be necessary for outgrowth from the plexus.

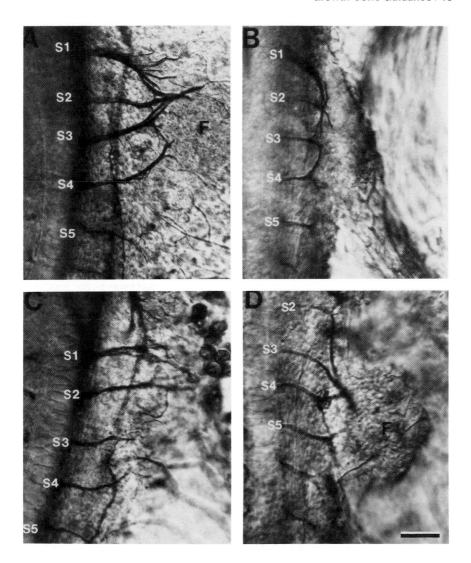

Figure 5. Trajectory of motor nerves from S1-S4 which
innervate the fin bud (F) labeled with an antibody against
acetylated tubulin. Anterior, up; lateral, right; scale,
50 μm. A. Wildtype embryo. B. P1 mutant embryo. C.
Embryo following ablation of fin bud. D. Embryo following
ablation of fin bud and transplantation of another fin bud
in a more posterior position.

In order to see if the early fin bud normally influences outgrowth by the fin motor axons, the fin bud was ablated or ablated and another fin bud transplanted to an ectopic location. The manipulations were performed 4 hr prior to the time motor axons normally made their turns, followed by culturing embryos without their yolk sacs. In control embryos fin motor axons made their normal turns and formed a plexus at the base of the fin bud. However, in the absence of fin buds axons from S1-S4 failed to make their normal turns and did not form a plexus. When fin axons were confronted with an ectopic fin bud, the axons turned towards the ectopic fin bud and formed a plexus at the base of the ectopic fin bud. These experiments suggest that fin motor axons are attracted by the early fin bud via a long-distance cue.

DISCUSSION

So far our analyses of mechanisms of growth cone guidance suggest that multiple mechanisms may be active during pathfinding by neurons in the fish embryo much like for motor axons in the chick (Landmesser, 1988; Tosney and Landmesser, 1984; Tosney, 1987; Tosney, 1988). Earlier experiments involving laser ablation of specific axons in the spinal cord of Medaka embryos demonstrated that specific cell-cell interactions were necessary for pathfinding by a certain class of spinal interneuron (Kuwada, 1986). In the absence of specific axons these interneurons failed to extend their growth cones normally. These results suggested that some growth cones decide which pathway to extend into by contact-mediated recognition of specific axons much like growth cones in the insect CNS (Raper et al., 1983; Harrelson et al., 1988). The description of pathfinding by identified neurons in the brain and spinal cord of zebrafish embryos is consistent with the contact-mediated actions of specific cells on their growth cones. Nuc PC growth cones may choose the TPOC over the MLF and ventral tegmental commissure by selectively fasciculating with the axons of the TPOC. Furthermore, these actions may be both attractive and inhibitory and mediated by the same set of cells. CoPA and VeLD growth cones may be, respectively, instructed to cross the midline and turn anterior or inhibited from crossing the midline and turn posterior by contact with the floor plate cells. In this case the hypothesized inhibition of growth cones is specific for some neurons but not others as with chick growth cones in vitro (Kapfhammer and Raper, 1986) and in vivo (Walter et al., 1987). Finally, the experiments involving the ablation and transplantation of limb buds indicate that long-distance cues also operate in the fish embryo. Limb buds attract fin motor axons at a distance to guide them to the base of the developing fin similar to the attraction of trigeminal axons by the maxillary arch in the mouse embryo (Lumsden and Davies, 1986). Ongoing analysis of the cyclops mutant and ablation and transplantation of floor plate cells in the spinal cord; and elimination of the TPOC axons and transplantation of clusters of brain neurons will test the hypothesized interactions in the CNS. In the future these highly detailed analyses of pathfinding should allow the delineation of many if not all the mechanisms which guide a single growth cone from its initial emergence from the cell body to its arrival at the target.

ACKNOWLEDGMENT

We thank H. Tomita and A. Shima for providing us with the pl mutant. This work was supported by grants from NIH, March of Dimes Birth Defects Foundation, and the Office of the Vice-President for Research of the University of Michigan.

REFERENCES

Bernhardt RR, Chitnis AB, Lindamer LA, Kuwada JY (submitted). Identification of spinal neurons in the embryonic and larval zebrafish. J. Comp. Neurol.
Chitnis AB, Kuwada JY (in press). Axonogenesis in the brain of zebrafish embryos. J. Neurosci.
Dodd J, Jessell T (1988). Axon guidance and the patterning of neuronal projections in vertebrates. Science. 242: 692-699.
Harrelson AL, Bastiani, MJ, Snow PM, Goodman CS (1988). From cell ablation experiments to surface glycoproteins: Selective fasciculation and the search for axonal recognition molecules. In S Easter, K Barald, B Carlson (eds): "From Message to Mind," Sunderlind, MA: Sinauer Assoc. Inc., pp. 96-109.

Kapfhammer JP, Grunewald BE, Raper JA (1986). The selective inhibition of growth cone extension by specific neurites in culture. J. Neurosci. 6: 2527-2534.

Kuwada JY (1986). Cell recognition by neuronal growth cones in a simple vertebrate embryo. Science. 233: 740-746.

Kuwada JY, Bernhardt RR, Chitnis AB (in press). Pathfinding by identified growth cones in the spinal cord of zebrafish embryos. J. Neurosci.

Kuwada JY, Bernhardt RR, Nguyen N (submitted). Development of spinal neurons and tracts in the zebrafish embryo. J. Comp. Neurol.

Landmesser LT (1988). Peripheral guidance cues and formation of specific motor projections in the chick. In S Easter, K Barald, B Carlson (eds): "From Message to Mind," Sunderlind, MA: Sinauer Assoc. Inc., pp. 121-133.

Lumsden AGS, Davies AM (1986). Chemotropic effect of specific target epithelium in the developing mammalian nervous system. Nature 323: 538-539.

Myers PZ, Eisen J, Westerfield M (1986). Development and axonal outgrowth of identified motoneurons in the zebrafish. J. Neurosci. 6: 2278-2289.

Raper JA, Bastiani MJ, Goodman CS (1983). Guidance of neuronal growth cones: Selective fasciculation in the grasshopper embryo. Cold Spring Harbor Symp. Quant. Biol. 94: 391-399.

Tessier-Lavigne M, Placzek M, Lumsden AGS, Dodd J, Jessell TM (1988). Chemotropic guidance of developing axons in the mammalian central nervous system. Nature. 336: 775-778.

Tomita H (1982). Gene analysis in the Medaka (Oryzias latipes). Medaka 1: 7-10.

Tosney KW, Landmesser LT (1984). Pattern and specificity of axonal outgrowth following varying degrees of chick limb bud ablations. J. Neurosci. 4: 2518-2527.

Tosney KW (1987). Proximal tissues and patterned neurite outgrowth at the lumbosacral level of the chick embryo: Deletion of the dermamyotome. Dev. Biol. 122: 540-588.

Tosney KW (1988). Proximal tissues and patterned neurite outgrowth at the lumbosacral level of the chick embryo: Partial and complete deletions of the somite. Dev. Biol. 127: 266-286.

Walter J, Henke-Fahle S, Bonhoeffer F (1987). Avoidance of posterior tectal membranes by temporal retinal axons. Development 101: 909-913.

**Advances in Neural Regeneration
Research, pages 17–32**
© 1990 Wiley-Liss, Inc.

TARGET REGULATION OF NEUROTRANSMITTER PHENOTYPE IN
DEVELOPING SYMPATHETIC NEURONS

Story C. Landis

Department of Neurosciences, Case Western Reserve
University School of Medicine, Cleveland, Ohio
44106

INTRODUCTION

The role of the target in determining the final number of
neurons during development of the vertebrate nervous system
is well established. In a variety of neuronal systems it has
been shown that more neurons are generated initially then
are present in adult animals. A number of experimental
studies have provided evidence that the size of the target
field is an important factor in regulating cell survival
(reviewed in Oppenheim, 1981). Although target regulation of
neuron number is regarded as a general phenomenon in the
developing nervous system, it is probably best understood at
the molecular level for peripheral sympathetic and sensory
neurons (reviewed by Thoenen and Barde, 1980; Levi-
Montalcini, 1987; Barde, 1989). In this case, targets
produce limiting amounts of an essential trophic factor,
Nerve Growth Factor (NGF), which binds to high affinity
receptors on responsive neurons, is internalized and
transported retrograde to the cell body where it appears to
prevent the activation of a death program (Martin et al.,
1988). In adult animals, NGF continues to exert a trophic
action on sympathetic and sensory neurons; for example,
treatment with exogenous NGF increases levels of transmitter
synthetic enzymes and neuropeptides while treatment with NGF
antibodies, which reduces endogenous levels of NGF, reduces
expression of these markers.

Not only may targets determine the number of neurons but
recent studies in several different experimental systems
demonstrate that targets can influence the phenotypic
properties of the surviving neurons. For example, the size
of sympathetic neuron cell bodies and the extent and

branching of their dendritic arbors is influenced by the
size of the target which they innervate during development
(Purves et al., 1988; Voyvodic, 1989). Frank, Smith and
Westerfield have suggested that the peripheral targets of
sensory neurons, cutaneous or muscle, determine the nature
and specificity of their central connections (Frank and
Westerfield, 1982; Smith and Frank, 1987). In the leech, the
morphology and central connections of Retzius cells in the
reproductive system differ from those of Retzius cells in
other segments. This difference develops after target
contact and is dependent upon innervation of the
reproductive organs (Glover and Mason, 1986; Macagno et al.,
1986; Jellies et al., 1987; Loer et al., 1987; Loer and
Kristan, 1989a,b). Finally, in the studies summarized below,
we have examined the developmental expression of
neurotransmitters in sympathetic neurons and found that
neurotransmitter choice in vivo is critically dependent
upon target derived factors.

ENVIRONMENTAL REGULATION OF TRANSMITTER CHOICE IN VITRO

Our interest in the possible role of the target in
determining neuronal phenotype arose from a series of cell
culture studies which have explored the cellular and
molecular mechanisms which regulate the transmitter choice
of sympathetic neurons in vitro. When neurons are
dissociated from the superior cervical ganglia of newborn
rats, all of them are noradrenergic (Mains and Patterson,
1973; Johnson et al., 1976; Patterson and Chun, 1977b;
Landis, 1980). If the neurons are grown in defined medium or
under conditions in which they are chronically depolarized,
they continue to develop as noradrenergic neurons (Walicke
et al., 1977; Iacovitti et al., 1982; Wolinsky et al., 1985;
Raynaud et al., 1987). If, however, they are grown in the
presence of certain types of nonneuronal cells or in medium
conditioned by such cells, the neurons acquire cholinergic
function and decrease their expression of noradrenergic
properties (Patterson and Chun, 1977a; Reichardt and
Patterson, 1977; Landis, 1980; Swerts et al., 1983; Potter
et al., 1986; Raynaud et al., 1987). In the case of heart or
skeletal muscle cells, the induction of cholinergic
properties does not require direct contact but can occur
through the release of a soluble cholinergic inducing
activity into the medium. The effect of this conditioned
medium or cholinergic differentiation factor (CDF) is
blocked when the growth conditions mimic neuronal activity,

such as the presence of elevated potassium (Walicke et al., 1977). Studies of neuron/heart microcultures in which the changing transmitter properties of single neurons were followed over time has shown unequivocally that the cholinergic factor produced by nonneuronal cells induces neurons that have already begun to differentiate along a noradrenergic pathway to become cholinergic (Furshpan et al., 1976; Landis, 1976; Potter et al., 1986).

Environmental factors can influence the choice not only of traditional neurotransmitters by cultured sympathetic neurons but they also affect the expression of neuropeptides. For example, coculture with nonneuronal cells increases the expression of Substance P while growth conditions which mimic activity decrease it (Kessler et al., 1984; Kessler, 1985). Fractionation of heart cell conditioned medium has revealed the existence of several different factors which affect peptide expression in cultured sympathetic neurons (Nawa and Patterson, 1990; Nawa and Sah, 1990).

Initially studies of the mechanism of cholinergic induction in cultured sympathetic neurons focussed on the role of CDF from heart cell conditioned medium. This factor is a relatively heat-stable 45kD glycoprotein with at least five glycosylation sites (Fukada, 1985; Weber et al., 1985). Removal of the carbohydrate yields a 22kD protein which retains biological activity. Antisera raised against a partial peptide sequence obtained for CDF both immuno-precipitate the 45kD protein and the cholinergic inducing activity (Rao et al., 1990; Yamamori et al., 1990). It is now clear, however, that a number of more or less well characterized environmental signals can induce cholinergic function in cultured sympathetic neurons. Ciliary neurotrophic factor (CNTF), originally identified because of its ability to support the survival of ciliary neurons in culture, has recently been found to induce choline acetyltransferase (ChAT, the synthetic enzyme for acetylcholine) and decrease tyrosine hydroxylase (TH, the rate limiting enzyme in the catecholamine synthetic pathway) activity in cultured rat sympathetic neurons (Saadat et al., 1989). Two membrane associated molecules which induce cholinergic function in cultured rat sympathetic neurons have recently been partially purified from spinal cord (Adler and Black, 1986; Kessler et al., 1986; Wong and Kessler, 1987; Adler et al., 1989). In addition, human

placental serum, rat serum , chick embryo extract and a
heparin binding activity in brain extract (Higgins et al.,
1981; Iacovitti et al., 1981; 1982; Wolinsky and Patterson,
1985; Kessler et al., 1986) induce cholinergic function,
although they do not appear to decrease noradrenergic
function. It remains to be determined whether these several
cholinergic-inducing factors and activities are the same or
different. Comparison of the biological and immunological
properties of three of the best characterized factors, CDF,
CNTF and MANS (membrane-associated neurotransmitter-
stimulating factor; Wong and Kessler, 1987), indicates that
CDF is different from CNTF and MANS (Rao et al., 1990).

The studies of the neurotransmitter properties of sympathetic neurons developing in cell culture yielded two
surprising findings. First, postnatal and postmitotic
neurons could alter their neurotransmitter functions in not
only a quantitative but also a qualititative manner;
noradrenergic neurons could become functionally cholinergic.
Second, the environment could play an important role in
determining a functionally important aspect of the final
phenotype of neurons, their choice of neurotransmitter. To
assess whether the plasticity and environmental instruction
revealed in the cell culture studies are part of the normal
developmental repertoire of neurons, we have examined the
development of cholinergic sympathetic neurons in developing
rats using the innervation of sweat glands as a model
system.

NEUROTRANSMITTER EXPRESSION IN DEVELOPING CHOLINERGIC SYMPATHETIC NEURONS

Although the majority of principal neurons in sympathetic
ganglia are noradrenergic, a small proportion are
cholinergic. The best characterized are those that innervate
sweat glands which, in rats as in other laboratory animals,
are concentrated in footpads. Several lines of evidence
indicate that the sweat gland innervation is cholinergic and
sympathetic in the rat. First, functional assays demonstrate
that transmission is cholinergic; sweating evoked by nerve
stimulation is blocked by local injections of atropine, a
muscarinic antagonist, and treatment with cholinergic
agonists elicits sweat secretion (Stevens and Landis, 1987).
Second, homogenates of footpad tissue contain high levels of
choline acetyltransferase (ChAT) activity, gland-containing
tissue pieces synthesize acetylcholine from choline and

store it, and ChAT immunoreactivity is present in nerve terminals in the glands (Leblanc and Landis, 1986). The sweat gland innervation also contains immunoreactivity for two neuropeptides, vasoactive intestinal peptide (VIP) and calcitonin gene related peptide (CGRP) (Landis et al., 1988). Following injection of fluorescent tracers in front or hind footpads, labelled neurons are present in the stellate or lower lumbar paravertebral ganglia respectively. Many of the retrogradely labelled neurons contain VIP-IR, which in the footpads is restricted to sweat gland innervation, and thus these doubly labelled cells must give rise to the sweat gland innervation.

The neurotransmitter properties expressed by the developing sweat gland innervation are strikingly different from those expressed by the mature innervation. When axons first contact the developing glands during early postnatal development, they exhibit only catecholaminergic markers (Landis and Keefe, 1983; Landis et al., 1988). In contrast, cholinergic and peptidergic markers are undetectable; ChAT activity, acetylcholinesterase, and both VIP and CGRP immunoreactivities are absent (Leblanc and Landis, 1986; Landis et al., 1988). The neurotransmitter properties that characterize the mature innervation appear during the second and third postnatal weeks. Acetylcholinesterase staining is first detectable between 7 and 10 days, VIP-IR at 10 days and ChAT activity at postnatal day 11. CGRP-IR, the last property to appear, becomes detectable between days 14 and 21. The relatively close correspondence in the appearance of ChAT, acetylcholinesterase and VIP raises the possibility that these properties are coordinately regulated during development while CGRP may be independently regulated. As the gland innervation acquires cholinergic and peptidergic markers, detectable stores of catecholamines disappear and immunoreactivity for the catecholamine synthetic enzymes, TH and dopamine β-hydroxylase (DBH), decreases.

Several lines of evidence indicate that the changes in transmitter properties observed in the development of the sweat gland innervation take place in a single population of fibers rather than the loss of an early arriving noradrenergic population and its replacement by a late arriving population of cholinergic fibers. First, ultrastructural studies of the developing innervation following fixation with potassium permanganate to localize vesicular stores of norepinephrine provide evidence for the presence of a single population of axons whose cytochemical properties change with time (Landis and Keefe, 1983). Second, even though catecholamines are not stored in detectable amounts in the sweat gland innervation of adult rats, the innervation does, in fact, possess immunoreactivity for TH and DBH and high affinity catecholamine uptake, although at significantly lower levels than previously (Landis and Keefe, 1983; Landis et al., 1988). A final line of evidence comes from studies using the adrenergic neurotoxins, 6-hydroxydopamine and guanethidine, which are taken up selectively by catecholaminergic neurons and when administered to neonatal rats cause the destruction of peripheral noradrenergic cell bodies and nerve terminals. Following treatment of neonatal rats with either 6-hydroxydopamine or guanethidine, no acetylcholinesterase, VIP-IR, ChAT and characteristic sympathetic varicosities are present in the glands, indicating that the mature cholinergic and peptidergic innervation is derived from the initial catecholaminergic innervation (Yodlowski et al., 1984).

The neurotransmitter plasticity displayed by the developing sweat gland innervation is not unique. Examination of the development of neurotransmitter properties has disclosed a number of examples of altered expression of transmitter synthetic enzymes and neuropeptides and suggest that not only quantitative but also qualitative changes in transmitter expression may be common. The most thoroughly studied example are the transient catecholaminergic cells of the gut (Cochard et al., 1979; Teitelman et al., 1979; Gershon et al., 1984; Jonakait et al., 1985). In the gut of embryonic but not postnatal rats, cells are present which express TH-IR, DBH-IR and catecholamine histofluorescence. Several lines of evidence indicate that these cells do not die but rather acquire a different transmitter phenotype. It has proven difficult in this system, however, to establish what the final phenotype is.

TARGET ROLE IN DETERMINING TRANSMITTER PROPERTIES

The question that follows logically from the observed changes in phenotype is what causes the change. Although in principle the alterations in neurotransmitter related properties could be intrinsically determined, the studies of sympathetic neurons developing in cell culture reviewed above suggest that environmental cues could play a role in specifying transmitter properties. In addition to their choice of transmitter, the sweat gland neurons are distinguished by their target. This raises the possibility that the sweat glands influence the transmitter choice of the neurons which innervate them. In an initial series of experiments, the normal developmental interaction between the glands and the neurons which innervate them was disrupted by a single dose of 6-hydroxydopamine on postnatal day 2 (Stevens and Landis, 1988). Following this treatment, the arrival of the innervation in the target tissue was delayed (most likely due to chemical axotomy by the adrenergic neurotoxin) and so was the normal decline in endogenous catecholamines and the appearance of cholinergic function. These findings are consistent with a target role but do not provide direct evidence.

In a second series of experiments, neonatal SCG were transplanted to the anterior chamber of the eye with either sweat glands, a cholinergic sympathetic target, or pineal gland, an adrenergic sympathetic target (Stevens and Landis, 1990). After four weeks in oculo, the neurons were examined for the target-appropriate expression of transmitter systems. In the SCG/sweat gland cotransplants, the surviving neurons lost catecholamine fluorescence and consistently acquired ChAT-IR. In contrast, surviving neurons in the SCG/pineal cotransplants maintained catecholamine fluorescence and inconsistently acquired ChAT-IR. Most interesting was the finding that peptide expression was also target-appropriate; many neurons cotransplanted with sweat glands contained VIP while neurons cotransplanted with pineal contained Neuropeptide Y (NPY), the peptide normally present in the sympathetic innervation of the pineal. Thus, in these experiments, several aspects of neuronal phenotype, catecholamine fluorescence and neuropeptide immunoreactivity were expressed in a target-appropriate fashion. Only a small number of neurons survived transplantation, raising the possibility of selective survival and thereby complicating the interpretation of the results.

The possible role of the target, the sweat glands, in inducing the observed change in neurotransmitter related properties has been tested directly in cross-innervation studies. These experiments took advantage of the topographical segregation of cholinergic and noradrenergic sympathetic targets in rat skin. Hairy skin normally receives noradrenergic sympathetic innervation, particularly of piloerectors and blood vessels, but not cholinergic sympathetic innervation (Schotzinger and Landis, 1990). In contrast, the sweat gland-containing glabrous skin of the footpads normally receives cholinergic sympathetic innervation. By transplanting sweat gland-containing skin to the lateral thorax of early postnatal inbred Lewis rats, the sympathetic neurons which would normally innervate noradrenergic targets in the hairy skin innervate sweat glands instead. Since piloerectors and their innervation, like sweat glands, develop postnatally, these transplantation studies involve the de novo growth of sympathetic fibers rather than regeneration. Further, the transplanted glands are innervated by middle thoracic ganglia which do not normally provide innervation to sweat glands.

The innervation of the transplanted sweat glands exhibits neurotransmitter related properties appropriate for the novel target rather than normal hairy skin targets (Schotzinger and Landis, 1988). Although catecholamine containing fibers have formed an intensely fluorescent plexus in the transplanted glands by three weeks, at six weeks only occasional faintly fluorescent fibers are present. Acetylcholinesterase, ChAT activity and VIP are initially absent but appear in the innervation of the transplanted glands between three and six weeks. These changes reflect a specific target influence since replacing hairy skin with hairy skin does not elicit them. Treatment of the rats with 6-hydroxydopamine before transplantation to eliminate catecholaminergic sympathetic fibers prevents both the ingrowth of catecholaminergic fluorescent fibers and the development of ChAT, acetylcholinesterase and VIP immunoreactivity. Thus, the observed changes are occurring in sympathetic fibers. These results indicate that sweat glands are capable of inducing neurons which would not ordinarily innervate them to express the transmitter properties that characterize the normal gland innervation.

In a recent series of experiments, we examined whether sweat glands induce the transmitter phenotype in the neurons which normally innervate them by replacing sweat gland primordia in early postnatal rats with parotid gland, a target which receives noradrenergic sympathetic innervation. The innervation of the transplanted parotid gland retains intense catecholamine fluorescence and fails to develop ChAT

activity. Thus, the presence of the sweat gland appears to
be required for the normal loss of catecholamines and
induction of cholinergic function (Schotzinger and Landis,
1989).

It is of interest to determine the molecular nature of
the signal between the sweat glands and the neurons which
innervate them. As a first step, we have made aqueous
extracts of footpads and found that extracts from
developing, adult and denervated glands induce choline
acetyltransferase activity in cultured sympathetic neurons.
Experiments are underway to compare the properties of the
activity in sweat gland extract with several of the factors
identified as inducing cholinergic function in cultured
sympathetic neurons, including CDF, CNTF and MANS, or
whether it is a novel factor.

EFFECTS OF THE ALTERATION IN TRANSMITTER PROPERTIES ON
TARGET FUNCTION

The development and maintenance of secretory responsiveness in sweat glands appear to depend upon the presence
of cholinergic innervation, and therefore upon the target
dependent induction of cholinergic function in the sweat
gland innervation. Functional transmission first becomes
detectable at 14 days; pharmacological studies with
cholinergic and adrenergic agonists and antagonists indicate
that even in developing animals whose sweat gland
innervation contains catecholamines, nerve evoked sweat
secretion is mediated by acetylcholine (Stevens and Landis,
1987). It is of interest that the onset of nerve and agonist
induced sweating lags behind the development of cholinergic
properties in the sweat gland innervation and that glands
which do not respond to nerve stimulation in developing rats
are also unresponsive to agonists. These observations raise
the possibility that the cholinergic responsiveness of the
gland cells is induced by the release of acetylcholine from
the gland innervation. Consistent with this hypothesis is
the finding that the glands of adult animals sympathetically
denervated at birth do not sweat in response to cholinergic
agonists (Stevens and Landis, 1987). In addition, when the
innervation of the sweat glands is delayed, the development
of responsiveness is also delayed and tightly linked to the
onset of secretion following nerve stimulation (Stevens and
Landis, 1988). Finally, others have shown when glands are
acutely denervated by cutting the sciatic nerve, the glands

become unresponsive to cholinergic agonists; thus, maintenance of secretory responsiveness is dependent upon cholinergic innervation (Hayashi and Nakagawa, 1963; Kennedy and Sakuta, 1984;). These observations indicate the changes in the developing sweat gland innervation that are required for functional transmission in this system. A likely candidate is acetylcholine although this remains to be demonstrated directly.

We have examined the expression of muscarinic ligand binding sites in sweat glands as a first step in determining how the innervation regulates secretory responsiveness in the target (Grant and Landis, 1990). Ligand binding, competition and autoradiographic studies reveal that mature innervated glands possess typical "glandular" receptors, most likely m3. There does not, however, appear to be a correlation between the presence of muscarinic binding sites and the ability of the glands to secrete in response to cholinergic agonists. During development, muscarinic binding sites appear before the onset of secretory responsiveness and they are expressed at close to normal levels on both uninnervated and acutely denervated glands which are nonresponsive. Thus, it seems likely that one or more steps in the coupling of ligand binding to sweat secretion is innervation dependent. In any case, the phenotypic alteration in the sweat gland innervation appears crucial for triggering and maintaining functional maturation of the target cells.

CONCLUSIONS

In sum, our studies indicate that the neurons which innervate developing sweat glands are noradrenergic at the time of innervation but that as the sweat glands and their innervation mature, both cholinergic and peptidergic properties appear. Although endogenous stores of catechol-amine become undetectable, at least three of the properties that comprise the noradrenergic phenotype continue to be expressed at a low level. Transplantation studies have demonstrated that interaction with the developing sweat glands is responsible for inducing the alterations in transmitter properties. Further, the target dependent changes in the properties of the innervation appear to be required for the final functional maturation of the sweat gland cells. Thus, the establishment of functional synaptic transmission in this system requires a series of complex developmental interactions.

The developmental strategy employed in this system, initial noradrenergic differentiation which is subsequently suppressed and the secondary acquisition of cholinergic and peptidergic functions which are maintained, appears at first to be an unwieldy mechanism for the establishment of a functionally appropriate choice of neurotransmitter by a population of neurons. An explanation may lie in the early developmental history of sympathetic neurons. Sympathetic precursors acquire noradrenergic neurotransmitter properties early in development; as soon as neural crest cells aggregate to form sympathetic ganglia, noradrenergic properties are expressed (Cochard et al., 1979; Teitelman et al., 1979). The minority population in the adult ganglia that are cholinergic could, in principle, be generated either through the failure to induce adrenergic properties in the entire population of presumptive sympathetic neuroblasts or through the secondary induction of cholinergic properties in a subset of adrenergic neurons. Our studies of the development of cholinergic sympathetic neurons indicate that the second strategy is used. It is possible that this strategy may be a common one; the commitment of a neuroblast to a particular class of neurons may involve the acquisition of a transmitter phenotype which functions as a "default" state which is maintained in the absence of other cues. With environmental instruction, however, this "default" phenotype could be modulated either through the induction of a different classical transmitter or of neuropeptides.

REFERENCES

Adler JE, Black IB (1985). Sympathetic neuron density differentially regulates transmitter phenotype expression in culture. Proc Natl Acad Sci USA 82:4296-4300.
Adler JE, Black IB (1986). Membrane contact regulates transmitter phenotypic expression. Dev Brain Res 30:237-241.
Adler JE, Schleifer LS, Black IB (1989). Partial purification and characterization of a membrane-derived factor regulating neurotransmitter phenotypic expression. Proc Natl Acad Sci USA 86:1080-108.
Barde Y-A (1989). Trophic factors and neuronal survival. Neuron 2:1525-1534.

Cochard P, Goldstein M, Black IB (1979). Initial development
of the noradrenergic phenotype in autonomic neuroblasts
of the rat embryo in vivo. Dev Biol 71:100-114.

Frank E, Westerfield M (1982). The formation of appropriate
central and peripheral connexions by foreign sensory
neurones of the bullfrog. J Physiol 324:479-494.

Fukada K (1985). Purification and partial characterization
of a cholinergic differentiation factor. Proc Natl Acad
Sci USA 82:8795-8799.

Gershon MD, Rothman TP, Joh TH, Teitelman G (1984).
Transient and differential expression of aspects of the
catecholaminergic phenotype during development of the
fetal bowel of rats and mice. J Neurosci 4:2269-2280.

Glover JC, Mason A (1986). Morphogenesis of an identified
leech neuron: segmental specification of axonal
outgrowth. Dev Biol 115:256-260.

Grant M, Landis SC (1990). Development and regulation of
muscarinic receptors in sweat glands. J Neurosci,
submitted.

Hayashi H, Nakagaw T (1963). Functional activity of the
sweat glands of the albino rat. J Invest Dermatol
41:365-371.

Higgins D, Iacovitti L, Joh TH, Burton H (1981). The
immunocytochemical localization of tyrosine hydroxylase
within sympathetic neurons that release acetylcholine in
culture. J Neurosci 1:126-131.

Iacovitti L, Joh TH, Park DH, Bunge RP (1981). Dual
expression of neurotransmitter synthesis in cultured
neurons. J Neurosci 1:685-690.

Iacovitti L, Johnson M, Joh TH, Bunge RP (1982). Biochemical
and morphological characterization of sympathetic neurons
grown in chemically defined medium. Neurosci 7:2225-2239.

Jonakait GM, Markey KA, Goldstein M, Dreyfus CF, Black IB
(1985). Selective expression of high affinity uptake of
catecholamines by transiently catecholaminergic cells of
the rat embryo: studies in vivo and in vitro. Dev Biol
108:6-19.

Jellies J, Loer CM, Kristan WB (1987). Morphological changes
in leech Retzius neurons after target contact during
embryogenesis. J Neurosci 7:2618-2629.

Johnson MI, Ross D, Myers M, Rees R, Bunge R, Wakshull E,
Burton H (1976). Synaptic vesicle cytochemistry changes
when cultured sympathetic neurons develop cholinergic
interactions. Nature 262:308-310.

Kennedy WR, Sakuta M (1984). Collateral reinnervation of
sweat glands. Ann Neurol 15: 73-78.

Kessler JA (1985). Differential regulation of peptide and catecholamine characters in cultured sympathetic neurons. Neurosci 15:827-839.

Kessler JA, Adler JE, Jonakait GM, Black IB (1984). Target organ regulation of Substance P in sympathetic neurons in cell culture. Dev Biol 103:71-79.

Kessler JA, Conn G, Hatcher VB (1986). Isolated plasma membranes regulate neurotransmitter expression and facilitate the effects of a soluble brain cholinergic factor. Proc Natl Acad Sci USA 83:3528-3532.

Landis SC (1976). Rat sympathetic neurons and cardiac myocytes developing in microcultures: correlation of the fine structure of endings with neurotranmitter function in single neurons. Proc Natl Acad Sci USA 73:4220-4224.

Landis SC (1980). Developmental changes in the neurotransmitter properties of dissociated sympathetic neurons: a cytochemical study of the effects of medium. Dev Biol 77:348-361.

Landis SC, Keefe D (1983). Evidence for neurotransmitter plasticity in vivo: Developmental changes in the properties of cholinergic sympathetic neurons. Dev Biol 98:349-372.

Landis SC, Siegel RE, Schwab M (1988). Evidence for neurotransmitter plasticity in vivo: II. Immunocytochemical studies of rat sweat gland innervation during development. Dev Biol 126:129-140.

Leblanc G, Landis SC (1986). Development of choline acetyltransferase activity in the cholinergic sympathetic innervation of sweat glands. J Neurosci 6:260-265.

Levi-Montalcini R (1987) The nerve growth factor: thirty-five years later. EMBO J 6:1145-1154.

Loer CM, Jellies J, Kristan WB (1987). Segment-specific morphogenesis of leech Retzius neurons requires particular peripheral targets. J Neurosci 7:2630-2638.

Loer CM, Kristan WB (1989). Peripheral target choice by homologous neurons during embryogenesis of the medicinal leech. II. Innervation of ectopic reproductive tissue by nonreproductive Retzius cells. J Neurosci 9:528-538.

Loer CM, Kristan WB (1989). Central synaptic inputs to identified leech neurons determined by peripheral targets. Science 244: 64-66.

Macagno E, Peinado A, Stewart R (1986). Segmental differentiation in the leech nervous system: specific phenotypic changes associated with ectopic targets. Proc Natl Acad Sci USA 83:2746-2750.

Mains RE, Patterson PH (1973). Primary cultures of dissociated sympathetic neurons. I. Establishment of long-term growth in culture and studies of differentiated properties. J Cell Biol 59:329-345.

Martin DP, Schmidt RE, DiStefano PS, Lowry OH, Carter JG, Johnson EM (1988). Inhibitors of protein synthesis and RNA synthesis prevent neuronal death caused by Nerve Growth Factor deprivation. J Cell Biol 106:829-844.

Nawa H, Patterson PH (1990). Separation and partial characterization of neuropeptide-inducing factors in heart cell conditioned medium. Neuron, in press.

Nawa H, Sah DWY (1990). Distinct factors in conditioned media control the expression of a variety of neuropeptides in cultured sympathetic neurons. Neuron, in press.

Oppenheim RW (1981). Neuronal cell death and some related regressive phenomena during neurogenesis: a selective historical review and progress report. In Cowan WM (ed): "Studies in Developmental Neurobiology," Oxford: Oxford University Press, pp 74-133.

Patterson PH, Chun LLY (1977a). Induction of acetylcholine synthesis in primary cultures of dissociated rat sympathetic neurons. I. Effects of conditioned medium. Dev Biol 56:263-280.

Patterson PH, Chun LLY (1977b). Induction of acetylcholine synthesis in primary cultures of dissociated rat sympathetic neurons. II. Developmental aspects. Dev Biol 60:473-481.

Potter D, Landis SC, Matsumoto SG, Furshpan EJ (1986). Synaptic functions in rat sympathetic neurons in microcultures. II. Adrenergic/cholinergic dual status and plasticity. J Neurosci 6:1080-1090.

Purves D, Snider W, Voyvodic JT (1988). Trophic regulation of nerve cell morphology and innervation in the autonomic nervous system. Nature 336: 123-128.

Rao MS, Landis SC, Patterson PH (1990). The cholinergic differentiation factor from heart cell conditioned medium is different from the cholinergic factors in sciatic nerve and spinal cord. Dev Biol, submitted.

Raynaud B, Clarous D, Vidal S, Ferrand C, Weber MJ (1987). Comparison of the effects of elevated K+ ions and muscle-conditioned medium on the neurotransmitter phenotype of cultured sympathetic neurons. Dev Biol 121:548-558.

Reichardt L, Patterson PH (1977). Neurotransmitter synthesis and uptake by isolated sympathetic neurons in culture. Nature 270:147-151.

Saadat S, Sendtner M, Rohrer H (1989). Ciliary neurotrophic factor induces cholinergic differentiation of rat sympathetic neurons in culture. J Cell Biol 108:1807-1816.

Schotzinger RJ, Landis SC (1988). Cholinergic phenotype developed by noradrenergic sympathetic neurons after innervation of a novel cholinergic target tissue in vivo. Nature 335:637-639.

Schotzinger RJ, Landis SC (1989) Target regulation of neurotransmitter phenotype of rat sympathetic neurons in vivo: evidence from parotid gland transplants. Soc Neurosci Abstr 15:1359.

Schotzinger RJ, Landis SC (1990) Postnatal development of autonomic and sensory innervation of thoracic hairy skin of the rat: a histochemical, immunocytochemical and radioenzymatic study. Cell Tiss Res, submitted.

Smith C, Frank E (1987). Peripheral specification of sensory neurons transplanted to novel locations along the neuraxis. J Neurosci 7:1537-1549.

Stevens LM, Landis S (1987). Development and properties of the secretory response in rat sweat glands: relationship to the induction of cholinergic function in sweat gland innervation. Dev Biol 123:179-190.

Stevens LM, Landis SC (1988). Developmental interactions between sweat glands and the sympathetic neurons which innervate them: effects of delayed innervation on neurotransmitter plasticity and gland maturation. Dev Biol 130:703-720.

Stevens LM, Landis SC (1990). Target influences on transmitter choice by sympathetic neurons develoing in the anterior chamber of the eye. Dev Biol 137, in press.

Swerts JP, Le Van Thai A, Vigny A, Weber MJ (1983). Regulation of enzymes responsible for neurotransmitter synthesis and degradation in cultured rat sympathetic neurons. Dev Biol 100:1-11.

Teitelman G, Baker H, Joh TH, Reis DJ (1979). Appearance of catecholamine synthesizing enzymes during development of the rat nervous system: Possible role of tissue enviroment. Proc Natl Acad Sci USA 76:509-513.

Thoenen H, Barde Y-A (1980). Physiology of nerve growth factor. Physiol Rev 60:1284-1335.

Voyvodic JT (1989). Peripheral target regulation of dendritic geometry in the rat superior cervical ganglion. J Neurosci 9:1997-2010.

Walicke PA, Campenot RB, Patterson PH (1977). Determination of transmitter function by neuronal activity. Proc Natl Acad Sci USA 74:3767-3771.

Weber MJ, Raynaud B, Delteil C (1985). Molecular properties of a cholinergic differentiation factor from muscle conditioned medium. J Neurochem 45:1541-1547.

Wolinsky E, Landis SC, Patterson PH (1985). Expression of noradrenergic and cholinergic traits by sympathetic neurons cultured without serum. J Neurosci 5:1497-1508.

Wolinsky E, Patterson PH (1985). Rat serum contains a developmentally regulated cholinergic inducing activity. J Neurosci 5:1509-1512.

Wong V, Kessler JA (1987). Solubilization of a membrane factor that stimulates levels of Substance P and choline acetyltransferase in sympathetic neurons. Proc Natl Acad Sci USA 84:8726-8729.

Yamamori T, Fukada K, Aebesold R, Korsching S, Fann M, Aranda M, Nawa H, Kent S, Hood L, Patterson PH (1990). The cholinergic neuronal differentiation factor is a hematopoietic regulator. Science, in press.

Yodlowski M, Fredieu JR, Landis SC (1984). Neonatal 6-hydroxydopamine treatment eliminates cholinergic sympathetic innervation and induces sensory sprouting in rat sweat glands. J Neurosci 4:1535-1548.

Advances in Neural Regeneration
Research, pages 33–41
© 1990 Wiley-Liss, Inc.

SYNAPTIC COMPETITION STUDIED AT DEVELOPING AND REGENERATED NEUROMUSCULAR JUNCTIONS IN LIVING MICE

Jeff W. Lichtman, Rita J. Balice-Gordon,
Junichi Nabekura, Peter van Mier and
Mark M. Rich

Washington University School of
Medicine Department of Anatomy & Neurobiology
Box 8108, St. Louis, MO 63110

INTRODUCTION

The final and functionally most critical step in neural regeneration is the re-establishment of synaptic connections between damaged neurons and their targets. In distinction to the rapidly growing body of information concerning the factors that regulate axon growth, synaptogenesis is still relatively mysterious. Part of the difficulty in understanding what regulates synapse formation stems from the fact that neurons must solve several different problems in order to establish appropriate connections. First the pre- and postsynaptic elements must be matched qualitatively. That is, neurons must innervate target cells of the right type. While axon guidance may bring neurons into proximity with their target cells, recognition of the appropriate site for synapse formation is also necessary. For example, the axons of α and γ motor neurons travel in the same nerves but within the muscle they innervate different types of muscle fibers. Synaptogenesis, however, must also be quantitatively appropriate. For example it is necessary that synaptic connections be of the appropriate strength (i.e. quantal content). It is also important that the number of target cells contacted by an axon (divergence) and the number of axons that innervate a target cell (convergence) be regulated as well. Quantitative matching is especially important because synaptic relays convey information by sending signals to many targets (divergence) and integrating information from many sources by convergent connections. Work at the neuromuscular junction and other simple synapses argues that it is unlikely that recognition mechanisms regulate these quantitative aspects. Rather it seems that relatively subtle interactive mechanisms titrate the number of axons that innervate target cell and the number of target cells each axon ultimately projects to. In skeletal muscle, for example, each muscle fiber is ultimately innervated by a single motor axon even though anyone of several different motor axons could have served equally well. Moreover, during early stages of synaptogenesis more than one axon does innervate each fiber, but competitive interactions eliminate this multiple innervation by causing the synapses of one or more axons to withdraw while the synapses of another axon are maintained or even grow (see Purves and Lichtman, 1985, for review).

STUDYING DYNAMIC EVENTS IN LIVING MICE

In order to explore the mechanisms underlying the loss of convergent innervation on target cells, we have observed the phenomenon as it occurs over time in living mice. Using vital dyes to innocuously stain living nerve terminals (Magrassi et al., 1987) and non-blocking doses of α-bungarotoxin to label postsynaptic sites (acetylcholine receptors), we have viewed synaptic loss during reinnervation in the living mouse sternomastoid muscle (Rich and Lichtman, 1989a). Synaptogenesis during reinnvervation recapitulates many of the developmental events that are far more difficult to study in very young animals. The results of these studies present, in many ways, a surprising picture about the events underlying synaptic competition.

Reoccupation of Endplate Sites During Nerve Regeneration

When crushed or laser ablated motor axons regenerate and reinnervate muscle they do so by retracing the pathway of the original innervation (Rich and Lichtman, 1989a; van Mier and Lichtman, 1989). Schwann cell tubes are reoccupied by motor axons which course back to the original synaptic sites. Because acetylcholine receptors precisely mark the former sites of synaptic contact and are quite stable over the 1 - 2 weeks between nerve damage and reinnervation, we were

able to see that when axons reoccupy endplate sites they
very accurately reoccupy all the original presynaptic
areas that had earlier overlain acetylcholine receptors
(see also Letinsky et al., 1976). We were intrigued,
however, by the fact that although all the former
synaptic sites were reoccupied, the branching pattern
that the regenerating axon used to reoccupy these sites
was sometimes different from the original pattern of
nerve terminal branches at the endplate before
denervation. This result argued that within the
endplate the pathway the axon took to get from one
synaptic site to another was not particularly important,
whereas irrespective of pathway taken the reoccupation
of receptor-rich areas of the postsynaptic membrane was
in each case precise. This suggested that areas of high
receptor density are particularly attractive to nerve
terminals and that the ability of nerves to retrace
former nerve pathways is not the reason for accurate
reoccupation of endplate sites. The attractiveness of
receptor rich sites has significance because during
synapse elimination in development and reinnervation
receptor sites disappear (see below).

Sprouts and Sprout Withdrawal Following Nerve Regeneration

Several days after axons first re-enter the muscle,
sprouts can be seen originating at many endplate sites.
The proportion of endplates with sprouts is related to
the duration of denervation. Thus crushing the nerve a
second time four days after the initial crush delays
axonal return by 3 days (from 4 days to 7 days) and
roughly doubles the number of endplates with sprouts.
These sprouts project in all directions, some running
along the length of their own muscle fiber, while others
cross muscle fibers. Some sprouts can be clearly seen
to course between endplates on nearby fibers to
interconnect them. In such cases it is not always easy
to tell which endplate is the source and which the
target of the sprout as each endplate is also occupied
by an axon reaching it through the original Schwann cell
tube. When we observed sprouts over time they could be
seen to be highly dynamic adding and losing branches
daily (Rich and Lichtman, unpublished).

Interestingly, with time virtually every sprout disappeared from reinnervated muscles. This withdrawal included the loss of sprouts that interconnected and probably provided multiple inputs to reinnervated endplates.

Multiple Innervation and its Elimination During Reinnervation

A number of investigators have noticed that muscle fibers and even some types of neurons are transiently multiply innervated following nerve regeneration (see for example McArdle, 1975; Lichtman, 1980; Gorio, et al., 1983). In the sternomastoid muscle, this is also the case (Rich and Lichtman, 1989a). The loss of multiple innervation and re-establishment of uniformly singly innervated muscle fibers parallels the loss of sprouts in this muscle suggesting that the transient sprouts are the source of the multiple innervation. In fact following double nerve crush both the incidence of sprouts interconnecting endplates and the amount of multiple innervation is twice that seen following single nerve crush. Thus, by following endplates as sprouts regressed we hoped to visualize the process of synapse elimination.

Synapse Elimination Occurs by Loss of Presynaptic Sites

An obvious question we were interested in answering was whether synapse loss was related to, or instigated by, competition between axons for the same synaptic site. Thus did one axon get eliminated because another axon captured the synaptic site it had been occupying? Following the loss of sprouts, however, it was clear that the remaining axon did not occupy the sites vacated by the other axon. Rather, synaptic terminal staining permanently disappeared from regions of the endplate near the area the sprout had entered. Even over long periods (months), the remaining axon never showed staining at these sites. Because when axons first reinnvervate endplates all of the postsynaptic receptors were reoccupied, we next determined what had happened to these vacated postsynaptic sites.

Synapse Elimination is Concurrent With the Loss of
Postsynaptic Acetylcholine Receptors

During the period when sprouts are retracting and
multiple innervation is diminishing we found that at
many endplates some of the sites containing a high
density of acetylcholine receptors were disappearing.
This loss of α-bungarotoxin binding was due to both the
lack of insertion of new receptors at these areas as
well as a selective loss of already inserted receptors
(Rich and Lichtman, 1989a). The loss of receptor sites
was dependent on reinnervation because chronically
denervated endplates, although atrophic, did not loose
sites. Furthermore the loss of receptor sites only
occurred early during reinnervation; after that time
endplates with missing sites remained stable without
additional loss or any new areas added for many months.

It was clear that the receptor sites that
disappeared were precisely subjacent to the regions of
nerve terminal withdrawal already described. Thus
endplates both before reinnervation and at long times
after synapse elimination maintained a precise alignment
between pre- and postsynaptic sites: all receptors
(remaining) were occupied and all nerve terminal
staining was adjacent to receptors.

From these and strikingly similar observations at
developing neuromuscular junctions followed over time as
convergent innervation is lost (Balice-Gordon and
Lichtman, 1989, in preparation), we concluded that
during synaptic competition both axon terminals and the
receptors in the underlying postsynaptic membrane are
eliminated. A question of considerable interest, then,
was whether receptor loss was the result of nerve
terminal loss or was it perhaps the cause?

Receptor Loss Precedes Nerve Terminal Loss

By viewing reinnervated junctions at the time
receptor staining was becoming faint we hoped to better
understand the timing of nerve and receptor loss. We
argued as follows: if nerve terminal loss is the cause
of the loss of underlying receptors then each
postsynaptic area with light receptors should no longer
have stained nerve terminal over it. However, when we

looked at light receptor areas we often found that nerve
terminal staining could still be seen over these sites.
With time, both the nerve terminal and receptor staining
at these sites completely disappeared, as described
above. Thus, the first anatomical evidence we found
anticipating synapse elimination was a drop in the
intensity of postsynaptic receptor staining. While such
a loss of receptor staining could have been due to a
subtle change in the innervating nerve terminal that was
not visible with the anatomical techniques we were
using, other results described below argued otherwise.

Taken at face value then, this result argued for a
postsynaptic change as antecedent to, and perhaps a
trigger for, nerve terminal loss. However, it was also
possible that the nerve terminal to be eliminated had
become functionally silent without a change in its
staining characteristics. The stain we used (4-di-2-
ASP) stains mitochondria in nerve terminals (Lichtman et
al., 1989) and thus might not be able to show changes
that are related to the function of terminals in the
process of being eliminated. For this reason we began a
study of the functional correlates of synapse
elimination.

Efficacy of Individual Quanta is Reduced at Synapses That Are Being Eliminated

Using a floating intracellular recording technique
to allow the amplitude of evoked and spontaneous
miniature endplate potentials to be measurerd without
the use of curare or other neuromuscular blocking
agents, we explored the strength of synapses that were
destined to be eliminated (Nabekura and Lichtman, 1989
and unpublished). In muscle fibers that were multiply
innervated by two inputs we occasionally found
spontaneous miniature endplate potentials of two
discrete amplitudes. By repetitively stimulating one of
the innervating axons we could elicit an increased
outflow of spontaneous miniatures from that axon. Using
this approach it was clear in some muscle fibers that
the spontaneous miniature endplate potentials
originating from the terminals of the more powerful axon
were in fact larger than the spontaneous miniatures
associated with the weaker input. The small size of the
quantal events from one axon relative to another could

be due to decreased acetylcholine packed in each
vesicle, a larger synaptic cleft width, or decreased
sensitivity of the postsynaptic membrane. However,
because we observed these small quanta at the very time
receptor sites were disappearing under normally stained
presynaptic terminals (see above) we favor the idea that
decreased receptor number under one of the competing
inputs is responsible for this difference in quantum
efficacy.

If our interpretation is correct this result
suggests that as competition between axons is occurring,
the postsynaptic cell is taking a very active role. By
selectivly deleting receptors under one axon the muscle
fiber tips the balance of influence progressively away
from one axon and towards the other. Because activity
is likely to be an important influence in synaptic
competition,the unequal influences of the axons due to
postsynaptic receptor loss may give rise to positive
feedback making the influences of the two axons
progressively more different and ultimately leading to
the complete silence of one input.

The Underlying Cellular Mechanism

The experiments described above suggest a plausible
sequence of events that occur during synaptic competition but do not explain why these events occur. Two
issues in particular are still poorly understood. The
first is why should receptor loss lead to the loss of
the overlying terminal. Receptor loss clearly would
cause a terminal to become functionally ineffective but
why should it retract? In order to get at that question
we began by testing the idea that something in the postsynaptic cell is necessary for the maintenance of nerve
terminals (Rich and Lichtman, 1989b). By causing muscle
fibers to degenerate without harming the nerve terminals
we found that synapses are eliminated from degenerated
fibers but promptly return as muscle fibers regenerate.
This seems to argue that postsynaptic factors do play an
important role in synapse maintenance. Further the consistent alignment of nerve terminal and receptor sites
implies that the maintenance factor must be colocalized
in the postsynaptic cell with the regions containing a
high density of acetylcholine receptors. As to what the
maintenance factor might be, our present view is that

presence or absence of adhesion between sites of pre-
and postsynaptic contact is a good candidate to be the
important factor in terminal maintenance and elimination
(Balice-Gordon and Lichtman, 1990).

The second issue that we do not understand at all
is why receptors are selectively lost under one nerve
terminal. It is attractive to suppose that one axon's
synaptic connection can destabilize the receptors under
another axon's terminals as first suggested by Stent
(Stent 1973; see also Lichtman and Balice-Gordon, 1990),
but we have no evidence on this point. We have begun to
get at this issue by selectively labeling the receptors
under a synapse that will be eliminated to see whether
or not these receptors migrate to lie beneath the
competing input (Balice-Gordon and Lichtman, 1989).

CONCLUSION

During reinnervation synapses go through a
recapitulation of the developmental phenomenon which
eliminates all but one axon at each neuromuscular
junction. Our work in living animals suggests an
interactive mechanism which diminishes the efficacy and
ultimately leads to the removal of one synapse at
multiply innervated endplates while another axon's
terminal thrives.

ACKNOWLEDGEMENT

This work is supported by grants from The National
Institutes of Health and The Muscular Dystrophy
Association.

REFERENCES

Balice-Gordon, R.J. and Lichtman, J.W. (1989) Competing
    motor nerve terminals and the acetylcholine
    receptors underlying them are rearranged during
    synapse elimination. Soc. Neurosci. Abs., 15: 165.
Balice-Gordon, R.J. and Lichtman, J.W. (1990) In vivo
    visualization of the growth of pre- and
    postsynaptic elements of neuromuscular junctions in
    the mouse. J. Neurosci. (in press).
Gorio, A., Carmignoto, G., Finesso, M., Polato, P. and
    Nunzi, M.G. (1983) Muscle reinnervation II:

sprouting, synapse formation and repression.
Neuroscience 8: 403-416.

Lichtman, J.W. and Balice-Gordon, R.J. (1990) Synaptic
competition in theory and in practice. J.
Neurobiol. 21: (in press).

Lichtman, J.W. (1980). On the predominantly single
innervation of submandibular ganglion cells in the
rat. J. Physiol. (Lond.) 302: 121-130.

Lichtman, J.W., Sunderland, W.J. and Wilkinson, R.S.
(1989) High resolution imaging of synaptic
structure with a simple confocal microscope. The
New Biologist 1: 75-89.

Magrassi, L., Purves, D. and Lichtman, J.W. (1987).
Fluorescent probes that stain living nerve
terminals. J. Neurosci. 7: 1207-1214.

McArdle, J.J. (1975) Complex endplate potentials at the
regenerating neuromuscular junction of the rat.
Exptl. Neurol. 49: 629-638.

Nabekura, J. and Lichtman, J.W. (1989) Progressive loss
of synaptic efficacy during synapse elimination.
Soc. Neurosci. Abs., 15: 165.

Purves, D. and Lichtman, J.W. (1985). Principles of
Neural Development. Sinauer Press: Sunderland
Mass. (Textbook).

Rich, M.M. and Lichtman, J.W. (1989a) In vivo
visualization of pre- and postsynaptic changes
during synapse elimination in reinnervated mouse
muscle. J. Neurosci. 5: 1781-1805.

Rich, M.M. and Lichtman, J.W. (1989b) Motor nerve
terminal loss from degenerating muscle fibers.
Neuron 3: (in press).

Stent, G.S. (1973) A physiological mechanism for Hebbs'
postulate of learning. Proc. Natl. Acad. Sci. USA
70: 997-1001.

van Mier, P. and Lichtman, J.W. (1989) Regeneration of
single laser-ablated motor axons and the
reoccupation of postsynaptic sites followed in
living mice. Soc. Neurosci. Abs., 15: 334.

**Advances in Neural Regeneration
Research, pages 43–55**
© 1990 Wiley-Liss, Inc.

SYNAPTIC REARRANGEMENT BY REGENERATING
OPTIC FIBERS IN THE ADULT GOLDFISH

Ronald L. Meyer

Developmental and Cell Biology,
Developmental Biology Center, University
of California, Irvine, California 92717

INTRODUCTION

When the optic nerve of a lower vertebrate is
severed, optic fibers will regrow back into
tectum to eventually reform a retinotopic
projection. In goldfish, the precision of
retinotopy can be nearly indistinguishable from
normal; behavioral recovery, including
restoration of color vision, is close to normal
and no retinal ganglion cells appear to be lost
(see Sperry, 1963; Meyer, 1990). The goldfish
visual system therefore provides an excellent
model for successful regeneration of a CNS system
which in adult mammals shows virtually no useful
regeneration. Understanding the underlying
cellular events may provide insight into
regenerative failure in mammals and can give us
a "wish list" of what we might hope to produce in
mammals.

After a nerve crush in goldfish, optic fibers
begin to invade the anterior end of tectum at
about 7-10 days and completely cover the
anterior-posterior extent of tectum, a distance
of several millimeters, in about 30 days. At
this time there is a rough order which gives
somewhat better than quadrant level retinotopy.
During the next month, retinotopy, improves
markedly to restore fine retinotopy, though at
the end of the second month the precision of the
map is still noticeably less precise than normal.
After several more months, there is a period of
slow improvement during which the map can become

indistinguishable from normal as assayed by both
electrophysiological and anatomical methods.
During this entire time, fibers are confined
to the appropriate optic lamina in tectum, but
they show permanent pathway abnormalities within
these layers, that is, many fibers traverse
highly abnormal routes to get to their correct
positions (Meyer, 1980; Meyer et al., 1985; Cook
and Rankin, 1986; Stuermer, 1988).

At least two kinds of processes are now
thought to mediate the restoration of topographic
order within tectum. One is a chemoaffinity type
of interaction which generates rough retinotopy
and the other an activity mediated ordering which
generates fine retinotopy. There is long-
standing evidence for chemoaffinity, that is, for
position specific markers in tectum and in retina
that generate selective axonal growth (see
Sperry, 1963; Meyer, 1990). Perhaps the most
dramatic demonstration of this selectivity is the
appropriate reinnervation of rotated fragments of
tectum (Yoon, 1975) and the corrective growth of
optic fibers surgically directed into the wrong
part of tectum (Meyer, 1984). These putative
markers appear to be quite stable in that optic
denervation for up to 18 months does not
diminish the corrective growth of the surgically
misdirected fibers. What these markers are and
how they function in cellular terms continues to
be a frustrating problem.

The main evidence for the role of activity
comes from experiments in which optic impulse
activity is eliminated by intraocular injections
of tetrodotoxin (TTX) (Meyer, 1983a; Schmidt and
Edwards, 1983). Under impulse blockade, fibers
reform their usual rough retinotopic projection
at one month but fail to subsequently refine this
projection while under blockade. This"refinement"
can be inhibited for at least 4 months and will
continue upon resumption of activity.
Stroboscopic illumination can also disrupt the
regeneration of fine retinotopy (Cook and Rankin,
1986). Related evidence comes from the formation
of "ocular dominance columns" by regenerating

fibers. Optic fibers normally project only to contralateral tectum, but it is possible to surgically redirect fibers to ipsilateral tectum. When both the redirected and host optic fibers are made to regenerate into one tectum simultaneously, they completely overlap at one month but then segregate out into discrete columnar domains at two months (Meyer, 1983b). This segregation is completely inhibited by TTX blockade (Meyer, 1982). This finding together with the evidence for the identity of chemo-affinity markers between the two eyes (Ide et al., 1983) indicate that this segregation is driven by activity.

The now widely held explanation for this activity mediated ordering is as follows: Ganglion cells which are next to each other in retina are known to have correlated impulse activity (Arnett, 1978). If optic fibers in the tectum preferentially terminated next to other optic fibers having correlated activity, then this would generate retinotopic order. Ocular dominance columns would similarly form since only fibers from the same eye would have tightly correlated activity. It seems likely that this activity dependent ordering is mediated through synaptic connections and for this reason much of our recent research has focused on the synaptic events associated with regeneration.

ULTRASTRUCTURAL ANALYSIS OF SYNAPSES

One of the most direct ways to study synapses is with ultrastructure. A series of electron micrographic studies was undertaken to explore the synaptic correlates associated with activity dependent ordering. The first project simply asked how many synapses optic fibers made at different times during regeneration. One can imagine several possibilities: Optic fibers might delay synaptogenesis until at their optimal sites, giving a progressive increase in synaptic number, a possibility favored by an earlier study (Murray et al., 1982). They might make many more synapses than needed and reduce this number so as to retain the appropriate ones, in a manner of reminiscent of synaptic loss during cortical and neuromuscular development. Or they may extensively rearrange connections while keeping the total number constant.

Answering this question turned out to be nontrivial. One problem was identifying optic fibers. Morphological criteria and degeneration labelling were unreliable for accurate quantization and regenerating optic fibers were very difficult to label with HRP. This was eventually solved with a simple "cold fill" method in which the nerve is sucked into a tube of HRP and the fish put in the refrigerator (Hayes and Meyer, 1988a). This produced dense fills of nearly all optic fibers while impeding degenration. Another problem was that the main optic innervation layer (stratum fibrosum et griseum superficiale, SFGS) shrinks and expands substantially during regeneration and the distribution of synapses within this layer shows sublaminar differences. To avoid the associated sampling problems, counts were made from montages of electron micrographs that spanned the entire radial extent of the SFGS, essentially a "core sample".

Using this method, synaptic and fiber counts were made in normal fish, and fish at 30, 60 and 120 days following intraorbital optic nerve crush (Hayes and Meyer, 1989a). Synaptic number was found to be restored to normal by 30 days and remained constant thereafter. Since most of the refinement takes place after 30 days, this implies that refinement is mediated by rearrangement of a constant number of synapses. Additional evidence for rearrangement came from counts of labelled fibers. The number of sampled optic fibers at 60 days fell to half that seen at 30 days, indicating that there was an initial exuberant production of branches followed by the elimination of many.

To obtain more direct evidence of rearrangement, fibers from both eyes were made to simultaneously regenerate into one tectum (Meyer and Kageyama, 1988). One nerve was labelled with HRP and the other with degeneration by removing this eye 1-2 days prior to the HRP labelling. At 30 days, fibers from both eyes formed terminals in the same region of tectum so that both were frequently seen in the same micrograph. At 60 days or later, samples taken in the middle of ocular dominance columns showed terminals from only one eye. This result, together with the below mentioned evidence that the total number of synapses in these doubly innervated tecta is normal, implies that at least half of all synapses are lost and remade during refinement. The actual number of remade synapses may be much higher.

We next asked whether activity regulates the reformation of this specific number of synapses. Does activity promote synaptogenesis or might it instead stimulate the net elimination of synapses? To test this, we blocked activity with intraocular injections of TTX and counted synapses and fibers at 30, 60 and 120 days of regeneration (Hayes and Meyer, 1989b). Somewhat to our surprise, there was no detectable effect of TTX on these measures. Synaptic numbers were normal and elimination of exuberant fibers occurred. This implies that activity does not regulate synaptic number but only synaptic distribution. It further implies that fiber elimination is an activity independent, endo-genous feature of regeneration.

If activity does not regulate synaptic number, then what does? Two general possibilities can be envisioned. Each optic fiber may make a fixed number of synapses or each tectal cell may only accept a fixed number of synapses. To test this, we took advantage of the retinotopic plasticity of the retinotectal projection. When the posterior half of tectum is removed and the optic nerve crushed, optic fibers will reform a "compressed" projection in which all optic fibers (no ganglion cells are lost) are squeezed onto the anterior remnant in retinotopic fashion

(Gaze and Sharma, 1970). If fibers make a fixed number of synapses, then the number of synapses in each tectal core sample would be twice normal. If tectal cells accept only a fixed number, then synaptic number per core sample would be normal. The number was normal, implying target regulation of synaptic number (Hayes and Meyer, 1988b). Interestingly, this was not a simple fixed density per unit tectal volume. The thickness of the SFGS nearly doubled, presumably due to the increase in the number of fibers. (This increase was restricted to the SFGS as determined by several cytological and cyto-chemical markers for its boundaries; Kageyama and Meyer, 1988b and unpublished.) The result was the number of synapses per unit volume was half normal. What was presumably normal was the number of synapses on each tectal cell, in line with earlier work by Murray et al. (1982), but not Marotte (1983).

This fixed number of synaptic sites suggests the possibility that a competition for limited synaptic sites may be a requirement for activity mediated synaptic rearrangement. We asked, therefore, if such rearrangement could occur under conditions in which one might expect competition to be minimized. Specifically, would refinement occur if only a small number of optic fibers are allowed to regenerate into tectum? This was accomplished by removing one eye and then surgically deflecting fibers from the innervated tectum into the denervated one. These deflected fibers were selected to originate from one retinal quadrant. From our previous work it was known that these deflected fibers would form an expanded projection over the general tectal region appropriate for the fibers. After several months, the deflected fibers were labelled with HRP and the usual core samples were taken (Hayes and Meyer, 1988a). In the most densely innervated regions of tectum, the number of synapses was almost half the normal number, indicating, not surprisingly, that fibers have an upper limit for the number of synapses they can support. The important implication for the present purposes was there are many "vacant" synaptic sites in these tecta.

Since this projection from deflected fibers is abnormally expanded, it is not trivial to show refinement, but a chance discovery from some previous work offered a convenient method for doing so. We had previously mapped the projection during regeneration by making small (1-2nl) spot injections of WGA-HRP into retina (Meyer et al., 1985). In normals, these spot injections always produce a single small clump of dense product that fills the SFGS. During regeneration, product is initially distributed over an order of magnitude larger area of tectum as a low density smear. By 2 months, product shrinks down but often into more than one clump. These multiple clumps resemble ocular dominance columns and can persist for several months. TTX blockade prevents much (but not all) of this shrinkage and completely eliminates the formation of multiple clumps, indicating these are generated by activity (Olson and Meyer, 1987). When this spot mapping method was used on fish with deflected fibers, fibers were observed to shrink down to form these multiple patches (Olson and Meyer, 1988). Thus activity dependent rearrangement can occur when there are "extra" synaptic sites. This implies that competition for a fixed number of sites is not needed for synaptic rearrangement and instead suggests the possibility that rearrangement may have a cooperative component rather than being strictly competitive.

The above findings as well as other observations give the impression that activity dependent synaptic rearrangement operates only late in regeneration and is limited to relatively short range topographic changes. To test whether this is true, the distribution of synaptic connections from a small region of retina was examined at early stages of regeneration. For this retinal spot injection of WGA-HRP was a sensitive method suitable for ultrastructure

(Kageyama and Meyer, 1988a). Contrary to expectation, regenerating fibers were found to make highly ectopic synaptic connections in early regeneration. At 3 weeks, fibers that normally terminate in posterior tectum made synaptic connections only in anterior tectum. At 5 weeks, synapses were found in both anterior and posterior tectum. After several months, synapses were restricted to their normal posterior tectum. At the light level, it was further found that TTX blockade delayed but did not prevent the transition to posterior innervation (Olson and Meyer, unpublished). Together these results imply that fibers can make and eliminate highly aberrant connections (large scale errors), and although this correction may not be directed by activity, it is accelerated by it.

PHARMACOLOGICAL ANALYSIS OF SYNAPTOGENESIS

The preceding studies point to the synapse as the major candidate for the cellular site of activity dependent ordering. To further dissect the responsible cellular mechanisms, we have recently turned to analyzing neurotransmission in this system. Some of the main findings will be briefly summarized here. There are two lines of evidence indicating that optic fibers use glutamate or related molecules as the primary neurotransmitter. One is immunohistochemistry (Kageyama and Meyer, 1989). With a double affinity purified antibody against gluteraldehyde conjugated glutamate made by Wenthold at NIH, strong immunoreactivity has been localized to retinal ganglion cells and optic fibers. Dense reactivity is associated with the main optic innervation layer, the SFGS, and this is greatly reduced 2 days after enucleation. At the EM level, reactive terminals were found in tectum which on the basis of position and cytological criteria are optic terminals.

The other evidence for glutamatergic trans-mission is pharmacologic (vanDeusen and Meyer, 1988). We developed an <u>in vitro</u> preparation in which the entire tectum together with the entire optic nerve is placed in a slice type recording chamber. This afforded very efficient stimulation of the nerve while permitting infusion of various pharmacologic probes. Kainate and quisqualate antagonists such as DNQX were highly effective in blocking the field potential. In addition, a slight decrement which included the earliest components of the potential was also seen with NMDA antagonists like APV and MK-801. Nicotinic cholinergic antagonists had no inhibitory effect, contrary to previous in vivo studies.

Since NMDA has been implicated in neuro-plasticity such as LTP (see Kennedy, 1989) and the development of visual cortex (Kleinschmidt et al., 1987) and tectum (Cline, et al., 1987), we asked whether NMDA might be involved in activity mediated ordering during nerve regeneration. Although previous studies had used direct infusion of APV with minipumps or slow release matrices, there were several reasons for not using this method. Specific antagonism of NMDA receptors with APV is concentration dependent. Infusion techniques usually produce a higher than optimal concentration at the infusion site and slow release matrices show an initial spurt followed by progressive decline. Recent reports also show that APV can have cytotoxic effects. To avoid these problems, we turned to MK-801, which is a highly potent NMDA antagonist that crosses the blood brain barrier. When fish were injected intraperitoneally with MK-801 beginning at 30 days, both the formation of ocular dominance columns and the late retinotopic refinement were prevented at 2-3 months (Meyer and Miotke, in preparation). This suggests that activity dependent synaptic rearrangement may be mediated via NMDA receptors.

CONCLUSIONS

Optic regeneration in goldfish is associated with a great deal of synaptic rearrangement. It seems likely that most early formed synaptic connections are eliminated in favor of more appropriate ones later. Activity plays an important role not only in directing the formation of the appropriate connection exemplified in fine retinotopy, but also appears to help speed the elimination of large scale errors involved in forming gross retinotopy. Strategies aimed at promoting mammalian regeneration may need to create conditions compatible with synaptic rearrangement within the target region in order to fully restore functional connectivity.

REFERENCES

Arnett DW (1978). Statistical dependence between neighboring retinal ganglion cells in goldfish. Exp Brain Res 32:49–53.

Cline HT, Debski EA, Constantine-Paton M (1987). N-methyl-D-aspartate receptor antagonist desegregates eye-specific stripes. Proc Natl Acad Sci USA 84:4342–4345.

Cook JE, Rankin EC (1986). Impaired refinement of the regenerated retinotectal projection of the goldfish in stroboscopic light: a quantitative WGA-HRP study. Exp Brain Res 63:421–430.

Gaze RM, Sharma SC (1970). Axial differences in the reinnervation of the goldfish optic tectum by regenerating optic nerve fibers. Exp Brain Res 10:171–181.

Hayes WP, Meyer RL (1988a). Retinotopically inappropriate synapses of subnormal density formed by surgically misdirected optic fibers in goldfish tectum. Dev Brain Res 38:304–312.

Hayes WP, Meyer RL (1988b). Optic synapse number but not density is maintained during regeneration onto surgically-halved tectum in goldfish: HRP-EM evidence that optic fibers compete for fixed numbers of postsynaptic sites on tectum. J Comp Neurol 274:539–559.

Hayes WP, Meyer RL (1989a). Normal numbers of retinotectal synapses during the activity sensitive period of optic regeneration in goldfish: HRP-EM evidence implicating synapse rearrangement and collateral elimination during map refinement. J Neurosci 9:1400–1413.

Hayes WP, Meyer RL (1989b). Impulse blockade by intraocular tetrodotoxin during optic regeneration in goldfish: HRP-EM evidence that the formation of normal numbers of optic synapses and the elimination of exuberant optic fibers is activity independent. J Neurosci 9:1414-1423.

Ide CF, Fraser SE, Meyer RL (1983). Eye dominance columns from an isogenic double-nasal frog eye. Science 221:293-295.

Kageyama GH, Meyer RL (1988a). Regenerating optic axons form transient topographically inappropriate synapses in goldfish tectum: a WGA-HRP EM study. Soc Neurosci Abstr 14:674.

Kageyama GH, Meyer RL (1988b). Laminar histochemical and cytochemical localization of cytochrome oxidase in the goldfish retina and optic tectum in response to deafferentation and during regeneration. J Comp Neurol 278:521-542.

Kageyama GH, Meyer RL (1989). Glutamate-immunoreactivity in the retina and optic tectum of goldfish. Brain Res 503:118-127.

Kennedy MB (1989). Regulation of synaptic transmission in the central nervous system: long-term potentiation. Cell 59:777-787.

Kleinschmidt A, Bear MF, Singer W (1987). Blockade of "NMDA" receptors disrupts experience-dependent plasticity of kitten striate cortex. Science 238:355-358.

Marotte LR (1983). Increase in synaptic sites in goldfish tectum after partial tectal ablation. Neurosci Lett 36:261-266.

Meyer RL (1980). Mapping the normal and regenerating retinotectal projection of goldfish with autoradiographic methods. J Comp Neurol 189:273-289.

Meyer RL (1982). Tetrodotoxin blocks the formation of ocular dominance columns in goldfish. Science 218:589-591.

Meyer RL (1983a). Tetrodotoxin inhibits the formation of refined retinotopography in goldfish. Brain Res 6:293-298.

Meyer RL (1983b). The growth and formation of ocular dominance columns by deflected optic fibers in goldfish. Dev Brain Res 6:279-291.

Meyer RL (1984). Target selection by surgically misdirected optic fibers in the tectum of goldfish. J Neurosci 4:234-250.

Meyer RL (1990). The case for chemoaffinity in the retinotectal system: recent studies. In Trevarthen C (ed): "Brain circuits and functions of the mind: essays in honor of R.W. Sperry," Cambridge: Cambridge University Press.

Meyer RL, Kageyama GH (1988): Synaptic overlap followed by segregation of differentially labeled optic terminals in the goldfish optic tectum. Soc Neurosci Abstr 14:674.

Meyer RL, Sakurai K, Schauwecker E (1985). Topography of regenerating optic fibers in goldfish traced with local wheat germ injections into retina: evidence for discontinuous microtopography in the retinotectal projection. J Comp Neurol 239:27-43.

Murray M, Edwards MA (1982). A quantitative study of the reinnervation of the goldfish optic tectum following optic nerve crush. J Comp Neurol 209:363-373.

Murray M, Sharma S, Edwards MA (1982). Target regulation of synaptic number in the compressed retinotectal projection of goldfish. J Comp Neurol 209:374-385.

Olson MD, Meyer RL (1987). Refinement of the goldfish retinotectal projection in the absence of activity and in the dark. Soc Neurosci Abstr 13:1418.

Olson MD, Meyer RL (1988). Retinotopic clustering in a low density tectal projection in goldfish: evidence against activity dependent competition. Soc Neurosci Abstr 14:674.

Schmidt JT, Edwards DL (1983). Activity sharpens the map during the regeneration of the retinotectal projection in goldfish. Brain Res 269:29-39.

Sperry RW (1963). Chemoaffinity in the orderly growth of nerve fiber patterns and connections. Proc Natl Acad Sci USA 50:703-710.

Stuermer CA, (1988). Trajectories of regenerating retinal axons in the goldfish tectum: I. A comparison of normal and regenerated axons at late regeneration stages. J Comp Neurol 267:55-68.

van Deusen EB, Meyer RL (1988). Different effects of KA/QA, NMDA and APB receptor antagonists on optic and toral afferent-stimulated activity of goldfish tectal neurons in vitro. Soc Neurosci Abstr 14:96.

Yoon M (1975). Readjustment of retinotectal projection following reimplantation of a rotated or inverted tectal tissue in adult goldfish. J Physiol 252:137-158.

Advances in Neural Regeneration
Research, pages 57–70

HORMONE AND LESION-INDUCED CHANGES IN SYNAPTIC INPUT TO SPINAL SOMATIC AND AUTONOMIC EFFERENT NEURONS IN ADULT MAMMALS

Jacqueline C. Bresnahan, Michael S. Beattie and M. Gail Leedy
Departments of Anatomy (JCB, MSB and MGL) and Surgery (MSB), and the Neuroscience Program (JCB and MSB), The Ohio State University, Columbus, Ohio 43210

INTRODUCTION

The anatomical correlates of behavioral alterations are difficult to discern but are beginning to be elucidated in simple organisms (e.g., Bailey and Chen, '89). Such correlates in complex mammalian forms are much more elusive, but may be approachable by examining reflex circuits, which are the most elemental components of behavior. It has long been thought that alterations in reflex circuitry underlie many of the observed behavioral consequences of spinal cord injury for example (Liu and Chambers, 1958; Goldberger and Murray, 1985), but definitive proof of such anatomical reorganization has been difficult to obtain (see Mendell, 1984; Pubols and Sessle, 1987). In this chapter, we will describe the results of several experiments designed to assess whether differences in anatomical organization can be demonstrated at the level of the motoneuron (MN) in response to lesions and hormonal manipulations which alter reflex function. The results of these studies suggest that synaptic growth processes are maintained in the adult mammalian spinal cord, and that they may be involved in reflex changes after injury associated with recovery or impairment of function, and may also participate in normal adaptations to the changing adult environment.

The reflexes that we have chosen to examine are the eliminative and sexual reflexes with afferent and efferent limbs located within the the sacral spinal cord. Like most behaviors, they have both somatic and autonomic components. These reflexes are important for the normal functioning of animals and are fundamental to a wide variety of complex social behaviors (e.g., territorial marking, sexual interactions). Further, the loss of voluntary control and maladaptive alterations of these reflex systems in humans with spinal cord injury constitutes an important and difficult clinical problem (Pedersen, 1983). Understanding the normal organization of these reflex pathways and their potential reorganization after CNS damage (Thor et al., 1986) is necessary to affect appropriate therapies to promote maximal recovery of function.

ORGANIZATION OF THE SACRAL SPINAL CORD

The sacral spinal cord of mammals contains both parasympathetic preganglionic neurons (PGNs) innervating the bowel, bladder, and sexual organs, and somatic motoneurons (MNs) innervating associated striated sphincters and pelvic musculature (e.g. Schroder, 1980; deGroat et al., 1981; Mawe et al., 1986; McKenna and Nadelhaft, 1986; Thor et al., 1989). Visceral and cutaneous afferents from sacral structures enter the cord at the same or closely adjacent segments containing the efferent neurons. Our morphometric analyses of synaptic changes in the adult female cat have concentrated on the sacral PGNs innervating the bladder ganglia of the cat, and on the somatic MNs innervating the external anal and urethral sphincters, located in Onuf's nucleus. During normal micturition and defecation, sacral PGNs are activated, promoting bladder or colon contractions while sphincteric MNs are inhibited, allowing for elimination. The sacral PGNs and Onuf's nucleus MNs send axons to the periphery via the pelvic and pudendal nerves respectively (deGroat et al., 1981), and can therefore be unequivocally identified as efferent neurons by making tracer injections into these nerves.

Our studies in the male rat have focused on the somatic MNs involved in penile reflexes and ejaculation. These MNs are located in a region homologous to Onuf's nucleus which has been called the spinal nucleus of the bulbocavernosus (SNB), or alternatively, the dorsomedial nucleus of the lumbosacral cord (Schroder, 1980; McKenna and Nadelhaft, 1986). The latter term is perhaps more appropriate, since this nucleus contains MNs innervating the external anal sphincter as well as the bulbocavernosus (BC) muscle. During penile erection and ejaculation, the BC and associated muscles are active, and essential for normal sexual function (Sachs, 1982; Hart and Melese-d'Hospital, 1983). Since both sphincteric and BC MNs project via the pudendal nerve, we have used injections of tracer into the BC muscle itself in order to unequivocally identify BC MNs in these studies.

The normal regulation of both eliminative and sexual

reflexes involves important ascending and descending components, as well as significant contributions from sympathetic efferents. Discussion of these aspects of the organization of sacral reflexes is beyond the scope of this chapter, but interested readers are referred to several comprehensive reviews (de Groat et al., 1981; Gorski, 1985; Hart and Leedy, 1985; Gonella, 1987).

SPINAL CORD TRANSECTION EFFECTS ON ELIMINATIVE REFLEXES AND EFFERENT NEURON INPUTS

In order to address the hypothesis that reflex changes after spinal cord transection are related to changes in synaptic inputs to reflex motoneurons, we examined the reflex behavior and sacral cord ultrastructure of adult female cats which had sustained acute (4 days) or chronic (10-11 weeks) complete (or nearly so) thoracic spinal cord transections, and compared them to normal animals (Bresnahan et al., 1987; Leedy et al., 1988). Horseradish peroxidase (HRP) applied to the pudendal or pelvic nerves 96 hrs prior to sacrifice was used to label efferent neurons. Labelled neurons were identified in 60 um thick vibratome sections treated with diaminobenzidine (DAB) and cobalt chloride and processed for sequential light and electron microscopy (Beattie, et al., 1978; Mawe et al., 1986; Leedy et al., 1987, 1988). This allowed detailed maps of the position of labelled neurons, as well as whole-cell measurements, to be made prior to thin-sectioning for electron microscopy. Large montages of labelled PGNs or Onuf's MNs were made at 23,100 X. Synaptic terminals contacting labelled MN profiles or attached proximal dendritic profiles were classified and measured as reported previously (Leedy et al.,1987, 1988; Mawe et al., 1986). That is, terminals were designated as containing round, pleomorphic, or flat vesicles, and the number of dense cored vesicles was noted; the cell membrane in apposition to glial and neuronal elements was determined; morphologically defined "active sites" were measured; and the number of terminals per unit membrane as well as the proportion of membrane apposed by terminals of various types and by synaptic active sites was derived.

Changes in Eliminative Reflexes

Cats in the chronic transection group were monitored daily for eliminative function. This was indeed necessary during the early postoperative period when spontaneous urination was severely compromised. Over the course of the 10-11 post-operative weeks, spontaneous defecation recovered rapidly but spontaneous urination recovered gradually. In addition, as reported by others (e.g., deGroat et al., 1981; Thor et al., 1986), it became possible to induce defecation and urination by cutaneous stimulation of the perigenital region which in normal adult cats inhibits eliminative reflexes. This tactile stimulation-induced elimination was evident in all animals by three weeks postoperatively. It should be noted however, that it took several weeks for most animals to release a good stream of urine.

Changes in Synaptic Input to Onuf's Nucleus MNs

The ultrastructural results for identified Onuf's nucleus MNs are shown in table 1, and provide evidence for both a rapid partial denervation of MNs, and a replacement of those lost inputs. While the overall numbers of synaptic terminals and the proportion of membrane apposed by terminals did not change as a result of transection, the size of synaptic terminals decreased as a result of the lesion. More importantly, the proportion of terminals exhibiting round synaptic vesicles increased after transection, suggesting that a lost population of large, pleomorphic vesicle containing terminals had been replaced by terminals from a different source.

Changes in Synaptic Inputs to Sacral PGNs

The results of spinal cord transection on inputs to identified sacral PGNs are shown in table 2. In contrast to Onuf's nucleus MNs, transection produced no change in the proportion of terminal types. Rather, there was evidence for chronic loss of input to the PGNs, with a concomitant increase in glial coverage. There was a significant decrease in the number of terminals per unit of PGN membrane and in the average size of the terminals in apposition to the PGNs in the chronic group. These results suggest that there is a loss of larger terminals on the PGNs in the chronic group, which are not replaced.

Lesion-induced plasticity in the adult mammalian spinal cord has been reported by some and denied by others (see discussions in Pubols and Sessle, 1987). Detailed ultrastructural studies have provided evidence for synaptic plasticity in the dorsal horn after rhizotomy in the cat (Murray and Goldberger, 1986), and more recently in the phrenic nucleus after spinal cord hemisection (Goshgarian et al., 1989). The results reported here suggest that synaptic replacement in response to denervation may occur in some spinal cord systems but not in others.

TABLE 1

Onuf's Nucleus Motoneurons

	Normal	Acute	Chronic
Synapses/100 um	(X ± s.e.m.)		
Somata	12.6±1.2	13.1±1.5	13.5±1.2
Dendrites	26.1±1.1	27.5±4.1	24.7±3.8
% membrane with terminals			
Somata	20.5±2.6	17.6±1.6	19.3±1.8
Dendrites	44.8±5.4	35.4±5.0	35.9±4.4
terminal area (um$_2$)			
Somata	1.04±.11*	0.88±.05	0.94±.11
Dendrites	1.38±.20*	0.95±.07	0.97±.06
active site length (um)			
Somata	0.39±.04***	0.30±.02	0.31±.03
Dendrites	0.40±.05***	0.20±.04	0.28±.05
% membrane with active sites			
Somata	1.36±.22**	0.97±.16	1.18±.22
Dendrites	3.74±.73**	1.84±.40	2.92±.68

---

* Overall ANOVA (somata + dendrites), $F_{2,92} = 3.60$, $p < 0.03$, post-hoc Scheffe: Normal > acute = chronic.

** Overall ANOVA (somata + dendrites), $F_{2,92} = 4.40$, $p < 0.02$, post-hoc Scheffe: Normal > acute = chronic.

*** Overall ANOVA (somata + dendrites), $F_{2,91} = 8.45$, $p < 0.0005$, post-hoc Scheffe: Normal > acute = chronic.

(Normal = no transection, Acute = 4 days post-transection, Chronic = 10-11 weeks post-transection.)

TABLE 2

SPN Preganglionic neurons

	Normal	Acute	Chronic
Synapses/100 um[@]	(X ± s.e.m.)		
Somata	10.64±1.18	11.93±1.12	9.26±2.00
Dendrites	18.87±4.38	19.30±3.25	11.22±1.94
% membrane with terminals[#]			
Somata	16.37±1.93	17.31±1.81	11.66±2.79
Dendrites	28.03±4.79	28.89±4.62	15.46±2.66

@ Overall ANOVA (somata + dendrites), $F_{2,105} = 2.91$, p < .059.

Overall ANOVA (somata + dendrites), $F_{2,105} = 5.70$, p < .005,

post-hoc Scheffe: Normal = Acute > Chronic, p < .005.

(Normal = no transection, Acute = 4 days post-transection,

Chronic = 10-11 weeks post-transection.)

HORMONAL EFFECTS ON SYNAPTIC INPUTS TO RAT SNB MOTONEURONS

Castration has been shown previously to eliminate penile reflexes in male rats in ex copula testing (Hart, 1967). Replacement therapy with implanted silastic tubes containing crystalline testosterone (T) reestablishes reflex activity within a short time (Gray et al., 1980; Hart et al., 1983; Hart and Meles-d'Hospital, 1983; Meisel et al., 1984). The motoneurons innervating the bulbocavernosus (BC) muscle, which is involved in penile erections, have been identified and it has been determined that these sexually dimorphic neurons are T-dependent during development (Breedlove and Arnold, 1983; Nordeen et al., 1985), and also that in the adult, they react to T deprivation (castration) by losing somatic size and dendritic arborization (Breedlove and Arnold, 1981; Breedlove, 1985; Kurz et al., 1986). We have examined the effects of castration and replacement therapy on the synaptic inputs to identified BC MNs in the rat using sequential light and electron microscopic techniques outlined above (Leedy et al., 1987a,b).

TABLE 3

Rat SNB Motoneurons

	No T	Short term T	Long term T
Synapses/100 um[@]	(X ± s.e.m.)		
Somata	19.7±1.6	22.6±2.3	21.9±1.9
Dendrites	15.3±1.7	20.9±1.9	24.5±2.4
% membrane with terminals[#]			
Somata	27.7±2.9	31.8±3.5	35.3±2.7
Dendrites	22.8±3.6	35.8±4.0	42.0±4.3

[@] Overall ANOVA (somata + dendrites), $F_{2,110} = 3.77$, $p < .05$,

   orthogonal comparisons: LONG TERM T > SHORT TERM T > NO T

[#] Overall ANOVA (somata + dendrites), $F_{2,110} = 6.61$, $p < .005$,

   orthogonal comparisons: LONG TERM T > SHORT TERM T > NO T

Male rats were screened initially for penile reflexes and those exhibiting erections were castrated and assigned to one of three groups: No T - no testosterone replacement for 6 weeks; Short-term T - no testosterone replacement for 6 weeks followed by 48 hrs of T replacement; and Long-term T - testosterone replacement for the entire 6 wk postcastration period. Two series of animals were prepared, one for behavioral analysis which received penile reflex testing at the end of the experiment, and one series for anatomical study which received BC muscle injections of HRP 48 hrs prior to the end of the experiment.

Reflex Alterations

In the test for penile reflexes, those animals receiving either 6 wks of post-castration androgen replacement, as well as those receiving only 48 hrs of replacement therapy, showed moderate to high levels of penile erections, while those with no exogenous androgen showed very low levels of reflexes. Only 2/9 animals in the No T group responded with a mean of 1.8 erections, compared to 8/9 responding in the Short-term T group with a mean of 25.3 erections, and 7/9 Long-term T animals with a mean of 11.4

erections.

Light Microscopic Measurements

At the light microscopic level, comparisons across groups were made for the somatic, nuclear, and nucleolar areas. The somatic size was significantly greater in the Long-term T group than in either the No T or Short-term T groups, and no increase in somatic area was noted after 48 hrs of T administration. Similar results were obtained when nuclear areas were compared. However, the relationship for nucleolar areas was quite different; the Short-term T group had the smallest mean area with no difference between the No T and Long-term T groups.

Synaptic inputs

Differences in synaptic inputs to SNB MNs are shown in Table 3. There were significant differences in the number of terminals per 100 um of MN membrane length, as well as the percent of the perimeter directly apposed by synaptic terminals. The Long-term T group had the highest level of terminal apposition, the No T group had the lowest level and the Short-term T group was intermediate, suggesting that 48 hrs of T exposure was enough to increase the synaptic inputs to the BC motoneuron surface. When the terminal types were compared, no differences were observed between groups with the exception that the Long-term T group had significantly more terminals containing dense cored vesicles (21% for the No T and Short-term T groups, and 26% for the Long-term T group).

These results suggest that synaptic inputs onto MNs in the penile reflex circuit are sensitive to T levels (see also Matsumoto et al., 1988). In addition, the inputs can be induced to change rapidly (within 48 hrs) in response to androgenic stimulation.

VARIABILITY OF SYNAPTIC INPUT IN INTACT ANIMALS

The rapid changes in synaptic inputs to MNs in response to lesions or hormone replacement suggest that synaptic populations in adult mammals may be normally sensitive to physiological stimuli, and indeed that such populations may be in flux, with their static number at any given sampling time (for morphological studies) regulated by the animal's physiological state. In extreme circumstances, such as denervation by lesioning, or complete removal of a trophic stimulus (e.g., testosterone), that regulation is observable by relatively crude morphometric analyses. A related question, however, and the one really addressed in the introduction to this chapter, is whether behavioral changes or states can be related to synaptic states as measured in static morphological studies. The following experiment was done to determine whether normal variations in reflex activity across a population of individuals is reflected in the synaptic inputs to relevant spinal cord MNs.

During screening for ex copula penile reflexes, wide variations in reflex responsiveness are encountered, such that some animals exhibit many erections while others exhibit none (Gray et al., 1980; Hart et al., 1983). (This is not to say that animals showing no reflexes are incapable of doing so. They simply do not during the test period. It may be concluded that the probability of reflex activity is being assessed.) We asked whether such spontaneous variations in reflex elicitability were related to the number or type of synaptic inputs to BC MNs.

An initial group of 40 animals were screened for penile reflexes and two groups of six rats were selected for comparison of synaptic inputs: a No Reflex group consisting of animals showing no reflexes during three 30 min. test periods; and a High Reflex group consisting of animals exhibiting the highest level of reflex activity during the testing periods. All animals received bilateral injections of cholera toxin conjugated HRP into the BC muscle to label the BC MNs 48 hrs. prior to sacrifice. At the time of sacrifice, blood was collected for T assays which showed no difference in circulating T levels between the two groups indicating that the difference in reflex levels was not T-dependent. Indeed, previous studies showing that penile reflexes can be maintained with T levels much lower than that those in the present study (Davidson et al., 1978; Hart et al., 1983). Thus, it appears that while T is a necessary factor for the normal operation of the system, the range of expressed behaviors may be dependent on other factors.

Synaptic Input Comparisons

The differences in synaptic input onto BC MNs in the No vs. High Reflex groups are shown in Table 4. Perhaps surprisingly, the No Reflex group had greater synaptic input than did the High Reflex group. The No Reflex group had significantly greater percent of the membrane contacted by terminals than did the High

Reflex group, as well as more terminals per unit membrane length, and greater active site coverage than did the High Reflex group. No differences in terminal types between groups were noted, but the High Reflex group had a greater proportion of terminals containing dense cored vesicles.

TABLE 4

No vs. High Reflex Groups

	No Reflexes	High Reflexes
Synapses/100 um		
Somata	19.4 ± 1.8	15.2 ± 7.0
Dendrites	24.7 ± 2.3	15.2 ± 8.3
	(F = 12.96, p < 0.001)	
% membrane with terminals		
Somata	30.3 ± 3.3	22.3 ± 2.6
Dendrites	41.0 ± 4.7	22.1 ± 3.2
	(F = 14.86, p < 0.0005)	
% membrane with active sites		
Somata	1.5 ± 0.3	1.2 ± 0.7
Dendrites	2.9 ± 0.6	1.6 ± 1.0
	(F = 4.95, p < 0.05)	

Such differences in synaptic input to BC MNs in these two behaviorally defined groups might be related to the types of synaptic input onto the MNs. For example, there may be less descending inhibitory input to the MNs in the High Reflex group. Such descending inhibition has been described from the brainstem (Marson and McKenna, 1989), and removal of descending input by spinal transection results in a release of the spinal reflex (Hart, 1968; Sachs and Garinello, 1979; Meisel and Sachs, 1980).

CONCLUSIONS

There are two basic conclusions that may be drawn from the data presented here:

First, it is possible to relate differences in reflex activity (behavior) to differences in the number or types of synaptic terminals found on MNs constituting the final common pathway for those reflexes. These differences in static samples of synaptic input can be detected whether the reflex alterations are consequent to radical assaults on the system, or represent naturally occurring variations in the normal population.

Second, it seems apparent that the synaptic inputs to adult mammalian spinal cord MNs are capable of new growth under some conditions. That capacity may reflect an ongoing regulation of synaptic numbers. The presence of growth and regulatory mechanisms even at the level of the final common reflex pathway suggests that such mechanisms might be recruited in strategies aimed at enhancing recovery of function after spinal cord injury.

The way in which such alterations in synaptic input occurs may be different for different systems. In the case of the sacral PGNs, lesions may produce differences related simply to removal of inputs, and whatever cellular or molecular compensation accompanies denervation. In the case of Onuf's nucleus MNs, lesions may result in the actual reorganization of inputs, with vacated synaptic sites occupied by different classes of synaptic terminals (i.e., "heterotypic sprouting"; see Goldberger and Murray, 1985). Trophic factors such as testosterone may alter the overall set-point of synaptic inputs without altering the relative contributions of different afferent systems. And finally, differences between individuals, which may be the consequence of different physiologic or developmental histories, may be reflected in both synaptic number and differences in the balance between different afferent systems.

At this point such conclusions are purely speculative, since the data take the form of simple morphological categories and measurements which relate only nominally to differences in reflex behavior. However, it would seem likely that further, more detailed studies of changes in afferent inputs to MNs of chemically and functionally defined afferents as they relate to reflex changes are feasible, and may provide insights into questions of both recovery of function and the basic relationship of brain to behavior.

Acknowledgments: These studies were supported by NIH Grants NS-10165 and NS-07747.

REFERENCES

Bailey CH, Chen M (1988). Long-term sensitization in Aplysia increases the number of presynaptic contacts onto the identified gill motor neuron L7. Proc Natl Acad Sci USA 85: 9356-9359.

Beattie MS, Bresnahan JC, King JS (1978). Ultra-structural identification of dorsal root primary afferent terminals after anterograde injury filling with horseradish peroxidase. Brain Res 153:127-134.

Breedlove SM (1985). Hormonal control of the anatomical specificity of motoneuron to muscle innervation in rats. Science 227:1357-1359.

Breedlove SM, Arnold AP (1981). Sexually dimorphic motor nucleus in the rat lumbar spinal cord: Response to adult hormone manipulation, absence in androgen-insensitive rats. Brain Res 225:297-307.

Breedlove SM, Arnold AP (1983). Hormonal control of a developing neuromuscular system. II. Sensitive periods for the androgen-induced masculinization of the rat spinal nucleus of the bulbocavernosus. J Neurosci 3:424-432.

Bresnahan JC, Leedy MG, Beattie MS (1988): Effects of spinal cord transection on Onuf's nucleus motoneurons of cats. Soc Neurosci Absts 13:165-165.

Davidson JM, Stefanick ML, Sachs BD, Smith ER (1978). Role of androgen in sexual reflexes of the male rat. Physiol Behav 21: 1441-146.

deGroat WC, Nadelhaft I, Milne RJ, Booth AM, Morgan C, Thor K (1981). Organization of the sacral parasympathetic reflex pathways of the cat. J Auton Nerv Sys 3:135-160.

Goldberger ME, Murray M (1985). Recovery of function and anatomical plasticity after damage to the adult and neonatal spinal cord. In Cotman CW (ed): "Synaptic Plasticity," New York: Guilford Press, pp 77-110.

Gonella J, Bouvier M, Blanquet F (1987). Extrinsic nervous control of small and large intestines and related sphincters. Physiol Rev 67: 902-961.

Gorski RA (1985). Gonadal hormones as putative neurotrophic substances. In Cotman CW (ed): "Synaptic Plasticity", Guilford Press: New York, pp 287-310.

Goshgarian H, Yu X, Rafols J (1989). Neuronal and glial changes in rat phrenic nucleus occurring within hours after spinal cord injury. J Comp Neurol 284: 519-533.

Gray GD, Smith ER, Davidson JM (1980). Hormonal regulation of penile erection in castrated male rats. Physiol Behav 24:463-468.

Hart BL (1967). Testosterone regulation of sexual reflexes in spinal male rats. Science 155: 1283-1284.

Hart, BL (1968). Sexual reflexes and mating behavior in the male rat. J Comp Physiol Psychol 65: 453-460.

Hart BL (1983). Role of testosterone secretion and penile reflexes in sexual behavior and sperm competition in male rats: a theoretical contribution. Physiol Behav 31: 823-827.

Hart BL, Leedy MG (1985). Neurological bases of male sexual behavior: a comparative analysis. In Adler N (ed): "Neurobiology of Reproduction" vol. 7, New York: Plenum Press, pp 373-422.

Hart BL, Melese-d'Hospital PY (1983). Penile mechanisms and the role of striated penile muscles in penile reflexes. Physiol Behav 31:807-813.

Hart BL, Wallach SJR, Melese-d'Hospital PY (1983). Differences in responsiveness to testosterone of penile reflexes and copulatory behavior of male rats. Horm Behav 17:274-283.

Kurz EM, Sengelaub DR, Arnold AP (1986). Androgens regulate the dendritic length of mammalian motoneurons in adulthood. Science 232:395-398.

Leedy MG, Beattie MS, Bresnahan JC (1987). Testosterone-induced plasticity of synaptic inputs to adult mammalian motoneurons. Brain Res 424:386-390.

Leedy MG, Beattie MS, Bresnahan JC (1988). Effects of spinal cord transection on synaptology of preganglionic neurons in the sacral parasympathetic nucleus of cats. Soc Neurosci Abstr 14:698-698.

Leedy MG, Bresnahan JC, Beattie MS (1987). Testosterone-dependent ultrastructural alterations in the spinal nucleus of the bulbocavernosus (SNB) in male rats. Soc Neurosci Abstr 13:166-166.

Leedy MG, Bresnahan JC, Mawe GM, Beattie MS (1988). Differences in synaptic inputs to preganglionic neurons in the dorsal and lateral band subdivisions of the cat sacral parasympathetic nucleus. J Comp Neurol 268:84-90.

Liu CM, Chambers WW (1958). Intraspinal sprouting of dorsal root axons. Arch Neurol 79:46-61.

Marson L, McKenna K (1989). A medullary site mediating inhibition of spinal sexual reflexes. Soc Neurosci Abstr 15:630.

Matsumoto A, Micevych PE, Arnold AP (1988). Androgen regulates synaptic input to motoneurons of adult rat spinal cord. J Neurosci 8:4168-4176.

Mawe GM, Bresnahan JC, Beattie MS (1986). A light and electron microscopic analysis of the sacral parasympathetic nucleus after labelling primary afferent and efferent elements with HRP. J Comp Neurol 250:33-57.

McKenna KE, Nadelhaft I (1986). The organization of the pudendal nerve in the male and female rat. J Comp Neurol 248:532-549.

Meisel RL, O'Hanlon JK, Sachs BD (1984). Differential maintenance of penile responses and copulatory behavior by gonadal hormones in castrated male rats. Hormones Behav 18:56-64.

Meisel RL, Sachs BD (1980). Spinal transection accelerates the developmental expression of penile reflexes in male rats. Physiol Behav 24: 289-292.

Mendell LM (1984). Modifiability of spinal synapses. Physiol Rev 64:260-324.

Murray M, Goldberger M (1986). Replacement of synaptic terminals in lamina II and Clarke's nucleus after unilateral lumbosacral dorsal rhizotomy in adult cats. J Neurosci 6: 3205-3217.

Nordeen EJ, Nordeen KW, Sengelaub DR, Arnold AP (1985). Androgens prevent normally occurring cell death in a sexually dimorphic nucleus. Science 229: 671-674.

Pedersen E (1983). Regulation of the bladder and colon-rectum in patients with spinal lesions. J Auton Nerv Sys 7:329-338.

Pubols LM, Sessle BJ (1987). "Effects of Injury on Trigeminal and Spinal Somatosensory Systems." New York: A.R.Liss.

Sachs BD (1982). Role of striated penile muscle in penile reflexes, copulation, and induction of pregnancy in the rat. J Reprod Fertil 66: 433-443.

Sachs BD, Garrinello LD (1979). Spinal pacemaker controlling sexual reflexes in male rats. Brain Res 171: 152-156.

Schroder HD (1980). Organization of the motoneurons innervating the pelvic muscles of the male rat. J Comp Neurol 192:567-587.

Thor K, Kawatani M, deGroat WC (1986) Plasticity in the reflex pathways to the lower urinary tract of the cat during postnatal development and following spinal cord injury. In Goldberger ME, Gorio A and Murray M (Eds) "Development and plasticity of the spinal cord", Padova, Italy: Liviana Press, pp. 65-80.

Thor K, Morgan C, Nadelhaft I, Houston M, deGroat WC (1989). Organization of afferent and efferent pathways in the pudendal nerve of the female cat. J Comp Neurol 288: 263-279.

**Advances in Neural Regeneration
Research, pages 71–86**
© 1990 Wiley-Liss, Inc.

MOLECULAR EVENTS DURING LESION-INDUCED SYNAPTOGENESIS

Oswald Steward, Enrique R. Torre, Linda L. Phillips,
and Patricia A. Trimmer

Departments of Neuroscience and Neurological Surgery,
University of Virginia Health Sciences Center,
Charlottesville, Virginia 22908

INTRODUCTION

A well characterized process of lesion-induced
synaptogenesis occurs in many brain regions after damage to
normal inputs. The cellular mechanisms of synapse
replacement following injury are of interest because they
may provide clues about how growth can be induced in the
mature CNS. The process is also inherently interesting
because lesion-induced growth may contribute to recovery of
function after brain injury (for a review, see Steward,
1989).

Lesion-induced synaptogenesis could occur in at least
three ways: 1) neurons may undergo a transformation to a
growth state in which there are general increases in the
synthesis of proteins for axons and dendrites; 2) there may
be a selective induction of "special" genes that are crucial
for the type of growth involved; or 3) synapse replacement
may occur as a result of a continuing process of synapse
turnover, so that no change in gene expression would be
required.

To begin to distinguish between these possibilities, we
have sought to identify the cellular and molecular events
that occur during lesion-induced synaptogenesis. We have
focused on the process of reinnervation that occurs in the
hippocampal dentate gyrus after removal of its normal
innervation from the entorhinal cortex. This system offers
special advantages because the events that occur have been

well characterized, and the cellular participants have been identified (for a review, see Steward, 1986).

The present study evaluates whether there are changes in gene expression in neurons that are being reinnervated (the dentate granule neurons). There are three reasons for this focus: 1) reinnervation of dentate granule neurons involves the degeneration and subsequent replacement of the majority of synaptic connections on these neurons (Matthews, et al., 1976; Steward and Vinsant, 1983); 2) there is a substantial dendritic remodeling during reinnervation that involves the deterioration and regrowth of dendrites and their spines (Caceres and Steward, 1983); and 3) there are increases in protein synthesis within the denervated dentate gyrus during the period of synapse replacement (Fass and Steward, 1983; and Phillips et al., 1987). The increase in protein synthesis occurs over the denervated neuropil, and is correlated with increases in the number polyribosomes beneath postsynaptic sites on dendrites (Steward, 1983). The close temporal relationship between the increases in protein synthesis and the early phases of the reinnervation process led us to propose that the increases in the synthesis of some protein(s) within the dendritic laminae play an important role in the reinnervation process.

The present study uses _in situ_ hybridization to evaluate whether there are changes in mRNA's for beta-actin, beta-tubulin, and the 68K neurofilament protein within the denervated dentate gyrus during the period of synapse replacement. We focused on these proteins to evaluate whether there is an increased synthesis of general cytoskeletal proteins for axons and dendrites during lesion-induced growth. We also evaluated the expression of glial fibrillary acidic protein (GFAP). We anticipated that GFAP would be a "positive control" for studies of changes in neuronal gene expression because there is a substantial hypertrophy of astrocytes in the denervated zone (Rose et al., 1976). As it turns out, the evaluation of GFAP expression revealed interesting new information about how the expression of GFAP is up-regulated following injury.

METHODS

A total of 34 adult male Sprague-Dawley rats (300-350g) received unilateral lesions of the entorhinal cortex using a procedure that has been described previously (Loesche and Steward, 1977). Animals were killed for in situ hybridization at 2,4,6,8,10,12,14, and 32 days postlesion (2 animals at each time point). Two control animals were also prepared. In situ hybridization was carried out on samples from all of these cases for the GFAP probe. For the actin, tubulin, and neurofilament probes, we focused on the 2-8 day postlesion interval, which spans the early phase of the reinnervation process.

Animals were perfused with with 4% paraformaldehyde in 0.1M phosphate buffer while deeply anesthetized with sodium pentobarbital. The brains were removed, and immersed in 15% sucrose in 4% paraformaldehyde/phosphate buffer for 1-4 hours. The brains were sectioned at 20um in the horizontal plane using a cryostat, and the sections were thaw mounted onto poly-lysine coated microscope slides. A total of 150-200 sections were collected throughout the dorso-ventral extent of the hippocampus. The sections were stored at -80°C prior to use. A 1 in 15 series of sections was used for each hybridization run.

The cRNA probes used in this study were derived from cDNA's that have been characterized previously. The probe for GFAP was derived from a cDNA clone characterized by Lewis et al. (1984). The probe for the 68K neurofilament protein was derived from a cDNA probe initially described by Lewis and Cowan (1985). The probes for beta-tubulin and beta-actin were derived from cDNA probes described by Cleveland et al. (1980). Fragments of these clones ranging in size from 1.2-2.2 kilobases were re-cloned into a Bluescript m13- vector by D. Chikaraishi (Tufts University). Samples of the Bluescript plasmid with the inserts were provided to us as a gift.

Large scale preparation of the plasmids with the cDNA inserts and production of labeled cRNA probes were carried out by the Molecular Probe Laboratory of the University of Virginia. Sense and antisense probes labeled with 35S were synthesized as described in Maniatis et al. (1983). Specificity of the 35S riboprobes was evaluated by Northern blot analysis using mRNA obtained from whole forebrain. All probes recognized a single band on the gels at an apparent molecular weight consistent with the respective mRNA's. There was no evidence of binding to either 18S or 28S rRNA.

In situ hybridization was carried out using the procedure described in Rosenthal et al. (1987).

RESULTS

Increases in mRNA for GFAP after Lesions of the Entorhinal Cortex

In tissue sections from control animals, the labeling for GFAP mRNA was fairly uniform throughout the brain (Fig. 1A). Grain density was slightly higher over the glia limitans at the brain surface, and over fiber tracts.

As illustrated in Figure 1B, there were very dramatic increases in labeling for the GFAP probe at 2 days postlesion. The increases in grain density were apparent in all regions that receive direct projections from the entorhinal cortex, and also in areas that would not contain terminal degeneration after such lesions. For example, there were increases in labeling throughout the hippocampus ipsilateral and contralateral to the lesion in both denervated and non-denervated laminae. There were also increases in labeling over the surface of the tectum, particularly ipsilateral to the lesion, and in periventricular zones throughout the brain.

A different pattern of labeling was observed at 4 days postlesion and thereafter. At 4 days postlesion, the labeling was highest in areas that would be expected to contain degeneration debris. Thus, within the hippocampus, grain density was highest in the molecular layer of the dentate gyrus ipsilateral to the lesion, and within stratum lacunosum moleculare bilaterally. There was still some

---

Figure 1. Increases in GFAP mRNA following unilateral destruction of the entorhinal cortex. A) Control; B) 2 days postlesion; C) 8 days postlesion. H=hippocampus; DG=dentate gyrus; Thal=thalamus, Sept=septum; ECL=lesion site in entorhinal cortex; SC and IC=superior and inferior colliculus; Cb=cerebellum; LD=lateral dorsal thalamus; slm=stratum lacunosum moleculare of the CA1 region of the hippocampus. From Steward et al. (submitted).

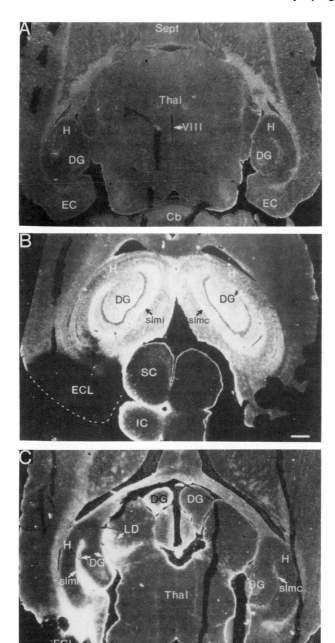

evidence of increased labeling in non-denervated zones (for example, in the hippocampus contralateral to the lesion); however, labeling within non-denervated zones was much lower than within the denervated laminae. By 6 days postlesion, the increases in labeling appeared to be restricted to the denervated zones (Fig. 1C).

Essentially the same pattern of labeling was evident between 6 and 14 days postlesion, except that the density of labeling within the denervated zone appeared to be higher at 8 days than at other intervals. This impression was confirmed by the quantitative analyses (see below). By 32 days postlesion, the levels of labeling over the denervated portions of the neuropil were only slightly higher than elsewhere within the section.

At 6-8 days postlesion, increased labeling for GFAP mRNA was also observed within the scar tissue at the boundary of the lesion. This increase was not apparent at 2 days postlesion when the increases in other areas were maximal. The levels of labeling remained high within the scar throughout the 6-14 day postlesion interval. By 32 days, labeling within the scar was near control levels.

Throughout the 4-14 day postlesion period, periventricular areas continued to exhibit increased labeling. The increases were restricted to a thin band of labeling adjacent to the ventricles. Qualitatively, the levels of labeling over periventricular zones did not appear to be as high between 4-14 days postlesion as at 2 days.

To define the time course of the increases in labeling revealed by _in situ_ hybridization, we evaluated grain density over the denervated laminae (the molecular layer of the dentate gyrus, and the stratum lacunosum moleculare of CA1). Grain density was also evaluated over the molecular layer of the dentate gyrus contralateral to the lesion, and over stratum radiatum of CA1. These latter areas contain little if any degeneration debris following unilateral entorhinal cortex lesions, and thus provide a measure of changes in grain density within non-denervated portions of the hippocampal neuropil. To provide an internal standard for variability in the extent of hybridization from case to case, grain density was evaluated over deep layers of the cerebral cortex.

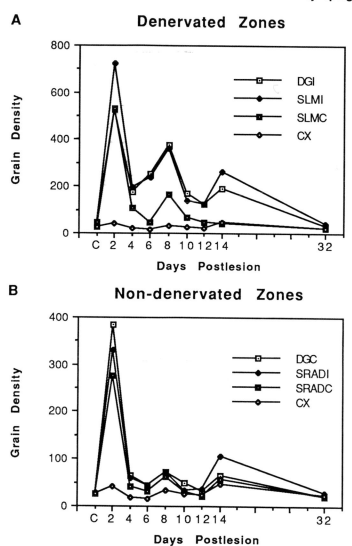

Figure 2. Quantitative analysis of the time course of increases in GFAP mRNA as revealed by in situ hybridization. A) Grain density in denervated zones; B) Grain density in non-denervated zones. DGI and DGC=molecular layer of the dentate gyrus ipsilateral and contralateral to the lesion; SLMi and SLMc=stratum lacunosum moleculare of the CA1 region ipsi- and contralateral to the lesion. Cx=cortex. From Steward et al. (submitted).

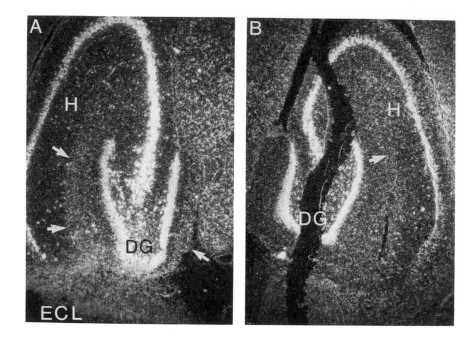

Figure 3. Distribution of beta-tubulin mRNA following unilateral destruction of the entorhinal cortex. A) 6 days postlesion; B) Control. Arrows indicate the denervated zones.   Abbreviations are as in Fig. 1.

        Figure 2A illustrates the time course of the changes in grain density within denervated zones. As expected, the increases in labeling were greatest at 2 days postlesion. The level of labeling decreased after 2 days postlesion, but remained much higher than control throughout the 4–14 day postlesion interval. There appeared to be a secondary peak in labeling between 6 and 8 days. By 32 days, the level of labeling was near control levels. Figure 2B illustrates the time course of changes in grain density in the non-denervated zones (the contralateral dentate gyrus, and stratum radiatum). Within the non-denervated zones, the levels of labeling were high at 2 days postlesion. Between 4 and 14 days postlesion, the levels of labeling in non-denervated zones were only slightly higher than control levels.

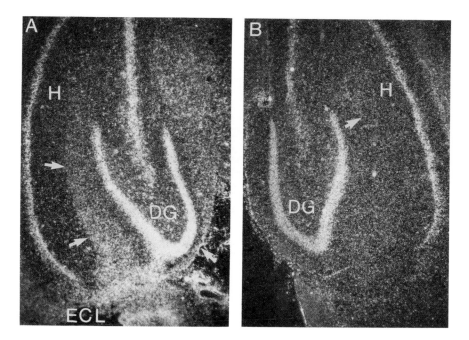

Figure 4.   Distribution of beta-actin mRNA following
unilateral destruction of the entorhinal cortex.   A)   6 days
postlesion; B) Control. Arrows indicate the denervated
zones.   Abbreviations are as in Fig. 1.

Beta-Actin and Beta-Tubulin

     In control animals, labeling for both beta-actin and
beta-tubulin was predominantly over neuronal cell bodies
(Figure 3A and 4A).   However, there was a diffuse labeling
of neuropil layers and fiber tracts.   This diffuse labeling
could reflect a high tissue background for these probes, or
could reflect the presence of low levels of the respective
mRNAs in glial cells and their processes or in dendrites.

     There was little change in the pattern of labeling for
tubulin and actin at 2 and 4 days postlesion.   However, at 6
and 8 days postlesion, there was an increase in labeling for
both probes over the denervated portions of the neuropil

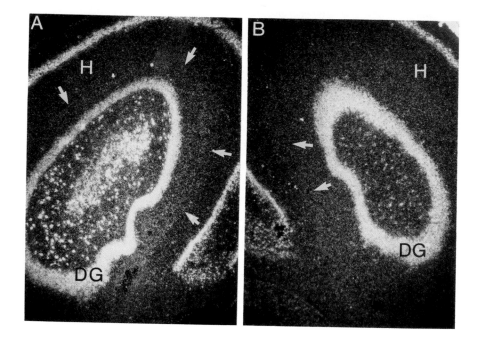

Figure 5. Distribution of neurofilament 68 mRNA following unilateral destruction of the entorhinal cortex. A) 6 days postlesion; B) Control. Arrows indicate the denervated zone. Abbreviations are as in Fig. 1.

ipsilateral to the lesion (Figure 3B and 4B). There was little increase in labeling in the terminal field of the crossed projection to the CA1 region of the hippocampus contralateral to the lesion (single arrows in Figs. 3B and 4B), and there were no increases in labeling over the dentate granule cell layer. There was an indication for an increase in labeling of neuronal cell bodies within the hilus of the dentate gyrus ipsilateral to the lesion. These neurons are the cells of origin of some of the fibers that reinnervate the granule cells.

There were also increases in labeling for both beta-actin and beta-tubulin mRNA within the scar tissue at the boundary of the lesion. These increases in labeling within the scar were not apparent at 2 days postlesion, but were prominent at 6 and 8 days.

Neurofilament

In control animals, labeling for the neurofilament probe appeared to be restricted to neuronal cell bodies (Fig. 5). Thus, in the hippocampus, the granule and pyramidal cell body laminae were heavily labeled, while labeling in the neuropil layers was light. There were a few labeled cells within the neuropil layers which presumably represent the isolated neuronal cell bodies that are present in these layers.

The neurofilament probe produced a different pattern of labeling after lesions than the probes for beta-actin and beta-tubulin. In particular, at 6-8 days postlesion, there was little if any increase in labeling over the denervated neuropil, at least in regions distant from the lesion site (Fig. 5). There did appear to be an increase in labeling of neuronal cell bodies within the hilus of the dentate gyrus ipsilateral to the lesion. In fact, the increase in labeling of neuronal cell bodies in the hilus was more obvious with the neurofilament probe than was true with the beta-actin and beta-tubulin probes.

DISCUSSION

The present study evaluated one mRNA that is specific to glia (GFAP), one mRNA that is specific to neurons (neurofilament 68), and two mRNAs that are present in both cell types (beta actin and beta tubulin). Our results reveal that there are dramatic increases in the levels of GFAP mRNA after unilateral entorhinal lesions. The increases are of three types: 1) a rapid transient increase in non-denervated zones in the hippocampus; 2) a sustained increase in denervated zones and in the glial scar bordering the lesion; 3) an increase in periventricular zones throughout the brain. In contrast, there were only modest increases in the levels of mRNAs for beta tubulin and beta-actin within the denervated zones and the scar. These increases were not evident until 6-8 days postlesion. There was little if any change in the pattern of labeling for the neurofilament probe in the denervated zones, however.

Relationship Between Increases in Particular mRNAs and Increases in Protein Synthesis in the Denervated Zone.

In our previous studies that revealed increases in protein synthesis within the denervated zone at 6-8 days postlesion, we speculated on the identity of the cells participating in the response (Fass and Steward, 1983). The parallels between the increased incorporation within the denervated neuropil and the increases in polyribosomes beneath synapses suggested an increased protein synthesis within dendrites. However, we could not exclude the possiblity that some or all of the increased incorporation reflected an increased synthesis of protein by reactive astrocytes.

The present results suggest that there is a dramatic increase in GFAP synthesis within the denervated neuropil. The question is whether this increase accounts for the increase in protein synthesis. If the increase in incorporation reflects synthesis by reactive astrocytes, then one would expect the time course of the increases in the mRNAs for glial proteins to be similar to the time course of increased incorporation. However, the increases in GFAP mRNA levels are most pronounced at 2 days postlesion, whereas the increases in synthesis are maximal at 6-8 days. It is possible that the increases in GFAP synthesis are delayed with respect to the increases in GFAP mRNA, so that levels of synthesis are actually maximal during the 6-8 day postlesion interval. This possibility does not seem likely because astrocyte hypertrophy is maximal at 1-2 days postlesion (Rose et al., 1976). It is also possible that there is a bi-phasic response of astrocytes, with one wave of increased GFAP synthesis occurring at 2 days postlesion, and a second wave at 6-8 days. If this is true then increases in GFAP synthesis cannot account for the increase in protein synthesis within the denervated zone, because there is no overall increase in protein synthesis when mRNA levels are at their highest.

The increases in mRNAs for beta tubulin and beta actin could reflect increased synthesis by either neurons or glia. However, circumstantial evidence suggests that the response is primarily glial. The increases within the denervated zone occur concurrently with increases in tubulin and actin mRNAs within the scar. The latter almost certainly reflect synthesis by astrocytes. Because of the similarities in the

time course of the increases in the denervated neuropil and
the scar, it seems most likely that the increases within the
scar also reflect synthesis by glia. The possibility cannot
be excluded, however, that the increases in beta-tubulin and
beta-actin mRNA reflect increased protein synthesis within
dendrites.

Our present results provide new insights into the
molecular events within reactive glia, and the signals that
regulate GFAP expression. The persistent increase in GFAP
mRNA within the denervated laminae presumably reflects
reactive gliosis in areas containing degeneration debris.
However, the increases in GFAP mRNA in areas that do not
contain degeneration must occur in response to some signal
other than degeneration debris. Possibilities for the
signal include: 1) release of a diffusable substance that
affects glial cells over a widespread area, or 2) changes
in activity produced by the lesion (transient increases in
activity at the time of the electrolytic lesion, or
persistent decreases in cellular activity thereafter).

In the case of the increases in GFAP mRNA in the
periventricular areas and over the surface of the tectum, a
diffusable factor seems most likely. A diffusable factor
would presumably be produced at the site of injury or within
areas that receive direct projections from the damaged
regions, and would diffuse throughout the ventricular
system. One would expect the effect of a diffusable factor
to be most pronounced in periventricular areas, and to
decrease with distance from the site of production. This is
essentially the pattern that was observed.

The increases in GFAP mRNA within the non-denervated
zones in the hippocampus were uniform throughout the depth
of the affected structure. There was no evidence of a
gradient with distance from the ventricular surface. Thus,
the pattern of increased labeling in the hippocampus is
different than would be expected in response to some
diffusable agent in the ventricular system. It is possible
that the increases in labeling within the hippocampus
reflect a change in activity that occurs as a result of the
lesion, or some other process related to the injury.

Gene Expression by Neurons participating in lesion-induced synaptogenesis

The present results permit us to refine our hypotheses about the mechanisms of lesion-induced synaptogenesis. Our results strongly suggest that there is no general increase in the production of cytoskeletal proteins by neurons that are being reinnervated. The changes in expression that we have observed most likely reflect events within reactive astrocytes. This leaves the other two possibilities: 1) that lesion-induced synaptogenesis involves an increased expression of some "special" growth related genes; or 2) that lesion-induced synaptogenesis can occur without any change in gene expression within the neurons being reinnervated.

Studies by Geddes et al. (1988) have provided evidence supporting the second possibility. These authors report substantial increases in the mRNA for the alpha-1 form of tubulin in the neurons being reinnervated. The significance of these increases for the lesion-induced growth process must still be established, because increases in labeling were also observed within granule cells on the side contralateral to the lesion. Nevertheless, the selective increases in particular classes of mRNA suggest that lesion-induced reinnervation involves an induction of "special" genes by neurons participating in the growth response.

It is important to note that the above conclusions apply only to the neurons being reinnervated. In fact, our results suggest that there may be an increase in synthesis of general cytoskeletal proteins within at least some of the neurons giving rise to reinnervating fibers. This conclusion is based upon the increased labeling for beta-tubulin, beta-actin, and neurofilament in the neurons in the hilus of the dentate gyrus ipsilateral to the lesion. Future studies will be required to address this issue.

Acknowledgements: Thanks to Leanna Whitmore and Paula Falk for their excellent technical help, and to N. Cowan and D. Chikaraishi for providing the plasmids used to produce cRNA probes. Thanks also to Ted Mifflin and the staff of the Molecular Probe Laboratory of the University of Virginia for producing the labeled cRNA probes used in this study. Supported by NIH grant NS12333 to O.S.

REFERENCES

Caceres AO, Steward O (1983) Dendritic reorganization in the denervated dentate gyrus of the rat following entorhinal cortical lesions: a Golgi and electron microscopic analysis. J Comp Neurol 214: 387-403.

Cleveland DW, Lopata MA, MacDonald RJ, Cowan NJ, Rutter WJ, and Kirschner MW (1980) Number and evolutionary conservation of alpha- and beta-tubulin and cytoplasmic beta- and alpha-actin genes using specific cloned cDNA probes. Cell 20: 95-105.

Fass B, Steward O (1983) Increases in protein precursor incorporation in the denervated neuropil of the dentate gyrus during reinnervation. Neurosci 9: 633-664.

Geddes JW, Cotman CW, Miller FD (1988) In situ hybridization of tubulin alpha-1 mRNA as a marker of neurons participating in reactive synaptogenesis. Neurosci Abs 14: 823.

Lewis SA, Cowan NJ (1985) Genetics, evolution, and expression of the 68,000-mol-wt neurofilament protein: isolation of a cloned cDNA probe. J Cell Biol 100: 843-850.

Lewis SA, Balcarek JM, Krek V, Shelanski M, and Cowan NJ (1984) Sequence of a cDNA clone encoding mouse glial fibrillary acidic protein: structural conservation of intermediate filaments. Proc Nat Acad Sci 81: 2743-2746.

Loesche J, Steward O (1976) Behavioral correlates of denervation and reinnervation of the hippocampal formation of the rat: recovery of alternation performance following unilateral entorhinal cortical lesions. Brain Res Bull 2: 31-40.

Maniatis T, Fritchs EF, Sambrook J (1983) Molecular Cloning. A Laboratory Manual. VI Ed. Cold Spring Harbor, New York. Cold Spring Harbor Laboratory.

Matthews DA, Cotman C, Lynch G (1976) An electron microscopic study of lesion-induced synaptogenesis in the dentate gyrus of the adult rat. I. Magnitude and time course of degeneration. Brain Res 115: 1-21.

Phillips LL, Nostrandt SJ, Chikaraishi DM, Steward O (1987) Increases in ribosomal RNA within the denervated neuropil of the dentate gyrus during reinnervation: evaluation by in situ hybridization using DNA probes complementary to ribosomal RNA. Mol Brain Res 2: 251-261.

Rose G, Lynch G, Cotman CW (1976) Hypertrophy and redistribution of astrocytes in the deafferented dentate gyrus. Brain Res Bull 1: 87–92.

Rosenthal A, Chan SY, Henzel W, Haskell C, Kuang W-J, Chen E, Wilcox JN, Ullrich A, Goeddel DV, Routtenberg A (1987) Primary structure and mRNA localization of protein F1, a growth-related protein kinase C substrate associated with synaptic plasticity. EMBO J 6: 3641–3646.

Steward O (1983) Alterations in polyribosomes associated with dendritic spines during the reinnervation of the dentate gyrus of the adult rat. J Neurosci 3: 177–188.

Steward O (1986) Lesion-induced synapse growth in the hippocampus: In search of cellular and molecular mechanisms. In: The Hippocampus. RL Isaacson and KH Pribram (Eds.) Plenum, pp. 65–111.

Steward O (1989) Reorganization of neuronal connections following CNS trauma: principles and experimental paradigms. J Neurotrauma 6: 99–152.

Steward O, Torre ER, Phillips LL, Trimmer PA (submitted) The process of reinnervation in the dentate gyrus of adult rats: time course of increases in mRNA for glial fibrillary acidic protein.

Steward O, Vinsant SV (1983) The process of reinnervation in the dentate gyrus of the adult rat. A quantitative electron microscopic analysis of terminal proliferation and reactive synaptogenesis. J Comp Neurol 214: 370–386.

**Advances in Neural Regeneration
Research, pages 87–102**

GROWTH PROMOTING AND INHIBITING FACTORS FOR NEURONS

Marston Manthorpe, David Muir, Theo Hagg
and   Silvio Varon

Department of Biology, M-001, School of
Medicine, University of California, San
Diego, La Jolla, California 92093

INTRODUCTION

The performance of each neuron within its own
community is regulated by exogeneous protein
"factors" contributed by adjacent cells,
extracellular matrices and surrounding fluids.
Neurons must possess receptor systems to bind these
factors and to transduce their binding into
cellular changes. Thus, each cellular performance
will be dictated by a particular combination of
factors available to the neuron as well as by the
neuron's own repertoire of receptors and
transducers. Neuronal cell performances
particularly pertinent to regeneration and subject
to regulation by proteins include cellular survival
and neurite elongation. Factor availability and
receptor repertoire may change after nervous tissue
damage or disease and the resulting dysfunctions
may be ameliorated by adminstration of the
corresponding exogneous factors. A better
understanding of the regulation of neuronal cell
health, growth and regeneration by exogenous
factors may provide rationale for their future
therapeutic applications. In this introductory
chapter to the session on growth promoting and
inhibiting factors, we will discuss influences of
selected factors on neurons in vitro and in vivo,
and relate some emerging concepts regarding their
potential physiological roles and clinical
utilities. Although this introductory chapter will

be intentionally restricted, further reading on this subject may be found in various reviews (Barde, 1989; Lipton, 1989; Manthorpe et al., 1986; 1989; 1990; Snider and Johnson, 1989; Varon et al., 1988a,b; 1989).

IN VITRO REGULATION OF NEURONAL SURIVIVAL AND GROWTH

During development, neurons survive and extend an axonal process toward their future innervation territory. The efferent axonal tip contacts and recognizes an appropriate target cell, axonal elongation ceases and functional synaptic associations are formed. Each developing neuron is being sought out, recognized as a target, and funtionally innervated by afferent neurons. Early in development, most neuronal populations are originally supernumerary. During a critical and defined period, neurons that apparently do not make successful target connections will die off. This form of "developmental neuronal death" prompted the hypothesis that cells in the target area supply the innervating neurons with neuronotrophic factors ("NTFs" or simply "trophic factors") which support the selective survival of the neurons (Landmesser and Pilar, 1978). This hypothesis has recently been extended to apply to the adult CNS where neurons retain NTF receptors and apparently continue to require the NTFs for neuronal performances (Varon et al., 1989). Other neuronal performances such as axonal growth, sprouting, guidance and synaptogenesis and plasticity may also be subject to factor regulation during maturation and aging.

Cell culture methods have been important for identifying and characterizing proteins potentially capable of regulating neuronal cell performances in vivo. In nearly all cases, cultures of regenerating embryonic neurons have been used because of the current lack of well-characterized in vitro preparations of purified adult neurons. A partial list of factors affecting the survival and axonal growth of cultured embryonic neurons is

presented in Table 1, along with a leading
reference for further reading. By far, the best
characterized NTF, nerve growth factor (NGF), was
discovered 40 years ago to be required for the in

TABLE 1. Neuronal growth promoting or inhibiting
factors

Factor   One Recent Reference

Neuronotrophic factors

Nerve Growth Factor   Levi-Montalcini,1987
Brain-Derived Growth Factor   Leibrock et al.,1989
Ciliary Neuronotrophic Factor   Manthorpe et al.,1989
Fibroblast Growth Factor   Walicke, 1988
Epidermal Growth Factor   Morrison et al.,1987

Neurite-promoting factors
in the Extracellular Matrix

Laminin   Manthorpe et al.,1990
Fibronectin   Rogers et al.,1987
Collagens   Pittman & Williams,1989
Proteoglycans   Chernoff,1988

Neuronotoxic Factors

Astroglial-derived toxicity   Lefebvre,et al.,1988
Brain-derived toxicity   Manthorpe,et al.,1982

Neurite-inhibitory Factors

Schwann cell inhibitor   Muir et al.,1989
CNS-derived inhibitor   Caroni & Schwab,1988
Inhibitor of outgrowth   Taniura et al.,1988

---

vitro and in vivo survival and general growth of
developing sympathetic and sensory neurons (Levi-
Montalcini, 1987). In contrast, cultured adult
peripheral neurons apparently do not require NGF
for their survival, although they do retain NGF

receptors and continue to respond to it (Lindsay et al., 1989). More recently NGF has been found to have trophic influences in vivo on adult peripheral (Snider and Johnson, 1989) and central neurons (Varon et al, 1989). Table 1 also lists other NTFs recognized within the past 10 years to support the in vitro survival of various developing peripheral (BDNF, CNTF, FGF) and/or central (FGF, EGF) neurons. Their roles within the adult nervous system in vivo remain to be established.

When proper in vitro precautions are taken to exclude trophic contributions from target and other supportive cells, cultured developing neurons will not survive without exogenous NTFs. In fact, NTFs are turning out to be quite ubiquitous in both their distribution and action. For example, the following general points about NTFs can be made at present: 1) the same NTF can act on different neuronal populations (eg., CNTF supports sensory, sympathetic and parasympathetic neurons; FGF can support both peripheral and central neurons; NGF can influence noradrenergic, cholinergic and GABAergic neurons), and the same neuron can be acted on by more than one NTF (eg., ciliary ganglionic motor neurons can be influenced by CNTF, FGF and NGF); 2) the same NTF can have more than one biological activity (eg., NGF can support neuronal survival and/or increase neurotransmitter enzyme synthesis), and one biological activity can be influenced by different NTFs (eg., CNTF and FGF support ciliary ganglion neuronal survival); 3) NTFs can also act on non neuronal cells (eg., FGF acts on fibroblasts; CNTF acts on oligodendroglial cell precursors; NGF may act on lymphocytes), and both neuronal and non-neuronal cells can produce NTFs (eg., NGF and CNTF are produced by Schwann, astroglial, muscle and fibroblastic cells); and finally 4) one cell type can produce multiple NTFs (eg., C-6 glial cells can produce NGF, CNTF and FGF).

This perplexing array of NTF features can be at least partially accomodated in a trophic hypothesis put forward over 10 years ago (Varon, 1977). The hypothesis assumes that neurons require more than one type of factor to function properly and to regenerate after injury. The NTFs act generically to upregulate overall anabolic processes that manifest themselves as general cellular growth capability. These general growth stimulating cell processes can be channeled into specific performances, (eg., axonal or dendritic elongation, neurotransmitter enzyme synthesis, synapse formation, etc.) if additional factors are available to the cell. Several candidate factors listed in Table 1 act in concert with NTFs to direct NTF supported cellular energies.

One type of factor, termed neurite promoting factor (NPF), stimulates neurite outgrowth. The most potent NPFs are widespread extracellular matrix components such as laminin, fibronectin, and the collagens and proteoglycans. The extracellular matrix NPFs appear to be somewhat universal in their action in that they stimulate neurite outgrowth from a wide variety of peripheral and central neurons. The NPFs, unlike the NTFs, do not support neuronal survival by themselves and NPFs are known to operate through different neuronal cell surface receptors (integrins) than those utilized by NTFs. The integrins are present on nearly all cells, whereas NTF receptors are much more specific and restricted in distribution. When neurons are supported in vitro by NTFs but not allowed an opportunity to interact with NPFs, neurite extension will not occur. The existence of NPFs fits the idea that neurons derive general support from one set of factors (NTFs) but rely on other factors such as NPFs to direct their NTF-stimulated energies into specific tasks such as formation of a growth cone and extension of neurite processes.

Two other categories of factors have been recognized that appear to antagonize the activities of the NTFs and NPFs. Glia- and brain-derived neuronotoxic (NXFs) and neurite inhibiting factors (NIFs) appear, respectively, to kill neurons supported by NTFs or inhibit neurites stimulated by NPFs.

The action of these four factors (NTFs, NPFs,
NXFs and NIFs) on a neuron is schematically
presented in Figure 1. Some neurons cultured in
the absence of adequate levels of NTF may survive,
albeit it in a somewhat atrophied state. With the
addition of more NTF, the general anabolic
reactions in the neuron increases. Without
specific instructions this increase only results in
general upregulation of many cellular processes and
hypertrophy of the somata. With the addition of a
neurite promoting factor, for example, this general
increase in anabolic metabolism is directed more
towards the expression of neurite extension. Thus,

FIGURE 1

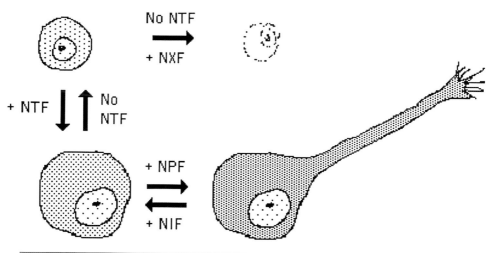

in order to extend an axon, a neuron must be
presented with both NTFs and NPFs and must possess
both NTF <u>and</u> NPF receptors. Both neuronal receptor
synthesis and factor production are themselves
likely to be under separate regulation. Even if
these requirements are met, cell survival or
neurite extension may not occur if the neuron is
presented with antagonistic factors. A neuron may
have adequate NTF and NPF supplies and still not
extend neurites or even may die if neurite

inhibitors (NIFs) or toxic factors (NXFs) are present, respectively. It has not yet been established whether antagonistic factors act on the neuron through distinct cell surface receptors or by modifying NTF/NPF molecules or their receptors. An example of the inhibition of neurite extension in the presence of adequate NPF is presented in Figure 2 (after Muir et al., 1989). In this case, a polyornithine substratum was prepared and coated with a purified rat NPF, laminin. A region of the laminin-polyornithine substratum was "painted" with a stripe of a neurite inhibitory factor (NIF) purified from rat RN22 Schwannoma cells. Embryonic day 8 chick ciliary motor neurons were cultured for one week on this substratum in the presence of excess CNTF to assure their survival. The neurons survived and extended

FIGURE 2.

+ CNTF
+ Laminin

+ CNTF
+ Laminin
+ NIF

+ CNTF
+ Laminin

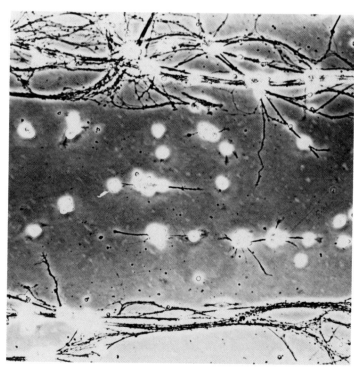

neurites into all areas except that treated with the NIF. Those neurons that attached directly to the NIF-coated region survived and exhibited very modest, if any, neurite outgrowth over the seven day period. Recent studies by us (unpublished observations) have suggested that the NIF can inhibit neurite growth in response to NPFs other than laminin. This suggests that this NIF interacts directly with the cell to inhihit some fundamental cellular process required for neurite extension. In vivo such NIFs could potentially prevent and confine neurite growth during target seeking and specification of terminal fields.

IN VIVO REGULATION OF NEURONAL SURVIVAL AND GROWTH

In vitro methods are useful in detecting and characterizing regulatory factors and in developing concepts about neuronal survival and neurite regulating factors. In vivo such factors may have roles in maintaining the cytoarchitecture in normal nervous tissue and in promoting tissue repair after trauma or disease. For reparative studies, one experimental approach is transection of adult axons followed by factor administration and assessment of factor-induced restorations. Specific factors may sustain neuronal health after axotomy and may promote axonal regeneration back into the disconnected target territory. An important concern in this field of research is the extent to which specific factors can be directed to specific cell populations given their often pluripotential influences.

One model for central nervous system regeneration utilizes the adult rat septo-hippocampal system (Varon et al., 1989). Neurons within the hippocampal formation produce and deliver NGF to innervating medial septum cholinergic neurons which are then generally sustained by the retrogradely acquired NGF (Whittemore and Seiger, 1987). In one experimental paradigm, aspiration of the dorsal fornix and fimbria pathways removes all dorsal cholinergic input to the hippocampal formation and deprives the corresponding afferent medial septum neurons of their putative supply of target-derived NGF. The axotomy causes a quantitative disappearance of cholinergic medial septum neurons detectable by their staining for acetylcholinesterase or choline acetyltransferase (ChAT). Intraventricular administration of purified NGF, intended to replace the lost hippocampal-derived NGF, prevents this axotomy-induced loss (Hefti, 1986; Kromer, 1987; Williams et al., 1986).

This loss of detectable cholinergic neurons was originally attributed to degeneration and death of the axotomized cell bodies which had become deprived of NGF supplied retrogradely by the hippocampus. However, when the target-deprived medial septum neurons are first allowed to disappear and then supplied with exogenous NGF, most of the missing neurons regain their cholinergic staining properties, even if the NGF administration delayed by as long as 3 months (Hagg et al., 1988). This suggests that a constant supply of hippocampal NGF is required to maintain the synthesis of the function related cholinergic enzymes, and that this requirement can be met artificially by providing NGF. It also suggests that hippocampal NGF is not required for the survival of these adult CNS neurons (see also Sofroniew et al., 1990).

Such studies with the adult rat septohippocampal system have encouraged suggestions that the loss of cholinergic neurons or their functions in humans, such as those associated with Alzheimer's disease, may be partially corrected by experimental treatments with intraventricular NGF (Phelps, et al., 1989). These studies also encourage the view that other neurodegenerative disorders and even trauma-induced degeneration may be susceptible to neuronotrophic and neurite promoting factor related therapies. Such therapies should be preceded by a detailed understanding of how such factors operate in the experimental models. We will use the adult rat septohippocampal model and NGF administration to illustrate considerations that should be entertained for human therapeutic application of neuron directed growth promoting or inhibiting factors.

FIGURE 3

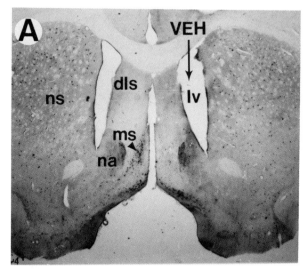

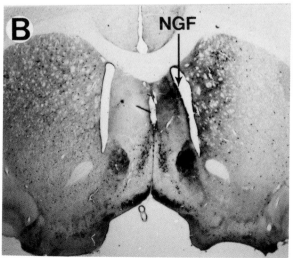

Figure 3 shows choline acetyltransferase (ChAT) immunostained coronal sections of an adult rat brain at the level of the medial septum. The animals had received a unilateral fimbria-fornix transection followed at two weeks by a two week intraventricular adminstration of vehicle (VEH) or vehicle-NGF (NGF) on the ipsilateral (right) side. Note that axotomized medial septal (ms) ChAT-positive cell bodies are nearly absent after transection and vehicle administration (Figure 3A) but retained after NGF treatment (Figure 3B).

Cross-sectional size distributions of the ChAT-positive medial septum cell bodies without or with restoration by delayed NGF administration shows that these neurons shrink considerably prior to their disappearance after axotomy, reappear in a shrunken state soon after delayed NGF administration and increase their size on further NGF treatment (Hagg et al, 1989a). Thus, these adult CNS cholinergic neurons display in vivo an authentic trophic response to NGF deprivation and administration, similar to that illustrated earlier for cultured peripheral neurons (see Figure 1). The NGF controlled size stimulation of the cholinergic neurons is presumably associated with increased synthesis of basic anabolic components, as well as that of function related ones such as the cholinergic enzymes.

In addition to its influences on ChAT staining and cell size, intraventricular admininstration of NGF elicits increases levels of acetyl-cholinesterase and NGF receptor and even other proteins in these same medial septum neurons (Hagg et al 1989a,b). In the NGF treated brain (Figure 3B), but not in the vehicle treated one (Figure 3A), a periventricular ChAT positivity appears in the dorso-lateral septum (dls) and laterally in the medial neostriatum (ns). Higher magnification analysis of these regions (Hagg et al., 1989c) indicates that the septal staining occurs as a new fine fiber plexus while the striatal staining occurs as an intensification of an existing diffuse area containing cholinergic structures including ChAT-positive cell bodies. The lateral septal staining may reside on sprouted septal axons. Some of the periventricular striatal ChAT staining appears in cell bodies that are 40% larger than those on the other side of the brain and in corresponding areas of vehicle treated animals. In addition, the nucleus accumbens (na) of NGF treated animals becomes increasingly ChAT-positive compared to vehicle treated animals. Since neither striatum nor nucleus accumbens are mechanically damaged by fimbria-fornix transection, their apparently normal, non-lesioned cholinergic neurons must have the capacity to respond to an exogenous supply of NGF, perhaps with an upregulation of their general anabolic reactions.

Several other adult CNS neuronal systems may also respond to intraventricular NGF administration. Other cholinergic neurons such as those in the nucleus basalis of Meynert may respond to NGF (Fischer et al., 1987). Fetal rat GABAergic medial septal neurons have been recently reported (Dreyfus et al., 1989) to have NGF receptors and to be supported by NGF in vitro, and they may retain the ability to respond to NGF in the adult. Even Purkinje neurons in the cerebellum are reported to contain NGF (Pioro and Cuello, 1988) and NGF receptors (Cohen-Cory et al., 1989). Thus, by attempting to direct NGF administration to one neuronal system, one may influence many other neuronal systems. Future therapeutic application of NTFs like NGF to the human nervous system will have to consider that the chronically applied NTF will likely have unwanted effects on many parts of the nervous system. An understanding of proper dosages and the effects co-admininstration of NTFs and/or the use of transiently applied factors may offer ways to better localize such NTF therapies, once such therapies are established to be beneficial in the nervous system.

REFERENCES

Barde Y-A (1989). Trophic factors and neuronal survival. Neuron 2:1525-1534.
Caroni P, Schwab ME (1988). Two membrane protein fractions from rat central myelin with

inhibitory properties for neurite growth and fibroblast spreading. J Cell Biol 106:1281-8.

Chernoff EA (1988). The role of endogenous heparan sulfate proteoglycan in adhesion and neurite outgrowth from dorsal root ganglia. Tissue and Cell 20:165-78.

Cohen-Corey S, Dreyfus CF, Balck IB (1989). Expression of high- and low-affinity nerve growth factor receptors by Purkinje cells in the developing cerebellum. Exp Neurol 105:104-109.

Dreyfus CF, Bernd P, Martinez HJ, Rubin SJ, Black IB (1989). GABAergic and cholinergic neurons exhibit high-affinity nerve growth factor binding in rat basal forebrain. Exp Neurol 104:181-185.

Fischer W, Wictorin K, Björklund A, Williams LR, Varon S, Gage FH (1987). Amelioration of cholinergic neuron atrophy and spatial memory impairment in aged rats by nerve growth factor. Nature 329:65-68.

Hagg T, Manthorpe M, Vahlsing HL, Varon S (1988). Delayed treatment with nerve growth factor reverses the apparent loss of cholinergic neurons after acute brain damage. Exp Neurol 101:303-12.

Hagg T, Fass-Holmes B, Vahlsing HL, Manthorpe M, Conner J. Varon S (1989a). Nerve Growth Factor (NGF) reverses axotomy-induced decreases in choline acetyltransferase, NGF-receptor and size of medial septum cholinergic neurons. Brain Res 505:29-38.

Hagg T, Muir D, Engvall E, Varon S, Manthorpe M (1989b). Laminin-like antigen in rat CNS neurons: Distribution and changes upon brain injury and nerve growth factor treatment. Neuron 3:721-732.

Hagg T, Hagg F, Vahlsing HL, Manthorpe M, Varon S (1989c). Nerve growth factor effects on cholinergic neurons of neostriatum and nucleus accumbens in the adult rat. Neurosci 30:95-103.

Hefti F (1986). Nerve growth factor promotes survival of septal cholinergic neurons after fimbrial transections. J Neurosci 6:2155-2162.

Kromer LF (1987). Nerve growth factor treatment after brain injury prevents neuronal death. Science 235:214-216.

Landmesser L, Pilar G (1978). Interactions between neurons and their targets during in vivo synaptogenesis. Fed Proc 37:2016-2021.

Lefebvre PP, Rigo JM, Leprince P, Rogister B, Delree P, Hans P, Born JD, Moonen G (1988). Demonstration of a neuronotoxic activity in the cerebrospinal fluid of severe head injured patients. Agressologie 29:241-2.

Leibrock J, Lottspeich F, Hohn A, Hofer M, Hengerer B, Masiakowski P, Thoenen H, Barde YA (1989). Molecular cloning and expression of brain-derived neurotrophic factor. Nature 341:149-52.

Levi-Montalcini R (1987). The nerve growth factor 35 years later. Science 237:1154-62.

Lindsay R (1989). Nerve growth factors (NGF, BDNF) enhance axonal regeneration but are not required for survival of adult sensory neurons. J Neurosci 8:2394-2405.

Lipton SA (1989). Growth factors for neuronal survival and process regeneration. Arch Neurol 46:1241-1248.

Manthorpe M, Longo FM, Varon S (1982). Comparative features of spinal neuronotrophic factors in fluids collected in vitro and in vivo. J Neurosci Res 8:241-250.

Manthorpe M, Rudge J. Varon S (1986). Astroglial cell contributions to neuronal survival and neuritic growth. In: Fedoroff S, Vernadakis A (eds): "Astrocytes", Vol 2, New York: Academic Press, pp 315-376.

Manthorpe M, Ray J, Pettmann B, Varon S (1989). Ciliary Neuronotrophic Factors. In Rush R (ed): "Nerve Growth Factors", New York: John Wiley & Sons Ltd, pp 31-56.

Manthorpe M, Muir D, Hagg T, Engvall E, Varon S (1990). Glial cell laminin and neurite outgrowth. In Levi G (ed.): "Differentiation and Functions of Glial Cells", New York: Alan Liss Inc, pp 135-146.

Morrison RS, Kornblum HI, Leslie FM, Bradshaw RA (1987). Trophic stimulation of cultured neurons from neonatal rat brain by epidermal growth factor. Science 238:72-75.

Muir D, Engvall E, Varon S, Manthorpe M (1989). Schwannoma cell-derived inhibitor of the neurite promoting activity of laminin. J Cell Biol 109:2353-2362.

Phelps CH, Gage FH, Growdon JH, Hefti F, Harbaugh R, Johnston MV, Khachaturian ZS, Mobley WC, Price DL, Raskind M et al. (1989). Potential use of nerve growth factor to treat Alzheimer's disease. Neurobiol Aging 10:205-207

Pioro EP, Cuello AC (1988). Purkinge cells of adult rat cerebellum express nerve growth factor receptor immunoreactivity: light microscopic observations. Brain Res 455:182-186.

Pittman RN, Williams AG (1989). Neurite penetration into collagen gels requires Ca2+-dependent metalloproteinase activity. Dev Neurosci 11:41-51.

Rogers SL, Letourneau PC, Peterson BA, Furcht LT, McCarthy JB (1987). Selective interaction of peripheral and central nervous system cells with two distinct cell-binding domains of fibronectin. J Cell Biol 105:1435-1442.

Sofroniew MV, Galletly NP, Isacson O, Svendsen CN (1990). Survival of adult basal forebrain cholinergic neurons after loss of target neurons. Science 247:338-342.

Snider WD, Johnson EM (1989). Neurotrophic molecules. Annals of Neurol 26:489-506.

Taniura H, Hayashi Y, Miki N (1988). An 82-kilodalton membrane protein that inhibits the activity of neurite outgrowth factor. J Neurochem 50:1572-1578.

Varon S (1977). Neural growth and regeneration: A cellular perspective. Exp Neurol 54:1-6.

Varon S, Manthorpe M, Davis GE, Williams LR, Skaper SD (1988a). Growth factors. Adv Neurol 47:493-521.

Varon S, Pettmann B, Manthorpe M (1988b). Humoral and surface-anchored factors in development and repair of the nervous system. Prog Brain Res 73:465-89.

Varon S, Hagg T, Manthorpe M (1989). Neuronal growth factors. In Seil FJ (ed): "Neural Regeneration and Transplantation: Frontiers of Clinical Neuroscience" Vol 6 New York: Alan R liss, pp 101-121.

Walicke PA (1988). Basic and acidic fibroblast growth factors have trophic effects on neurons from multiple CNS regions. J Neurosci 8:2618-2627.

Williams LR, Varon S, Peterson GM, Wictorin K, Fisher W, Björklund A, Gage FH (1986). Continuous infusion of nerve growth factor prevents basal forebrain neuronal death after fimbria fornix transection. Proc Natl Acad Sci USA 83:9231-9235.

Whittemore SR, Seiger Å (1987). The expression, localization and functional significance of ß-nerve growth factor in adult rats with fimbria-fornix lesions. Behav Brian Res 17:17-24.

**Advances in Neural Regeneration
Research, pages 103–114
© 1990 Wiley-Liss, Inc.**

FIBROBLAST GROWTH FACTOR (FGF): A MULTIFUNCTIONAL
GROWTH FACTOR IN THE CNS

Patricia Ann Walicke

Department of Neuroscience, University of
California San Diego, La Jolla, CA 92093

The modern history of trophic factors commenced
with the discovery and purification of nerve growth
factor (NGF). Since then numerous trophic factors
have been purified for non-neuronal cells. Some,
such as erythropoietin and granulocyte-monocyte
colony stimulating factor, have already been
successfully tested in human diseases and will soon
enter general clinical use. Studies with NGF have
led to significant insights into the growth regulation of neurons in sympathetic and sensory ganglia
and the nucleus basalis, but NGF appears to address
less than 1% of CNS neurons. It has long been
proposed that most other neurons also use neurotrophic factors (NTF), but purification of these
factors has advanced slowly.

As other trophic factors were purified, it
became apparent that many of them were found in the
CNS. At least one and often several members of the
following families of trophic factors have been
found in brain or cultured glial cells: insulin-
like growth factors (IGF), fibroblast growth
factors (FGF), tumor necrosis factors (TNF),
interleukins (IL), colony stimulating factors
(CSF), transforming growth factor alpha (TGFa),
transforming growth factor beta (TGFb) (Walicke,
1989). Another theme that has emerged in growth
factor research is multifunctionality (Sporn and
Roberts, 1988). Although each factor was initially
identified by its effects on one cell type, further

studies have usually shown influences on multiple cell types. These factors are most often ascribed a role in regulation of non-neuronal CNS cells, but at least some of them could also have NTF activity. This chapter will focus on one of these multifunctional factors (MF), basic fibroblast growth factor (bFGF). The approaches and models discussed are applicable to other MFs found in brain, and hopefully more of these will be examined as potential NTFs.

As a starting point, criteria for identification of a MF as a NTF are proposed in Table 1. Together these constitute a rigorous test, and several were only rather recently fulfilled for NGF, especially in the CNS. With the exception of the third criterion, they essentially use the type of logic employed in Koch's postulates. The third criterion is included because of the stress on the role of retrograde transport in the actions of NGF. It is listed only as probable to avoid exclusion of glial derived factors which might act directly on the neuronal soma. The criteria can be useful in providing an outline for design of experiments to test the hypothesis that a MF might be a NTF.

TABLE 1. Criteria for a Neurotrophic Factor

1. Stimulates neuronal survival and/or growth in vitro
2. Acts through specific receptors on neurons
3. Probably internalized and retrogradely transported
4. Exogenous administration increases neuronal survival and\or growth in vivo
5. Depletion of endogenous stores decreases neuronal survival and\or growth in vivo

---

bFGF AS A NTF

bFGF is a 16 kD peptide which was the first member of the FGF family to be sequenced and cloned. More recently it has become clear that there are also larger products of the bFGF gene in brain tissue. It is highly pleiotropic, stimulating many types of mesenchymal cells, endocrine cells and glia. So far four other homologous proteins have been identified and grouped in the FGF family. These are acidic FGF (aFGF), hst/KS-FGF, int-2 and FGF-5. All of these may be present in the brain (Folkman et al., 1988; Baird & Walicke, 1989).

bFGF has been reported to increase the survival of at least some neurons present in cultures obtained from a variety of cortical regions, hippocampus, striatum, thalamus, septum, mesen-cephalon, cerebellum, spinal cord and parasym-pathetic ganglia. It is not a universal NTF since it fails to support sympathetic neurons or periphe-ral sensory neurons. Since many of these studies were conducted in cultures with less than 1% glial contamination, it is likely that bFGF directly stimulates neurons. In addition, bFGF increases neurite growth and levels of transmitter related products. It is not specific for one transmitter phenotype, but affects cholinergic, dopaminergic or GABAergic markers as appropriate (Unsicker et al., 1987; Hatten et al., 1988; Walicke, 1988). The effects of bFGF and NGF on responsive neurons in vitro appear similar, except that bFGF is more broad spectrum.

bFGF receptors have been characterized in cultures of fetal hippocampal neurons. Like fibroblasts, neurons have two binding sites: 1) a high capacity, low affinity system likely related to heparan sulfate; 2) a saturable, high affinity membrane receptor. The Kd of the receptor is about 0.2 nM. Affinity labeling studies suggest the presence of two glycoprotein receptors of about 135 and 90 kD (Walicke et al., 1989). Similar recep-tors have been purified from adult brain tissue.

bFGF has been purified from brain tissue and identified by both immunological markers and N-amino terminal sequencing. bFGF mRNA can be extracted from many brain regions including cortex, hippocampus, hypothalamus and pons. In vitro, astrocytes are capable of synthesizing bFGF. Although bFGF mRNA is barely detectable in cul-

tures of telencephalic neurons, in situ hybridization studies show a few hippocampal neurons with
high levels of bFGF mRNA (Hatten et al., 1988;
Emoto et al., 1990). Immunohistochemistry localizes
bFGF protein in the somata of large pyramidal
neurons of the cortex and hippocampus (Pettmann et
al., 1986). Since few neurons possess bFGF mRNA on
in situ hybridization, the source of this bFGF
protein is as yet uncertain.

bFGF has been applied in several experimental
models of neural injury in vivo. One of these is
the fimbria-fornix transection model widely used in
CNS research with NGF. Like NGF, bFGF increases
the survival of injured septal cholinergic neurons,
but the effect is less than with NGF (Anderson et
al., 1988). However, bFGF appears to stimulate
areas where NGF is not active. bFGF enhances
peripheral nerve regeneration, including axons from
spinal cord motoneurons. It has been reported to
enhance regeneration of dopaminergic fibers in the
striatum and to increase survival of retinal
ganglion cells after optic nerve lesion (Sievers et
al., 1987; Baird & Walicke, 1989). It remains to
be established whether these effects are produced
by direct action of bFGF on neurons as in vitro, or
indirectly through stimulation of other responsive
cell types.

In summary, the available experimental data
present a reasonable case for consideration of bFGF
as a NTF. The first criterion has been satisfied
by studies in multiple laboratories. There is
probable evidence to support the second, fourth and
fifth criteria, although many important questions
remain. Among these might particularly be mentioned
the cellular source of bFGF in intact brain and the
mechanism by which bFGF is released from cells.
Since some of the other forms of FGF in the brain,
such as hst/KS-FGF and FGF-5, may be more easily
released, they might mediate some of the actions
proposed for bFGF.

MFS AND NTFS

To call bFGF a NTF probably underestimates and

unrealistically simplifies its true range of action. Besides neurons, bFGF stimulates astrocytes, immature oligodendrocytes, endothelial cells, fibroblasts, and some pituitary cells. Based on its activities in vitro, bFGF might be predicted to play a role in a number of events which occur after brain injury, including neuronal sprouting and plasticity, gliosis, neovascularization, and connective tissue scar formation. Since bFGF is a MF, there is no a priori reason why it cannot participate in all of these processes, although its relative importance undoubtedly varies. This potential plethora of activities suggests a fundamentally different mode of action of bFGF from NGF.

The theoretical model of NTF function derived from NGF is based on the frequently unstated assumption that a NTF acts solely on neurons. As usually presented, the model contains two elements, the "target cell," which produces NTF, and the neuron. This simplification of a tissue to two lone cell types is permissible only with the assumption that none of the other cellular constituents interact significantly with the trophic factor. Furthermore the factor is assumed to act in only one direction, often represented by an arrow from the target cell to the neuron. For a MF, possible autocrine actions on the target cell would need to be added. New, more general models of NTF function need to be constructed for use with MFs. At a minimum, these must include all of the potentially responsive cellular elements present in a tissue. Since the cellular composition of a tissue inevitably changes with injury or inflammation, separate models may be needed for intact and damaged tissue.

Since MFs contradict the assumption of neuron specificity, it would not be surprising if they did not conform to other predictions of the NGF derived model. Nonetheless, deviations from predicted properties have been used to argue against identification of MFs as NTFs. For example, it has been stated that bFGF is not a NTF because its concentration in brain extracts is too high to limit neuronal survival. But bFGF is likely involved in multiple regulatory processes with non-neuronal cells as well as neurons. Additionally basement membranes around capillaries contain relatively inert stores of bFGF. The fraction of total brain bFGF which participates in NTF function is as yet unknown, but would be the only portion relevant to the preceding argument.

MODELS FOR MFS IN THE CNS

Too little is known about control of MF action for proposal of a detailed model, but some thoughts can be suggested. Certainly appropriate models will need to include all of the responsive cells present in a tissue. But perhaps the division of a tissue into a disconnected series of different cell types is itself misleading. It is possible that MFs might be designed to address structural or functional units containing more than one cell type. For example, the basic unit regulated by bFGF might be a neuron with its required support cells. Its ability to stimulate neurons, glial cells and blood vessels would then appear logical rather than surprising.

It has been suggested that each MF might be an element in a code for growth control (Sporn and Roberts, 1988). The code consists of combinations of growth factors and other elements which together control ordered growth. To make the analogy more concrete, trophic factors as a means of intercellular communication can be compared to written language. A MF is analogous to a letter of the alphabet, which must be combined with others to form a meaningful word. In contrast, NGF as usually modeled is more analogous to an ideogram or hieroglyphic symbol. The presence of a molecule of NGF in a tissue is a highly specific command for growth of a certain type of neuron. In contrast, the presence of a molecule of bFGF is highly ambiguous. It might be there to command neurite outgrowth or capillary formation. The significance of a molecule of bFGF is likely dependent on the context in which it appears.

To a considerable extent, the context for a MF is likely set by other available growth factors, both inhibitory and stimulatory. But other types of signals are also undoubtedly important. For neurons, these are likely to include: 1) extracellular matrix; 2) traditional hormones like thyroxine and gonadal steroids; 3) neurotransmitters acting locally on the terminal or growth cone; 4) neurotransmitters acting on the soma to produce electrical activity; 5) proteases and protease inhibitors. The suggestion that all of these play a role in growth control is far from new. The proposed model does perhaps differ in implicitly suggesting that the specificity and informational content of the whole is greater than simply the sum of its parts. To further complicate matters, the timing and sequence of the signals is probably also important, since the first agent might alter the range of cellular responses available for those following.

Combinations of Growth Factors

A culture system of hippocampal neurons and astrocytes provides a simple model system for examining modulation of bFGF selectivity by addition of a second MF. EGF is a mitogen for astrocytes that does not increase hippocampal neuronal survival. Since bFGF and EGF have additive effects on glial proliferation, the presence of EGF enhances glial but not neuronal response to bFGF. Thus EGF and bFGF together are relatively more glial-specific. In contrast, TNFa inhibits glial proliferation but does not influence neuronal survival. In this system, the combination of TNFa and bFGF is relatively more neuron-specific. Although it is easy to examine combinations of factors in vitro, caution must be applied in extrapolation to cocktails for use in vivo. Since there is already a network of MFs present in intact tissue, the context for growth factor action will necessarily be different in vivo than in vitro.

The effects of a combination of bFGF and TGFb1 in hippocampal cultures provide several interesting points for discussion. By itself, TGFb1 does not alter neuronal survival or glial proliferation (Fig. 1). When it is examined in the presence of bFGF, however, TGFb1 decreases glial proliferation and increases neuronal survival. The recognition of TGFb1 activity in this system is dependent on the context provided by bFGF. It may appear surprising that a single factor, TGFb1, is acting concurrently to stimulate one cell population and to inhibit the other. It is not uncommon for a MF to be either a growth inhibitor or enhancer depending on the cell population and the context. Since TGFb1 also inhibits endothelial proliferation in response to bFGF in vitro, TGFb1 and bFGF appears to be the most neuron-specific of the three examples.

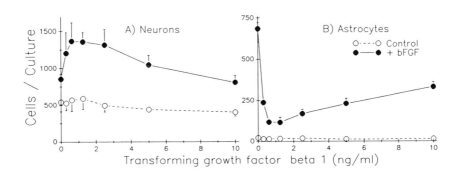

Figure 1. Neuronal survival (A) and astrocyte proliferation (B) in hippocampal cultures grown for 1 week with 5 ng/ml bFGF and indicted concentration of TGFb1.

But when purified cultures of hippocampal neurons or astrocytes were affinity labeled with TGFb1, receptors were detectable on astrocytes but not on neurons. Therefore the apparent stimulatory effects of TGFb1 on neuronal growth must be mediated indirectly through glial cells. This raises a second theme which may be important in MF action:

competitive and/or cooperative interactions among responsive cell types.

Competition and Cooperation among Different Cells

The results obtained with bFGF and TGFb1 are open to several interpretations. The most usual would be that a second factor released by the astrocytes mediated changes in neuronal survival. Since the proportion of astrocytes is smallest when neuronal survival is highest, this would have to be a toxic or inhibitory factor. However, when two cell types both use the same factor, more direct competition is possible. Perhaps as the numbers of astrocytes increased, they simply used up the available bFGF and starved out the neurons.

A model with direct competition for a MF between neurons and other cells, like astrocytes, has some interesting properties. Generally cells do not need MFs in the resting state, but only for mitosis. If neurons need a constant supply simply to survive, they start out in a tenuous position. If the factor acts at the distal end of a neurite, geometry creates further disadvantages. By the time the neuron has retrogradely transported the factor and then anterogradely transported cytoskeletal elements and grown a fraction of a millimeter, astrocytes can potentially complete several rounds of mitosis with significantly greater expansion. As the non-neuronal cell population increases, available MF would be used at an accelerating rate. In the case of bFGF, the affinity of the neuronal receptor is only about 1/5 that of receptors on astrocytes. Therefore, supplies of bFGF would effectively be exhausted sooner for neurons. Inherent cellular characterstics may make neurons relatively poor competitors for MFs, which may be relevant to their limited recovery after CNS injury.

Competitive or cooperative interactions could also be mediated more indirectly. Since the affinity of some growth factor receptors is regulated by phosphorylation, receptor state could be modified by neurotransmitters or other factors released by surrounding cells. Or cells could release additional MFs or other agents to alter the growth potential of their competitors.

Interactions between Cell and Factor

The NGF model assumes that the only parameters regulating cell response are the presence of receptors and the concentration of NGF. The neuron is passive, simply waiting for NTF to appear. Other models suggest, however, that cells can play an active role in obtaining their trophic stimulation. Whether a cell possesses the machinery to mobilize or activate a factor may be as important as whether it possesses receptors. In the case of the FGFs, mobilization of stores bound to heparan sulfate in the basement membrane may be an important regulatory step (Baird and Walicke, 1989; Folkman et al., 1988). Heparinases and proteases might be secreted to break down the matrix and release bFGF. Secretion of small carrier molecules of heparan sulfate has also been proposed. Many cells responsive to other MFs secrete binding or carrier proteins for the factor. The functional role of these carriers is not well understood, but they could participate in strategies to mobilize or protect the MF.

A variety of mechanisms probably also exist for altering MF structure to regulate MF activity. The principle of proteolytic activation was first demonstrated for the zymogens, but is also important in the regulation of angiotensin. Recently evidence has accrued for the possible existence of small trophic peptides within larger proteins like the beta amyloid precursor protein. It would not be surprising if proteolysis partially regulates activation and release of these trophic fragments. Phosphorylation presents another method for altering the activity of growth factors. After bFGF is phosphorylated by cAMP dependent kinase, its potency for stimulation of endothelial cell proliferation is increased (Feige and Baird, 1989).

These various mechanisms for mobilizing or

activating a MF can then be the basis for cooperative or competitive strategies among cell types
sharing the factor. For example, there might be
several cell types in a tissue which bear receptors
and are capable of responding to a single factor,
but only one cell type might have the activating
mechanism. This cell would be able to compete for
a much larger share of factor. But diffusion would
likely provide some activated factor to the surrounding cell types, resulting in cooperative
enhancement of their growth.

The models presented for action of MFs in this
discussion are not intended to be exhaustive. The
goal is simply to try to outline some of the
differences from the traditional NGF-derived model
which may prove important for MFs. These models
will necessarily be considerably more complex than
the NGF model. Development of appropriate models
for MF action provides a significant challenge, not
only in terms of data collection but also in terms
of synthesizing the information into a meaningful
theoretical framework.

REFERENCES

Anderson KJ, Dam D, Lee S, Cotman CW (1988). Basic
    fibroblast growth factor prevents death of
    lesioned cholinergic neurons in vivo. Nature
    332:360-361.
Baird A, Walicke PA (1989). Fibroblast growth
    factors. Brit Med Bull 45:438-452.
Emoto N, Walicke P, Baird A, Simmons D (1990).
    Expression of basic FGF mRNA in brain. Growth
    Factors (In Press).
Feige J, Baird A (1989) Basic fibroblast growth
    factor is a substrate for protein phoshorylation
    by capillary endothelial cells in culture. Proc
    Natl Acad Sci USA 86:3174-3178.
Folkman J, Klagsbrun M, Sasse J, Wadzinksi M,
    Ingber D, Vlodavsky I (1988). A heparin-binding
    angiogenic protein--basic fibroblast growth
    factor--is stored within basement membrane. Am J
    Pathol 130:393-400.
Hatten ME, Lynch M, Rydel RE, Sanchez J, Joseph-

Silverstein J, Moscatelli D, Rifkin DB (1988). In vitro neurite extension by granule neurons is dependent upon astroglial-derived fibroblast growth factor. Dev Biol 125:280-289.

Pettmann B, Labourdette G, Weibel M, Sensenbrenner M (1986). The brain fibroblast growth factor (FGF) is localized in neurons. Neurosci Lett 68:175-180.

Sievers J, Hausmann B, Unsicker K, Berry M (1987). Fibroblast growth factors promote the survival of adult rat retinal ganglion cells after transection of the optic nerve. Neurosci Lett 76:157-162.

Sporn MB, Roberts AB (1988). Peptide growth factors are multifunctional. Nature 332:217-219.

Unsicker K, Reichert-Preibsch H, Schmidt R, Pettmann B, Labourdette G, Sensenbrenner M (1987). Astroglial and fibroblast growth factors have neurotrophic functions for cultured peripheral and central nervous system neurons. Proc Natl Acad Sci USA 84:5459-5463.

Walicke PA (1988). Basic and acidic fibroblast growth factors have trophic effects on neurons from multiple CNS regions. J Neurosci 8:2618-2627.

Walicke PA, Feige JJ, Baird A (1989). Characterization of the neuronal receptor for basic fibroblast growth factor (bFGF): Comparison to mesenchymal cell receptors. J Biol Chem 264:4120-4126.

Walicke PA (1989). Novel neurotrophic factors, receptors and oncogenes. Ann Rev Neurosci 12:103-126.

Advances in Neural Regeneration
Research, pages 115–124
© 1990 Wiley-Liss, Inc.

BASIC FGF, LESION-INDUCED NEURON DEATH AND NEURAL
REGENERATION

D. Otto and K. Unsicker

Department of Anatomy and Cell Biology,
University of Marburg, Robert-Koch-Str. 6
3550 Marburg, FRG

INTRODUCTION
Neural pathway lesions in the adult mammalian CNS usually
lead to an irreversible loss of function. This results from
the destruction of neurons, their connectivities, glial scar
formation and aborted attempts of axons to regenerate. The
sparse regenerative potential of the adult mammalian CNS,as
opposed to the peripheral neurous system, is apparently
determined by environmental rather than genetic cues (Aguayo
1985). However, molecules and regulatory mechanisms involved are only beginning to be identified and understood.Both
a lack of factors that facilitate survival of lesioned
neurons and promote axonal regrowth, and the presence of inhibitory cues may be conceived to contribute to preventing
reconstruction of circuitries and functional recovery
(Schwab and Caroni 1988). Trophic factors, which regulate
neuronal development, survival and axonal growth in vivo and
in vitro (Levi-Montalcini 1987) appear to be important in
controlling post-injury responses in the CNS and peripheral
nervous system (Logan et al. 1985; Whittemore and Seiger
1987; Finklestein et al. 1988). Understanding of how these
factors operate in physiological and pathophysiological
situations is a major long-term goal in neurotrauma research.
Clinical benefit, however, may already result from finding
ways to administer these factors in vivo and manipulate
their expression and that of their receptors in the CNS
environment after injury.

Basic FGF is a member of a family of heparin binding growth
factors with proliferative, differentiative and regulatory
effects on many mesodermal and neuroectodermal cells (Lobb

1988; Böhlen 1989). Its amino acid sequence has been determined and found to share 55% structural homology with acidic FGF. Basic FGF including several closely related trunca-
ted and N-terminally extended forms has a widespread tissue
distribution (Lobb 1988). It also occurs in the brain and
appears to be specifically regulated in response to CNS
lesions (Finklestein et al. 1988). It has been immunocytochemically localized in neurons of the CNS and PNS (Pettmann et al. 1986; Janet et al. 1988), and also been found
in astrocytes (Ferrara et al.1987; Hatten et al. 1988).
Moreover, neurons have been shown to possess receptors for
FGFs (Walicke et al. 1988). With regard to possible functions in the nervous system, the potency of bFGF as a neuronal survival and axonal growth promoting protein (Morrison
et al. 1986; Walicke et al. 1986; Unsicker et al. 1987), a
mitogen and differentiation inducing agent for astroglial
cells (Pettmann et al. 1985) and an angiogenic factor
(Risau et al. 1988) suggest a multifunctional role in neural
embryogenesis and trauma.
This article summarizes evidence from our laboratory suggesting that bFGF stabilizes the survival of axotomized
neurons and enhances regenerative responses in the adult
CNS, which is the initial crucial prerequisite for all subsequent regenerative steps.

THE FIMBRIA-FORNIX LESION PARADIGM
The fimbria-fornix pathway connecting the septal and hippocampal areas is a widely used CNS lesion model. Interruption of this pathway provokes cell death of cholinergic
neurons in the medial septum, which can be prevented by
intraventricular infusion or local gelfoam application of
the neurotrophic protein nerve growth factor (NGF; Hefti
1986; Williams et al. 1986; Otto et al. 1989). The rescue
effect of NGF, along with its established presence and
synthesis in the hippocampus (Ayer-LeLievre et al. 1988)
and retrograde transport in axons (Seiler and Schwab 1984)
having the specific receptros for NGF (Hefti et al. 1986)
strongly suggest a physiological role of NGF in this system.

Localization of immunoreactive bFGF (Pettmann et al. 1986)
and its mRNA (Gonzalez et al. Soc. Neuroscience 1989) in
hippocampal neurons as well as the documented survival,
neurite growth and transmitter promoting effects of bFGF on
cultured septal neurons (Walicke 1988; Grothe et al. 1989)
might argue in favor of a trophic function of bFGF similar
to NGF. We therefore administered bFGF(8µg) soaked in gel-

foam to the unilaterally transected fimbria-fornix (Otto et
al 1989). In parallel experiments NGF (20µg or 4µg, respectively) and cytochrome C (as a non-trophic control protein)
were applied. Basic FGF rescued approximately one fifth of
those axotomized medial septal neurons that died when a cytochrome C containing gelfoam was implanted. NGF applied at
4µg had an identical effect; at 20µg, however, it maintained a greater number of neurons than bFGF and also, in
contrast to bFGF, prevented cell shrinkage. Coronal sections
of the medial septal area stained for choline acetyltransferase revealed similar numbers of cholinergic neurons in
animals treated with bFGF or NGF (20µg). Thus, both intraventricular infusions (Anderson et al. 1988) and application in gelfoam of bFGF can prevent the degeneration of
cholinergic neurons in the medial septum following a fimbria-
fornix transection. Our studies, like those of Anderson
and collaborators (1988), did not reveal any overt vascular
sprouting or glial cell proliferation, two conceivable responses to an application to bFGF. This issue, however,
requires further investigation, since Barotte et al. (1989)
have reported a gliosis reaction following fimbria-fornix
transection and administration of bFGF to the lesion site.
It also remains to be investigated whether, in the complex
in vivo situation, bFGF may act on neurons both directly
and indirectly, i.e. via stimulating glial cells or affecting the inflammatory reaction.

ANIMAL MODELS OF PARKINSON'S DISEASE
Parkinson's disease is a neurodegenerative disorder of unknown etiology. The death of most dopaminergic cell bodies
in the substantia nigra, which project to the striatum, results in a dramatic loss of striatal dopamine (DA) and
severe impairment of motor skills. Substitution of transmitter by application of precursor analogues, the most
widely therapeutic approach, often yields unsatisfactory
results. Attempts to replace the drug therapy by transmit-
ter-releasing transplants of adrenal medullary chromaffin
or embryonic dopaminergic mesencephalic neurons to the
striatum have failed to produce a major therapeutic break-
through(cf. Goetz et al. 1989). However, the transplation
experiments in animal models of neurotoxin-induced Parkin-
sonism were useful in that they suggested an involvement of
transplant-derived trophic agents in the axonal sprouting
response of the few surviving nigrostriatal neurons that was
observed (Bohn et al. 1987; Fiandaca et al. 1988). Moreover,
they launched speculations that the degeneration of nigro-

striatal neurons might be the result of an imbalance of
toxic influences (perhaps provided by the environment;
Tanner 1989) and trophic support for nigral neurons provided by (a) striatal neurotrophic factor(s). In fact, a neurotrophic protein has been isolated from bovine striatum and
found to promote differentiation of cultured mesencephalic
neurons (DalToso et al.1988), an effect that is mimicked
by bFGF (Ferrari et al. 1989).

Chromaffin cells used in grafts to Parkinsonian animals and
humans contain several trophic factors stimulating survival,
neurite growth and transmitter syntheses of neurons in
vitro (Unsicker et al.1988,1989,1990). Basic FGF, which is
apparently contained in chromaffin cells (Blottner et al.
1989; Grothe and Unsicker 1989; Westermann et al.1990) was
applied in two animal models of Parkinon's disease (Otto
and Unsicker 1989; Otto et al.in preparation). In 1-methyl-
4-phenyl-1,2,3,6-tetrahydropyridine (MPTP) treated young
adult C57BL/6 mice (3x30mg/kg in 24 hours intervals), a
bFGF containing gelfoam (4µg) was transplanted into the
right caudate nucleus. Morphological as well as chemical
parameters of dopaminergic innervation of both striata were
studied two weeks after surgery. The bFGF treatment led to
a partial restoration of striatal DA levels on both sides
which were reduced to about 80% in mice carrying a gelfoam
implant containing cytochrome C as a non-trophic control
protein. Tyrosine hydroxylase (TOH),the rate-limiting enzyme
in DA synthesis, had restored its enzymatic activity in
striata to control levels. Somewhat surprisingly, TOH-immu-
noreactive fibers, which could not be visualized after the
MPTP treatment, reappeared in bFGF treated animals in the
ipsilateral striatum only (Fig.1). The fiber density was
especially high close to the bFGF-containing implant within
a zone of 150-200µm and decreased further away from it. The
contralateral side displayed sparse or no TOH-positive
fibers. These findings were in line with semiquantitative
data obtained from TOH-westernblots, which indicated that
striata ipsilateral to bFGF treatment contained more TOH-
protein than contralateral striata. As the DA turnover, reflected by the striatal levels of the DA metabolite 3,4-
dihydroxyphenylacetic acid (DOPAC), was higher on the contralateral than on the ipsilateral side, we assume either an
increase in the molar TOH-activity or an increased ratio of
phosphorylated/non-phosphorylated TOH on the contralateral
side in order to provide equal levels of the transmitter DA
in both striata.

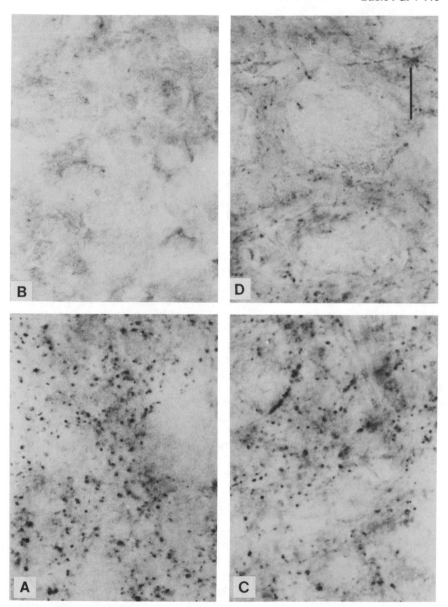

Fig.1 Striatal peroxidase-stained TH-IR fibers are visible as spotlike structures two weeks after implantation of a cyt C gelfoam (A). TH-IR fibers have disappeared in UPTP/cyt C treated mice (B). Treatment with bFGF caused reappearance of TH-IR fibers on the ipsilateral side only. The density was highest close to the implant (C),but was still increased further away from it (D). Bar = 2.5μm.

The potency of bFGF to overcome the consequences of a nigro-striatal lesion, was further underscored in experiments, in which a stereotactic unilateral lesion with 6-OHDA in adult rats was used to destroy more than 90 percent of dopaminergic nigral neurons leading to severe motor impairment (Otto et al. in preparation). Chronic intraventricular infusions of bFGF in this lesion model improved the pathological rotatory behavior as compared to an infusion of cytochrome C.

Although the mechanisms underlying the curative effects of bFGF still have to be explored, these initial experiments have provided encouraging results and are currently being expanded towards investigating the long-term effects of trophic factors such as bFGF, included in biocompatible polymers and implanted into the Parkinsonian brain.

BASIC FGF AND NEURAL REGENERATION: SUMMARY AND OUTLOOK
The two CNS lesion models presented in this article have clearly revealed the in vivo potency of bFGF as an important trophic factor that is capable of ensuring the first step in neural regeneration, the maintenance of the neuronal perikaryon after a surgical or toxic lesion. Moreover, the neuritogenic and axonal sprouting effects induced by bFGF in vitro (Walicke et al. 1986) and in vivo (Blottner and Unsicker 1989) indicate that exogenously applied bFGF may also promote the second regenerative step, the outgrowth and guidance of axons towards their target.

To date , it is not clear whether FGF is responsible for glial scar formation. It would seem that an involvement of bFGF in regeneration and scarring would have to put special emphasis on studies aiming to clarify relative contributions of different molecular weight forms to the spectrum of FGF functions.

Given the multifunctionality of the FGFs it is probably safe to assume that each individual function may be regulated separately, e.g. by interaction with other enhancing or inhibitory growth factors, stabilizing agents, by interference with receptor binding and transduction pathways, or by modulation of enzymatic inactivation. Irrespectively how complex a picture for the various functions of bFGF may eventually emerge, bFGF has already become established as an important trophic molecule for neurons, possibly belonging to a class of neurotrophic factors that are conceptually different from NGF.

Supported by Deutsche Forschungsgemeinschaft (Un 34/13-1)

REFERENCES

Barotte C, Eclancher F, Ebel A, Labourdette G, Sensenbrenner M, Will B (1989). Effects of basic fibroblast growth factor (bFGF) on choline acetyltransferase activity and astroglial reaction in adult rats after partial fimbria transection. Neuroscience Letters 101: 197-202.

Blottner D, Westermann R, Grothe C, Böhlen P, Unsicker K (1989). Basic fibroblast growth factor in the adrenal gland: Possible trophic role for preganglionic neurons in vivo. Eur J Neurosci 1: 471-478.

Blottner D, Unsicker K (1989).Maintenance of intermediolateral spinal cord neurons by basic fibroblast growth factor administered medullorectomized rat adrenal gland. Dependence on intact adrenal innervation and cellular organization of implants. Eur J Neurosci (in press).

Böhlen P (1989). Fibroblast growth factor. In: Sorg C (ed) Macrophage-Derived Cell Regulatory Factors. Cytokines. Basel, Karger, vol. 1, pp 204-222.

Bohn MC, Cupit L, Marciano F, Gash DM (1987). Adrenal medulla grafts enhance recovery of striatal dopaminergic fibers. Science 237: 913-916.

DalToso R, Giorgi O, Soranzo C, Kirschner G, Ferrari G, Favaron M, Benvegnù D, Presti D, Vicini S, Toffano G, Azzone GF, Leon A (1988). Development and survival of neurons in dissociated fetal mesencephalic serum-free cell cultures: I. Effects of cell density and of an adult mammalian striatal-derived neuronotrophic factor (SDNF). J Neurosci 8: 733-745.

Ferrara N, Ousley F, Gospodarowicz D (1988). Bovine brain astrocytes express basic fibroblast growth factor, a neurotrophic and angiogenic mitogen. Brain Res 462: 223-232.

Ferrari G, Minozzi UC, Toffano G, Leon A, Skaper SD (1989). Basic fibroblast growth factor promotes the survival and development of mesencephalic neurons in culture. Dev Biol 133: 140-147.

Fiandaca MS, Kordower JH, Hansen JT, Jiao SS, Gash DM (1988) Adrenal medullary autografts into the basal ganglia of Cebus monkeys: Injury-induced regeneration. Exp Neurol 102: 76-91.

Finklestein SP, Apostolides PJ, Caday CG, Prosser J, Philips MF, Klagsbrun M (1988). Increased basic fibroblast growth factor (bFGF) immunoreactivity at the site of focal brain wounds. Brain Res 460: 253-259.

Goetz CG, Olanow CW, Koller WC, Penn RD, Cahill D, Moratz R, Stebbins G, Tanner CM, Klawans HL, Shannon KM, Comelia CL, Witt T, Cox C, Waxman M, Gauger L (1989). Multicenter study of autologous adrenal medullary transplantation to the corpus striatum in patients with advanced Parkinson's disease. N Engl J Med 320: 337-341.

Gonzalez AM, Emoto N, Walicke P, Shimasaki S, Baird A (1989). The distribution of basic fibroblast growth factor mRNA in the adult rat brain. Soc Neurosci Vol 15, Abstr 287.17.

Gospodarowicz D, Neufeld G, Schweigerer L (1986). Molecular and biological characterization of fibroblast growth factor, an angiogenic factor which also controls the proliferation and differentiation of mesoderm and neuro-ectoderm derived cells. Cell Differentiation 19: 1-17.

Grothe C, Unsicker K (1989). Immunocytochemical localization of basic fibroblast growth factor in bovine adrenal gland, ovary and pituitary. J Cytochem Histochem In press.

Hatten ME, Lynch M, Rydel RE, Sanchez J, Joseph-Silver-stein J, Moscatelli D, Rifkin DB (1988). In vitro neurite extension by granule neurones is dependent upon astro-glial-derived fibroblast growth factor. Dev Biol 125: 280-289.

Hefti F (1986). Nerve growth factor promotes survival of septal cholinergic neurons after fimbrial transections. J Neurosci 6: 2155-2162.

Hefti F, Hartikka J, Salvatierra A, Weiner WJ, Mash DC (1986). Localization of nerve growth factor receptors in cholinergic neurons of the human basal forebrain. Neurosci Lett 69: 37-41.

Janet T, Grothe C, Pettmann B, Unsicker K, Sensenbrenner M (1988). Immunocytochemical demonstration of fibroblast growth factor in cultured chick and rat neurons. J Neurosci Res 19: 195-201.

Levi-Montalcini R (1987). The nerve growth factor 35 years later. Science 237: 1154-1162

Lobb RR (1988). Clinical applications of heparin-binding growth factor. Europ J Clin Invest 18: 321-336.

Logan A, Berry M, Thomas GH, Gregson NA, Logan SD (1985) Identification and partial purification of fibroblast growth factor from the brains of developing rats and leucodystrophic mutant mice. Neurosci 15: 1239-1246.

Morrison RS, Sharma A, deVellis J, Bradshaw RA (1986). Basic fibroblast growth factor supports the survival of cerebral cortical neurones in primary culture. Proc Natl Acad Sci USA 83: 7537-7541.

Otto D, Unsicker K (1989). Basic FGF reverses chemical and morphological deficits in the nigrostriatal system of MPTP treated mice. J Neurosci , submitted.

Otto D, Frotscher M, Unsicker K (1989). Basic fibroblast growth factor and nerve growth factor administered in gel foam rescue medial septal neurons after fimbria fornix transection. J Neurosci Res 22: 83-91.

Pettmann B, Weibel M, Sensenbrenner M, Labourdette G. (1985) Purification of two astroglial growth factors from bovine brain. FEBS Lett 189: 102-108.

Pettmann B, Labourdette G, Weibel M, Sensenbrenner M (1986). the brain fibroblast growth factor (FGF) is localised in neurones. Neurosci Lett 69: 175-180.

Risau W, Gautschi-Sova P, Böhlen P (1988). Endothelial cell growth factors in embryonic and adult chick brain are related to human acidic fibroblast growth factor. EMBO 7: 959-962.

Schwab ME, Caroni P (1988). Oligodendrocytes and CNS myelin are nonpermissive substrates for neurite growth and fibroblast spreading in vitro. J Neurosci 8: 2381-2393.

Seiler M, Schwab ME (1984). Specific retrograde transport of nerve growth factor (NGF) from neocortex to nucleus basalis in the rat brain. Brain Res 300: 33-39.

Tanner CM (1989). The role of environmental toxins in the etiology of Parkinson's disease. TINS 12: 49-54.

Unsicker K, Blottner D, Gehrke D, Grothe C, Heymann D, Stögbauer F, Westermann R (1988). Neuroectodermal cells: Storage and release of growth factors. In NATO ASI Series, H22, Neural Development and Regeneration (eds A Gorio et al). Springer, Berlin-Heidelberg.

Unsicker K, Gehrke D, Stögbauer F, Westermann R (1989). Characterization of trophic factors from chromaffin granules that promote survival of peripheral and central nervous system neurons. J Neurosci Submitted.

Walicke P, Cowan WM, Ueno K, Baird A, Guillemin R (1986). Fibroblast growth factor promotes survival of dissociated hippocampal neurones and enhances neurite extension. Proc Natl Acad Sci USA 83: 3012-3016.

Walicke PA, Feige JJ, Baird A (1988). Characterization of
  the neuronal basic fibroblast growth factor (bFGF)
  receptor. Soc Neurosci Vol 14, Abstr 149.10.
Westermann R., Johannsen M, Unsicker K, Grothe C (1989).
  Basic fibroblast growth factor (bFGF) immunoreactivity
  is present in chromaffin granules. Submitted.
Whittemore SR, Seiger A (1987). The expression, localization and functional significance of ß-nerve growth factor
  in the central nervous system. Brain Res Rev 12: 439-464.
Williams LR, Varon S, Peterson GM, Wictorin K, Fischer W,
  Bjorklund A, Gage FH (1986). Continuous infusion of nerve
  growth factor prevents basal forebrain neuronal death
  after fimbria fornix transection. Proc Natl Acad Sci USA
  88: 9231-9235.

Advances in Neural Regeneration
Research, pages 125–145
© 1990 Wiley-Liss, Inc.

MECHANISMS LEADING TO INCREASES IN NERVE GROWTH
FACTOR SYNTHESIS AFTER PERIPHERAL NERVE LESION

Rolf Heumann, Bastian Hengerer, Dan
Lindholm, Michael Brown[1] and Hugh Perry[1]

Max-Planck-Institute for Psychiatry,
Department of Neurochemistry, Am
Klopferspitz 18a, 8033 Martinsried,
F.R.G. and Department of Experimental
Psychology, South Parks Road, Oxford
OX1 3PT, Great Britain[1]

INTRODUCTION

The multiple actions of nerve growth factor
(NGF) on responsive neurons include the promotion
of neuronal cell survival, induction of fiber
outgrowth or axonal branching, and the regulation
of neurotransmitter enzyme and neuropeptide
synthesis (Levi-Montalcini and Angeletti, 1968;
Thoenen and Barde, 1980; Korsching, 1986).
Although such neuronal functions are regulated
during neuronal repair after lesion, the role of
NGF in regeneration is still a matter of
discussion (Diamond et al., 1987; Rich et al.,
1989a).

Here, we elaborate on the chain of events
finally leading to long-term alterations in NGF
and NGF receptor synthesis in the peripheral
nerve sheath, which may influence the regrowth
and functional recovery of NGF responsive
neurons. We will first discuss the rapid initial
changes occurring within minutes and hours after
lesion. We demonstrate that the cellular
immediate-early genes (see Ryseck et al., 1989)
may be involved in the transcriptional activation
of the NGF gene. Secondly, the mechanisms of
long-term changes of NGF synthesis after peri-

pheral nerve lesion will be elaborated by emphasizing the specific role of macrophages in vivo (Heumann, 1987b). Thirdly, we discuss the possible physiological relevance of the macrophage dependent NGF synthesis for the process of peripheral nerve regeneration.

RESULTS AND DISCUSSION

NGF may not only be involved in long-term neurotrophic events like fiber density stabilization and promotion of survival; after dissecting rat iris or sciatic nerve segments and putting them into culture, a rapid increase of NGF-mRNA levels within hours has been demonstrated (Heumann and Thoenen, 1986; Heumann et al., 1987a). After 12 hours, NGF-mRNA decreased, reaching persistently low (but still elevated) levels after 24 to 48 hours. This time-course of changes in NGF-mRNA levels was reminiscent of that found for the mRNAs encoding the cellular immediate-early genes (Greenberg et al., 1986). We then started to investigate the possible relationship between inflammatory-like early reactions (see Caput et al., 1986) and NGF synthesis after nerve lesion (Heumann et al. 1987a).

Changes of Cellular Immediate-Early Gene mRNA Levels After Sciatic Nerve Lesion

Disturbing the local environment of a tissue by mechanical, chemical or electrical lesions leads to a rapid and transient increase in the mRNA levels coding for c-*fos* and c-*jun* (Kruijer et al., 1984; Verrier et al., 1986; Sagar et al., 1988). The protein products of these genes form a transcriptionally active complex termed AP-1, which is thought to act as an intermediate in coupling extracellular signals to changes in the cellular protein synthesis machinery regulating the expression of specific target genes (Curran and Franza, 1988). Here we investigate the possibility whether the NGF gene is one of the targets of Fos, thereby suggesting a link between lesion-induced reactions and trophic support of NGF responsive neurons.

Is the NGF-gene a novel target of Fos? Transection of the sciatic nerve leads to an immediate increase of the mRNAs coding for the nuclear proto-oncogenes c-*fos* (Fig. 1) and c-*jun* (not shown), followed by the increase in NGF-mRNA.

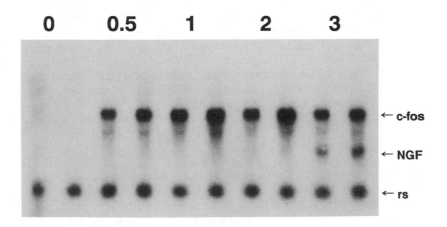

Figure 1. Northern blot showing the time course of changes of the mRNAs coding for c-*fos* or NGF. Rs: RNA-recovery standard added before RNA extraction to allow quantification of the mRNA levels. Duplicate samples were taken at 0, 0.5, 1, 2, and 3 hours as indicated. Note that NGF-mRNA appears 2.5 hours later than c-*fos* at this exposure time of the autoradiogram. Taken from Hengerer et al., 1990, with permission.

The increase in c-*fos* mRNA appears to be independent of protein synthesis because, in agreement with previous studies (Müller et al., 1984), the protein synthesis blocker cyclo-heximide does not prevent but rather potentiates the increase of c-*fos* mRNA when sciatic nerves are put into culture. In contrast, the subsequent increase of NGF-mRNA is greatly inhibited by cycloheximide (added at the beginning of the culture). These experiments suggested a protein synthesis dependent regulation of the transient increase(s) in NGF-mRNA levels (Hengerer et al., 1990).

The cellular immediate-early gene products Fos and Jun combine to form a heterodimer by means of their leucine-zipper regions (Landschulz et al., 1988). The complex specifically interacts with the AP-1 binding site (consensus sequence TGAG/CTCA) and thereby transactivates the corresponding target gene (Angel et al., 1987; Chiu et al., 1988). Inspection of the 5'-regions of the NGF gene (-1000 to +289) revealed that a perfect AP-1-like consensus sequence is located in the first intron of the NGF gene at a site which is immediately adjacent to the first exon. There are 7 additional AP-1 like sequences which have only one base exchanged within the AP-1 consensus sequence (Fig. 2).

In a recent investigation by Risse et al. (1989), the bases in an AP-1 consensus sequence have been permutated and the AP-1 complex did not efficiently bind to certain variant sites in vitro. According to this study the AP-1-like sequences located in the 5'-promoter region of the NGF gene are not expected to bind to the AP-1 complex. On the other hand, the mere presence of an AP-1 consensus sequence does not necessarily mean that it is functional: in the SV40 enhancer the AP-1 site neither regulates basal expression nor is it involved in the induction of gene expression by the tumor-promoting phorbol ester (Chiu et al., 1987).

In order to investigate the possible functional interaction between Fos and the NGF gene, we made use of transgenic mice produced by Rüther et al. (1987). These mice carry an exogenous heavy metal inducible *fos* gene construct which is expressed in most of the tissues. Preliminary experiments had shown that specific induction of the exogenous *fos* by

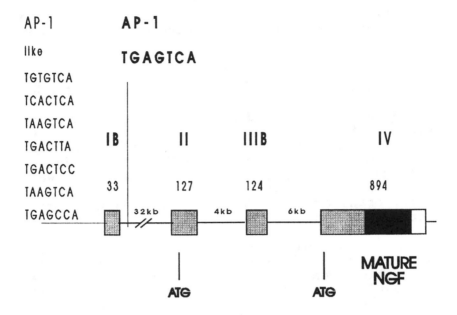

Figure 2. Simplified structure of the NGF gene. Boxes: exons; lines: introns. The number of bases per exon/intron are as indicated. The designation of the exons are shown according to Selbey et al. (1987).

cadmium chloride (Cd^{2+}) led to an increase in NGF-mRNA in the sciatic nerve <u>in vivo</u>. These results could be confirmed and extended in primary fibroblast cultures taken from the transgenic animals: the Cd^{2+}-induced exogenous *fos*-mRNA resulted in a nearly concomitant increase of the endogenous c-*jun*-mRNA (Hengerer et al., 1990), similar to the situation after transection of the sciatic nerve. Thus, the increased c-*fos* levels found in the cultured nerve segments could lead to a transactivation of c-*jun* mRNA by the AP-1 complex, although other mechanisms cannot be excluded yet. Interestingly, a rapid positive regulation of c-*jun* by its own protein product has been recently described in Hela cells resulting from an autoregulation of c-*jun* via the AP-1 protein complex (consisting of Fos and Jun; Angel et al., 1988).

The Cd^{2+}-induced increases in c-*jun* and c-*fos* mRNAs were followed by a 6-fold increase in NGF-mRNA in these transgenic fibroblasts. No such increases were found in Cd^{2+}-treated control fibroblasts, indicating the specificity of the observed changes. In order to investigate if this effect of *fos* expression on NGF-mRNA was due to a transcriptional activation, assays were performed using NGF-promoter/chloramphenicol acetyltransferase (CAT)-reporter fusion constructs (Fig.3).

After transfecting the transgenic fibroblasts with such a fusion construct, the Cd^{2+}-induced *fos* expression caused a strong transcriptional activation of the NGF-promoter (Fig. 3). Subsequently, we tested if the transactivation of the NGF gene is correlated with the protection of one or several of the AP-1 (-like) binding sites. DNAse footprint analysis of the 5'-region of the NGF gene was performed using nuclear extracts obtained from transgenic fibroblasts expressing low or high Cd^{2+}-induced levels of *fos*. A selective protection was only found in the region between +33 to +55, where the perfect AP-1 consensus sequence is located (Fig. 2). Other regions like the TAATA-box were constitutively occupied. This selective protection of the intron-located AP-1 site suggested but did not prove its functional involvement in the transcriptional regulation of the NGF gene (Hengerer et al., 1990).

Is the AP-1 binding site of the NGF gene essential for the lesion-induced changes in NGF synthesis? We isolated sciatic or skin fibroblasts of normal mice and used them as a paradigm for the investigation of lesion-induced changes in gene expression. The fibroblasts were cotransfected with the Cd^{2+} inducible *fos* expression vector together with various NGF-promoter constructs coupled to a CAT-reporter

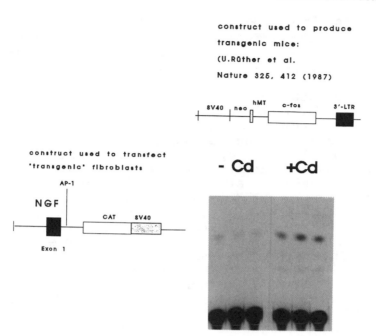

Figure 3. NGF promoter activity measured in transfected transgenic fibroblasts in the absence or presence of Cd^{2+}. Top: Structure of the *fos* gene construct used to generate transgenic mice: SV40, enhancer and promoter. neo: G418 resistance gene . hMT: human metallothionein IIa promoter. 3'-LTR: long terminal repeat of the proviral FBJ-MuSV (according to Rüther et al., 1985). Left: Structure of the NGF promoter/CAT reporter construct. (Modified from Hengerer et al., 1990 with permission).

gene. The results show that the presence of the AP-1 site located in the first intron of the NGF gene is essential for the inducibility of the NGF promoter by Fos. This is supported by site-directed mutagenesis of the intron-AP-1 site which results in reduced basal transcription and abolishes the inducibility by Fos (Hengerer et al., 1990). Thus, the Fos-mediated regulation of NGF synthesis is functionally channeled through the single AP-1 recognition site located within the first intron of the NGF gene.

These studies in the peripheral nervous system lead to the question about the possible function of the AP-1 site of the NGF promoter in the central nervous system. After eliciting convulsions, e.g., by unilateral electrolytic lesions in the dentate gyrus hilus (Gall and Isackson, 1989), or after application of metrazol (R. Heumann, unpublished), NGF-mRNA levels are increased in the hippocampus within hours and this increase is paralleled or preceded by increases of c-*fos* and c-*jun* (Saffen et al., 1988). Interestingly, neuronal c-*fos* has been shown to be increased by noxious stimuli or by electrical stimulation (Hunt et al., 1987; Morgan et al., 1987, Sagar et al., 1988; Menetrey et al., 1989). It has been speculated that NGF is a candidate as target for *fos* in the hippocampus and that there is a possible link to the seizure-evoked elaboration of axonal branches in the hippocampus (Sonnenberg et al., 1989a).

Physiological Relevance of the Changes in NGF and NGF Receptor Synthesis After Sciatic Nerve Lesion

Functional recovery after nerve lesion requires that neurons are capable of surviving axotomy and subsequently regrowing the lesioned axons into a "permissive" environment promoting their elongation. Both trophic support at the proximal stump and "permissiveness" of the distal nerve will be considered in the context of the role played by NGF and its receptors.

Trophic supply at the tip of the proximal stump. We have previously shown that there is a "substitute" synthesis of NGF by non-neuronal cells in the peripheral nerve, thereby partially compensating the injury-induced interruption of the target-derived neurotrophic supply. The site of the new NGF synthesis was the neuroma-like structure developing at the tip of the proximal stump after sciatic nerve transection (Heumann et al., 1987a). Although this newly synthesized NGF was retrogradely transported through the proximal segments of the proximal nerve, the amount of NGF synthesized was found not to be sufficient to fully compensate the interrupted target-derived trophic supply. Consistent with this finding, it has been reported that the number of NGF high affinity receptors located on the preserved axons and the neuronal retrograde transport of NGF receptor (as measured by accumulation at the site of an additional crush lesion) was typically reduced after peripheral transection (Raivich and Kreuzberg, 1987; Verge et al., 1989). Although a substantial loss of sensory dorsal root ganglion neurons (DRG) has been documented after peripheral sciatic transection (Johnson and Yip, 1985; Schmalbruch, 1987), it needs to be clarified whether or not this is due to a deprivation of NGF or NGF related factors. Rescue of DRG neurons by application of large doses of NGF may possibly be due to a "pharmacological" effect (Rich et al., 1987), because the sensory DRG neurons, once mature, appear not to depend on NGF for survival (see Lindsay and Harmar, 1989).

Trophic supply by the peripheral stump. Comparison between crush and cut lesions. In contrast to the cut lesion, after crush lesion the regenerating axonal tips may gain access to the NGF which is newly synthesized along the distal nerve sheath. The lesion-induced expression of NGF low affinity receptors on the Schwann cells located in the distal nerve sheath (Taniuchi et al., 1986; Heumann et al., 1987b) may enable these Schwann cells to accumulate NGF (Rush, 1984), thereby serving as a favorable substrate promoting axonal elongation. An increased mean area of the cell bodies of the dorsal root ganglion (DRG) neurons (Rich et al., 1989b) and an increased number of axonally transported NGF receptors (Raivich and Kreutzberg, 1987) were found after crush lesions as opposed to the situation after cut lesions.

This supports the suggestion of an enhanced trophic supply of fibers actively regenerating through the distal nerve sheath which synthesizes NGF and NGF receptor.

After interaction with regenerating nerve fibers, the Schwann cell NGF receptor mRNA and the receptor protein are rapidly down-regulated, presumably by direct cell surface interactions (Heumann et al., 1987b; Taniuchi et al., 1988). Notably, NGF has no regulatory influence on the Schwann cell low affinity NGF receptor synthesis (Lemke and Chao, 1988), and a response of Schwann cells to NGF has not been demonstrated.

Similarly, spinal motor neurons have not been described to be responsive to NGF, although there is a transient increase in levels of low affinity NGF receptors after sciatic nerve transection. The low unlesioned control levels are reached again after advent of fibers at the target muscle (Ernfors et al., 1989).

In contrast, on PC12-cells, on cultured adult sensory neurons and on cholinergic neurons of the septum or neostriatum, the NGF receptors are up-regulated by the ligand, NGF (Doherti et al., 1988; Cavicchioli et al., 1989; Higgins et al., 1989; Gage et al., 1989; Lindsay et al., 1990), and thereby NGF may act to enhance its own action. Thus, the changes in levels of high affinity sensory neuron NGF receptors found after lesion may possibly reflect the changes in local trophic supply of these neurons (see Verge et al., 1989). It has to be assumed that the regulation of a transmembrane signal transduction mechanism for NGF, and not the expression of a low affinity receptor protein per se, ultimately determines and amplifies the physiological response to NGF.

The role of macrophages in the regulation of NGF or NGF receptor synthesis in vivo. Macrophages are known to invade the distal nerve stump within several days after peripheral nerve section and they are important for induction of

Schwann cell mitosis and the degradation of myelin (Beuche and Friede, 1986). In our previous investigations, the stimulatory effect of activated macrophages on NGF synthesis had been demonstrated (Heumann et al., 1987b). The major secretory substance responsible for the NGF-mRNA changes was the cytokine, interleukin-1 (Il-1)(Lindholm et al., 1987). While this was shown in cultured nerve segments, the in vivo evidence for a role of macrophages in regulating NGF synthesis remained to be determined. Recently, Lunn et al. (1989) described a mouse strain (C57Bl/6 Ola) where Wallerian degeneration following axotomy was nearly absent for at least 7 days and there was a strongly delayed recruitment of myelomonocytic cells. The morphological and functional intactness of the transected axons has been shown by the preservation of the myelin structure and by their ability to conduct compound action potentials (Lunn et al., 1989). In these mice we challenged our hypothesis about the role of macrophages on NGF and NGF receptor mRNA synthesis, which was based previously on in vitro experiments (Heumann et al., 1987b).

Initially we tested the response to lesion and to macrophages in the cultured nerve segments; the rapid and transient increase of NGF-mRNA was identical in the macrophage invasion delayed strain (C57Bl/6 Ola) as compared to the wild type (C57Bl/6j) mice. Importantly, the response of the nerve segments to macrophage conditioned medium was also the same in the C57Bl/6 Ola and in the wild type, indicating that the defect of the C57Bl/6 Ola strain does not reside in the general inability of Schwann cells or sciatic fibroblasts to synthesize NGF when exposed to macrophages. Next, we tested if the absence of macrophage recruitment would result in a reduced level of interleukin-1ß (Il-1ß) mRNA in the C57Bl/6 Ola. At two days after lesion the Il-1ß mRNA levels were 7-fold lower in the C57Bl/6 Ola as compared to the wild type (Fig. 4), and this corresponded well to the virtual absence of immigrated macrophages (Lunn et al.,

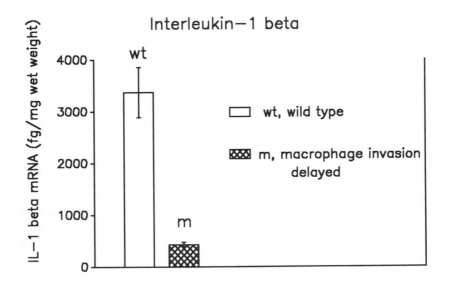

Figure 4. Levels of interleukin-1ß mRNA established 2 days after lesion by quantitative Northern blotting.

1989). Thus the increase in levels of Il-1ß mRNAs found in the distal nerve segment 2 days after sciatic lesion of normal animals appears to be directly coupled to the invasion of macrophages.

Our finding that NGF-mRNA levels are also 6-fold lower in the macrophage delayed strain as compared to the wild type supports the view that it is the recruitment of macrophages into the distal nerve that determines the synthesis of NGF, at least up to the 2 days measured after lesion (Brown et al., 1990).

It was evident from our previous studies that the Schwann cell NGF receptor expression was not regulated by the presence of macrophage conditioned medium in cultured nerve segments (Heumann et al., 1987b). Interestingly, in the macrophage invasion delayed mouse strain C57Bl/6

O1a, the Schwann cell NGF receptor mRNA levels remained very low at the 2 days measured after lesion, indicating that the macrophages could be involved in the regulation of the NGF low affinity receptor expression (Brown et al., 1990). The mechanism of its regulation is apparently not based on the release of soluble substances from macrophages as in the case of regulation of NGF synthesis, but probably due to the ability of macrophages to disturb the intimate Schwann cell-neuron interaction.

Mechanism suppressing the increase in NGF. The intracellular signal(s) leading to the IL-1-induced responses in the distal segment of the sciatic nerve is thought to be related to inflammatory mechanisms, because phospholipase-A2 inhibitors and glucocorticoids are able to prevent the Il-1-induced increases of NGF-mRNA (Lindholm et al., 1988). In monocytes, glucocorticoids are known to exhibit their anti-inflammatory effects by multiple mechanisms, such as inhibition of IL-1 synthesis at the transcriptional or post-translational level and by preventing the cellular release of this cytokine (Knudson et al., 1987; Kern et al., 1988).

In the case of peripheral nerves, glucocorticoids could have either an indirect negative regulatory action on NGF-gene transcription, e.g., by inhibition of Il-1 synthesis, or alternatively, by direct interaction with the NGF gene promoter. Such a negative regulation of NGF-mRNA levels by glucocorticoids (Lindholm et al., 1988) may explain the lower absolute increases in NGF-mRNA levels after nerve transection as compared to those of the in vitro cultured nerve segments (Heumann et al., 1987b). Thus, endogenous anti-inflammatory mechanisms may be involved in the "dampening" of the lesion-induced changes in NGF synthesis.

Is NGF involved in promoting recovery of neuronal functions after peripheral nerve lesion? Early experiments involved the investigation of fiber regrowth of sympathetic nerve terminals after application of 6-OH-dopamine and showed that NGF antibodies could transiently inhibit regeneration (Bjerre et al., 1974). More recently, the collateral reinnervation from sensory nerves could be specifically blocked in the presence of NGF antibodies (Owen et al., 1989).

While these and a number of additional observations (see Rich et al., 1989a) support a role for NGF in regeneration, others have questioned this suggestion because they were unable to block regeneration by NGF antibodies. After sciatic nerve crush lesion experiments in autoimmune animals synthesizing functional NGF-antibodies (as evidenced by the successful immuno-sympathectomy), the rate of regeneration of sensory fibers was not impeded as compared to the controls (Rich et al.,1984). Furthermore, the regrowth of sensory nerve fibers after crush lesions at a site before the nerve reaches the skin was not affected by the NGF antibodies (Diamond et al., 1987). The authors claim that penetration of antibodies was not a problem because expansion of sensory fields of innervation in the rat skin, i.e., sprouting of sensory axons, could be prevented by NGF antibodies.

Using the macrophage invasion delayed mouse strain C57Bl/6 01a, we were able to test the role of NGF in promoting fiber regrowth. The regeneration of motor neurons which express apparently "non-responsive" NGF receptors (see above) was found not to be impeded in the macrophage invasion delayed C57Bl/6 01a mice. After crush lesions, the motor neuron axons extended their tips along the unmyelinated Schwann cells at the same rate as within the Schwann cells of control animals (Lunn et al., 1989; Brown et al., 1989). In contrast, the long-term extension of NGF responsive sensory fibers was greatly reduced in the macrophage invasion delayed strain (Brown et al., 1990). The identity of the trophic substances responsible for a successful functional reinnervation, i.e., NGF, NGF-like substances, or lesion specific factors, needs still to be clarified.

CONCLUDING REMARKS

The above described transient increases in c-*fos* and c-*jun* mRNAs after sciatic nerve lesion may be sufficient to mediate short-term changes in NGF-mRNA levels. However, in order to promote functional regeneration, the macrophage dependent signals have to be transduced into changes of the intracellular protein synthesis machinery leading to persistent increases of NGF (or NGF receptor) synthesis. The interplay of the products of the immediate-early genes Fos and Jun and their relatives Fra, Jun-B and Jun-D (Chiu et al. , 1989; Sonnenberg et al., 1989b) have to be investigated as candidates contributing to the integration of inflammatory or anti-inflammatory signals rendering a target field permissive for axonal growth.

Acknowledgements: We thank Christl Lütticken for technical assistance and Dr. Patrick Carroll for reading the manuscript.

REFERENCES

Angel P, Imagawa M, Chiu R, Stein B, Imbra RJ, Rahmsdorf HJ, Jonat C, Herrlich P, Karin M (1987). Phorbol-ester inducible genes contain a common cis element recognized by a TPA-modulated transacting factor. Cell 49: 729-739.
Angel P, Hattori K, Smeal T, Karin M (1988). The *jun* proto-oncogene is positively autoregulated by its product, *jun*/AP-1. Cell 55: 875-885.
Beuche W, Friede RL (1986). Myelin phagocytosis in Wallerian degeneration of peripheral nerves depends on silica-sensitive, bg/bg-negative and Fc-positive monocytes. Brain Res 378:97-106.
Bjerre B, Bjorklund A, Stenevi U (1974). Inhibition of the regenerative growth of central noradrenergic neurons by intra-

cerebrally administered anti-NGF serum. Brain Res 74:1-18.

Brown MC, Lunn ER, Perry HV (1989). The route taken by axons growing down an intact distal nerve stump in mice. J Physiol 418:148P.

Brown MC, Perry HV, Lunn ER, Heumann R, Gordon S (1990). Consequences of non-degeneration of the distal nerve segment for survival and regeneration of afferent nerve fibers. In press.

Caput D, Beutler B, Hartog K, Thayer R, Brown-Shimer S, Cerami (1986). Identification of a common nucleotide sequence in the 3' untranslated region of mRNA molecules specifying inflammatory mediators. Proc Natl Acad Sci USA 83:1670-1674.

Cavicchioli L, Flanigan TP, Vaniti G, Fusco M, Polato P, Toffano G, Walsh FS, Leon A (1989). NGF amplifies expression of NGF receptor messenger RNA in forebrain cholinergic neurons of rats. Europ J Neurosci 1:258-262.

Chiu R, Imagawa M, Imbra RJ, Bockoven JR, Karin M (1987). Multiple cis- and transacting elements mediate the transcriptional response to phorbol esters. Nature (London) 329:648-651.

Chiu R, Boyle WJ, Meek J, Smeal T, Hunter JB, Karin M (1988). The c-fos protein interacts with c-jun/AP-1 to stimulate transcription of AP-1 responsive genes. Cell 54:541-552.

Chiu R, Angel P, Karin M (1989). Jun-B differs in its biological properties from, and is a negative regulator of c-Jun. Cell 59:979-986.

Curran T, Franza BR (1988). Fos and Jun: the AP-1 connection. Cell 55:395-397.

Diamond J, Coughlin M, MacIntyre L, Holmes M, Visheau B (1987). Evidence that endogenous beta nerve growth factor is responsible for the collateral sprouting but not the regeneration of nociceptive axons in adult rats. Proc Natl Acad Sci USA 84:6596-6600.

Doherty P, Seaton P, Flanigan TP, Walsh FS (1988) Factors controlling expression of NGF receptor in PC12 cells. Neurosci Lett 92:222-227.

Ernfors P, Henschen A, Olson L, Persson H (1989). Expression of nerve growth factor receptor mRNA is developmentally regulated and increased after axotomy in rat spinal cord motoneurons. Neuron 2:1605-1613.

Gage FH, Batchelor P, Chen KS, Chin D, Higgins GA, Koh S, Deputy S, Rosenberg MB, Fischer W, Bjorklund A (1989). NGF receptor reexpression and NGF-mediated cholinergic neuronal hypertrophy in the damaged adult neostriatum. Neuron 2:1177-1184.

Gall CM, Isackson PJ (1989). Limbic seizures increase neuronal production of messenger RNA for nerve growth factor. Science 245:758-761.

Greenberg ME, Hermanowsky AL, Ziff EB (1986). Effect of protein synthesis inhibitors on growth factor activation of c-*fos*, c-*myc* and actin gene transcription. Mol Cell Biol 6: 1050-1057.

Hengerer B, Lindholm D, Heumann R, Rüther U, Wagner EF, Thoenen H (1990). Lesion induced increase in nerve growth factor mRNA is mediated by c-*fos*. In press.

Heumann R, Thoenen H (1986). Comparison between the time course of changes in nerve growth factor protein levels and those of its messenger RNA in the cultured rat iris. J Biol Chem 261:9246-9249.

Heumann R, Korsching S, Bandtlow C, Thoenen H (1987a). Changes of nerve growth factor synthesis in non-neuronal cells in responses to sciatic nerve transection. J Cell Biol 104:1623-1631R.

Heumann R, Lindholm D, Bandtlow C, Meyer M, Radeke MJ, Misko TP, Shooter E, Thoenen H (1987b). Differential regulation of nerve growth factor (NGF) and NGF receptor mRNA in the rat sciatic nerve during development, degeneration and regeneration; role played by macrophages. Proc Natl Acad Sci USA 84: 8735-8739.

Higgins GA, Koh S, Chen KS, Gage F (1989). NGF induction of NGF receptor gene expression and cholinergic neuronal hypertrophy within the basal forebrain of the adult rat. Neuron 3:247-256.

Hunt SP, Pini A, Evan G (1987). Induction of c-fos-like protein in spinal cord neurons following sensory stimulation. Nature (London) 328:632-634.

Johnson EM, Yip HK (1985). Central nervous system and peripheral nerve growth factor provide trophic support critical to mature sensory neuronal survival. Nature (London) 314:751-752.

Kern JA, Lamb RJ, Reed J, Daniele RP, Nowell PC (1988). Dexamethasone inhibitition of interleukin 1 beta production by human monocytes. J Clin Invest 81:237-244.

Knudson PJ, Dinarello CA, Strom TB (1987). Glucocorticoids inhibit transcriptional and posttranscriptional expression of interleukin 1 in U937 cells. J Immunol 138:4129-4134.

Korsching S (1986). The role of nerve growth factor in the CNS. Trends Neurosci 9:570-573.

Kruijer W, Cooper JA, Hunter T, Verma I (1984). Platelet-derived growth factor induces rapid but transient expression of the c-fos gene and protein. Nature (London) 312: 711-716.

Landschulz WH, Johnson PF, McKnight SL (1988). The leucine zipper: A hypothetical structure common to a new class of DNA binding proteins. Science 240: 1759-1764.

Lemke G, Chao M (1988). Axons regulate Schwann cell expression of the major myelin and NGF receptor genes. Development 102:499-504.

Levi-Montalcini R, Angeletti PU (1968). Nerve growth factor. Physiol Rev 48:534-569.

Lindholm D, Heumann R, Meyer M, Thoenen H (1987). Interleukin 1 regulates synthesis of nerve growth factor in non-neuronal cells of rat sciatic nerve. Nature (London) 330: 658-659.

Lindholm D, Heumann R, Hengerer B, Thoenen H (1988). Interleukin 1 increases stability and transcription of mRNA encoding nerve growth factor in cultured rat fibroblasts. J Biol Chem 263:16348-16351.

Lindsay RM, Harmar AJ (1989). Nerve growth factor regulates expression of neuropeptide genes in adult sensory neurons. Nature (London) 337:362-364.

Lindsay RM, Shooter EM, Radeke MJ, Dechant G, Thoenen H, Lindholm D (1990). Nerve growth factor regulates expression of the nerve growth factor receptor gene in adult sensory neurons. In press.

Lunn ER, Perry HV, Brown MC, Rosen H, Gordon S (1989). Absence of Wallerian degeneration does not hinder regeneration in peripheral nerve. Europ J Neurosci 1:27-33.

Menetrey D, Gannon A, Levine JD, Basbaum AI (1989). Expression of c-*fos* protein in interneurons and projection neurons of the rat spinal cord in response to noxious somatic, articular, and visceral stimulation. J Comp Neurol 285: 177-195.

Morgan JI, Cohen DR, Hempstedt JL, Curran T (1987). Mapping patterns of c-*fos* expression in the central nervous system after lesion. Science 237: 192-197.

Müller R, Bravo R, Burckhardt J, Curran T (1984). Induction of c-*fos* gene and protein by growth factors precedes activation of c-myc. Nature (London) 312: 716-720.

Owen DJ, Logan A, Robinson PP (1989). A role for nerve growth factor in collateral reinnervation from sensory nerves in the guinea pig. Brain Res 476:248-255.

Raivich G, Kreutzberg GW (1987). Expression of growth factor receptors in injured nervous tissue. I. Axotomy leads to a shift in the cellular distribution of specific beta-nerve growth factor binding in the injured and regenerating PNS. J Neurocytol 16:689-700.

Rich KM, Yip HK, Osborne PA, Schmidt RE, Johnson EM (1984). Role of nerve growth factor in the adult dorsal root ganglia neuron and its response to injury. J Comp Neurol 230:110-118.

Rich KM, Luszcynski JR, Osborne PA, Johnson EM (1987). Nerve growth factor protects adult sensory neurons from cell death and atrophy caused by nerve injury. J Neurocytol 16:261-268.

Rich KM, Alexander TD, Pryor JC, Hollowell JP (1989a). Nerve growth factor enhances regeneration through silicone chambers. Exp Neurol 105:162-170.

Rich KM, Dish SP, Eichler ME (1989b). The influence of regeneration and nerve growth factor on the neuronal cell body reaction to injury. J Neurocytol 18:569–576.

Risse G, Jooss K, Neuberg M, Brüller HJ, Müller R (1989). Asymmetrical recognition of the palindromic AP1 binding site (TRE) by Fos protein complexes. EMBO J 12:3825–3832.

Rüther U, Wagner EF, Müller R, (1985). Analysis of the differentiation-promoting potential of the inducible c-*fos* genes introduced into embryonal carcinoma cells. EMBO J 4:1775–1781.

Rüther U, Garber C, Komitowsky D, Müller R, Wagner EF (1987). Deregulated c-*fos* expression interferes with normal bone development in transgenic mice. Nature (London) 325:412–416.

Rush RA (1984). Immunohistochemical localization of endogenous nerve growth factor. Nature (London) 312:364–367.

Ryseck RP, Hirai SI, Yaniv M, Bravo R (1989). Transcriptional activation of c-*jun* during the G_0/G_1 transition in mouse fibroblasts. Nature (London) 334:535–537.

Saffen DW, Cole AJ, Worley PF, Christy BA, Ryder K, Barbaran JM (1988). Convulsant-induced increase in transcription factor messenger RNAs in rat brain. Proc Natl Acad Sci USA 85:7795–7799.

Sagar SM, Sharp FR, Curran T (1988). Expression of c-*fos* protein in the brain: metabolic mapping at the cellular level. Science 240:1328–1330.

Schmalbruch H (1987). Loss of sensory neurons after sciatic nerve section in the rat. Anat Rec 219:323–329.

Selby MJ, Edwards R, Sharp F, Rutter WJ (1987). Mouse nerve growth factor gene: Structure and expression. Mol Cell Biol 7:3057–3064.

Sonnenberg JL, Rauscher FJ, Morgan JI, Curran T (1989a). Regulation of proenkephalin by Fos and Jun. Science 246:1622–1625.

Sonnenberg JL, Macgregor L, Curran T, Morgan JI, (1989b). Dynamic alterations occur in the level and composition of transcription factor AP-1 complex after seizure. Neuron 3:359–365.

Taniuchi M, Clark HB, Johnson EM (1986). Induction of nerve growth factor receptor in Schwann cells after axotomy. Proc Natl Acad Sci USA 83:4094-4098.

Taniuchi M, Clark HB, Schweitzer JB, Johnson M (1988). Expression of nerve growth factor receptors by Schwann cells of axotomized peripheral nerves: Ultrastructural location, suppression by axonal contact, and binding properties. J Neurosci 8:664-681.

Thoenen H, Barde Y-A (1980). Physiology of nerve growth factor. Physiol Rev 60:1284-1335.

Verge VMK, Riopelle RJ, Richardson PM (1989). Nerve growth factor receptors on normal and injured sensory neurons. J Neurosci 9:914-922.

Verrier B, Müller D, Bravo R, Müller R (1986). Wounding a fibroblast monolayer results in the rapid induction of the c-*fos* proto-oncogene. EMBO J 5:913-917.

Advances in Neural Regeneration
Research, pages 147–159
© 1990 Wiley-Liss, Inc.

ASTROGLIAL FACTORS SUPPORTING NEURITE GROWTH AND LONG-TERM
NEURONAL SURVIVAL

H.W. Müller, H.P. Matthiessen and C. Schmalenbach

Molecular Neurobiology Laboratory, Department of
Neurology, University of Düsseldorf, D-4000
Düsseldorf, F.R.G.

INTRODUCTION

Considering the complexity of the three-dimensional
architecture of functionally integrated neuronal networks in
the central nervous system (CNS) several questions arise:
What are the specific molecular and cellular conditions
provided within the CNS necessary to promote differentiation
of neurons into tight neuritic networks, to support
prolonged neuronal survival, or to stabilize synaptic
organization of functional circuitries. Knowledge of
endogenous neurotrophic survival factors and neurite
promoting or sprouting factors acting in the mammalian CNS
may be particularly useful to create supportive
environmental conditions for damaged nerve cells to enhance
their recovery and possibly restore their function
following injury or disease.

In the present paper we will provide evidence that
the astrocyte is a potential candidate cell to release
neuritogenic factors and neurotrophic proteins which may
promote (a) axonal and dendritic outgrowth and (b) support
"long-term" survival of central neurons derived from rat
brain. Data are presented (i) on the identification of two
major neurite-promoting factors produced by cerebral
astrocytes in culture and (ii) on the release of astroglial
protein with neurotrophic activity supporting "long-term"
survival of hippocampal neurons in vitro and (iii) on the
importance of neuronal cell/contact density for the
maintenance of neuronal networks.

NEURITE-PROMOTING FACTORS RELEASED BY IMMATURE ASTROCYTES IN CULTURE

Cultured astrocytes from neonatal mammalian central nervous system release neurite-promoting activities stimulating neuritic growth of peripheral and central neurons in vitro (Banker, 1980; Lindsay, 1979; Müller and Seifert, 1982). Furthermore, expression of the extracellular matrix glycoproteins laminin (LN) and fibronectin (FN) by cultured astrocytes has been described previously (Liesi et al., 1983; Price and Hynes, 1985; Selak et al., 1985; Matthiessen et al., 1989). When attached to the culture substratum both proteins purified from mouse EHS tumor or human serum, respectively, stimulate neurite outgrowth of peripheral neurons in vitro (Manthorpe et al., 1983a) and LN further promotes neuritic growth of cultured CNS neurons (Manthorpe et al., 1983a; Rogers et al., 1983; Beckh et al., 1987). Purified FN has been reported earlier to support neurite extension of retinal ganglion cells to some degree (Adler et al., 1985; Hall et al., 1987). Very recently additional evidence from our laboratory demonstrated a marked neurite promoting activity of FN for primary cultures of embryonic rat hippocampal neurons (Matthiessen et al., 1989) as well as highly enriched neuronal cultures from embryonic rat cortex (unpublished observation).

In this section we describe (i) the depletion of neurite-promoting activity from serumfree astroglia conditioned medium (ACM) by repetitive transfer through poly-L-lysine (PLL)-coated culture plastic dishes and the concomitant loss of LN and FN immunoreactivity from ACM; (ii) the fractionation of ACM by means of FPLC-anion exchange chromatography on Mono Q and specific precipitation of the neurite promoting activities from the most active peak fractions by anti-LN antibodies or gelatin agarose (to remove FN); (iii) evidence for the association of LN with proteoglycans is provided.

Serumfree conditioned medium was obtained from primary or secondary cultures of cerebral astrocytes derived from newborn rat. Fig. 1 (top) shows the depletion of neurite-promoting activity from ACM following the repetitive transfer of ACM to PLL-coated culture dishes. At each of the four transfer steps an aliquot of the medium was removed and tested for the remaining neurite promoting activity in a quantitative bioassay as described (Müller and Seifert,

1982; Matthiessen et al., 1989). This depletion experiment lead to removal of approximately 80-90% of neuritogenic activity from ACM. It is interesting to note that anti-LN and anti-FN immunoreactivities in ACM (Fig. 1, middle and bottom) were removed at a very similar degree by binding to PLL-coated substrate.

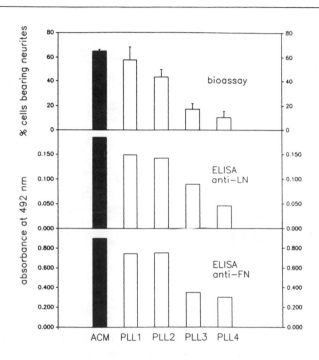

Figure 1. Depletion of neurite-promoting activity, anti-LN and anti-FN immunoreactivities of ACM by repetitive incubation with PLL-coated polycationic culture substratum. Top: neuritogenic activity, mean ± S.D. (n=3); middle: ELISA to detect anti-LN immunreactivity using a rabbit antiserum to purified mouse EHS-tumor LN (Gibco-BRL); bottom: ELISA to detect anti-FN immunoreactivity using a rabbit antiserum to purified human plasma FN (Calbiochem).

FPLC-fractionation of ACM on a Mono Q anion exchange chromatography column is presented in Fig. 2a. By means of the bioassay for neurite promoting activity of combined double-fractions two activity peaks could clearly be identified (Fig. 2b). The maximum biological activity was eluted at approx. 1,000 mM NaCl (fractions 34-35) indicating a high negative charge associated with the active molecule(s). A smaller peak of neurite promoting activity appeared at 2-300 mM NaCl (fractions 14-19).

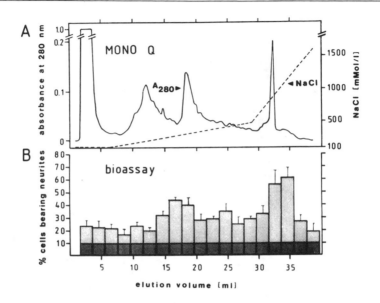

Figure 2. FPLC-anion exchange chromatography of ACM on Mono Q. (A) Protein profile: 7.2 mg of dialyzed and lyophilized ACM was resolved in 500 µl of 50 mM Tris-HCl buffer (pH 7.4, 100 mM NaCl) and separated on a Mono Q column (HR 5/5, Pharmacia). The bound material was eluted with a linear NaCl gradient ranging from 100 to 2,000 mM in the same buffer and the absorption at 280 nm was detected. (B) Neurite-promoting activity profile: Every two fractions (each of 1 ml) were pooled, dialyzed and added in triplicates of 500 µl to PLL-coated glass coverslips. The neurite-promoting activity was assayed using hippocampal neurons from embryonic (E18) Whistar rat and determined by counting the number of viable cells bearing neurites >2 cell diameters and given as percentage of the total number of viable cells. Five randomly chosen visual fields were counted.

In order to test whether the neurite promoting activities separated by anion exchange chromatography are related to either LN and/or FN we carried out specific precipitation of LN and FN immunoreactivity by means of anti-LN antibodies coupled to protein A-agarose and gelatin-agarose to remove FN, respectively (Fig. 3). Immunoprecipitation of fractions 15-16 by anti-LN antibody protein A-agarose complex diminished the neurite-promoting activity by 10-30% whereas treatment by gelatin-agarose to precipitate FN removed at least 50% of the biological activity in these fractions. A combination of both the LN- and FN-precipitating agents appeared to be additive in its effect. However, when fractions 33-34 of the major peak of neurite-promoting activity were treated in the same way, anti-LN protein A-agarose removed most of the biological activity (>50%) whereas the FN selective affinity gel had very little effect.

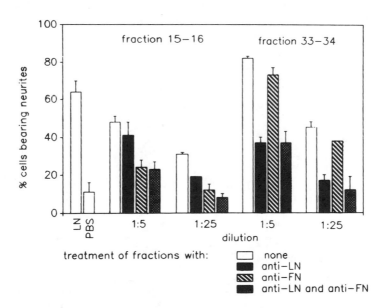

Figure 3. Specific precipitation of neurite-promoting activity from ACM. Aliquots of 500 µl of pooled fractions 15-16 or 33-34 obtained after anion exchange chromatography (see Fig. 2) were treated (a) with 200 µl (packed gel) of anti-LN antiserum bound to protein A-agarose, (b) with 200 µl of gelatin-agarose (to selectively precipitate FN) or (c) 200 µl of unloaded protein A-agarose. Supernatants were diluted 1:5 or 1:25 with N2 medium, respectively, and tested for remaining neurite-promoting activity on hippocampal

neurons. Mean ± S.D. (n=3). LN: neurite-promoting activity
in presence of purified mouse EHS-tumor LN (Gibco-BRL, 10
µg/ml PBS) bound to PLL-coated glass coverslips.

When the major peak of LN-containing neurite-
promoting activity (fractions 34-35 of Mono Q column, see
fig. 2b and 3) was treated with glycosaminoglycan degrading
enzymes the LN elution profile was modified (Fig. 4).
Heparitinase treatment degraded approx. 80% of the total LN-
proteoglycan complex, since the major neurite-promoting
activity peak associated with LN immunoreactivity was
shifted to lower salt concentrations following re-
chromatography on Mono Q. On the other hand, chondroitinase
ABC treatment had comparatively little effect suggesting
that LN in ACM is predominantly associated with a heparan
sulfate proteoglycan and to a lower degree to chontroitin or
dermatan sulfate proteoglycan.

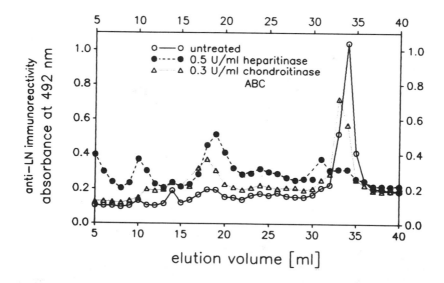

Figure 4. Sensitivity of LN immunoreactivity in ACM to
glycosaminoglycanases. ACM was lyophilized and fractionated
by anion exchange chromatography on a Mono Q column (see
Fig. 2). Pooled fractions 33-34 containing both the maximum
of LN immunoreactivity and neurite-promoting activity were
desalted and dialyzed against 50 mM Tris-HCl buffer (pH 7.4)
containing 100 mM NaCl and aliquots were treated in the

presence of 0.01% bovine serum albumin in a total vol. of
600 µl with Tris-buffer containing (a) 40 mM sodium acetate
and 2.5 mM calcium chloride for 3 h at 37 °C, (b) 0.5 U/ml
heparitinase (Seikagaku Kogyo Co.) and 2.5 mM calcium
chloride for 2 h at 43 °C or (c) 0.3 U/ml chondroitinase ABC
(Boehringer-Mannheim) in the presence of 40 mM sodium
acetate for 3 h at 37 °C. After incubation aliquots of 500
µl were rechromatographed on Mono Q and the fractions
obtained were assayed for shifts in LN immunoreactivity.

NEUROTROPHIC SURVIVAL ACTIVITY IN ASTROGLIAL CONDITIONED MEDIUM

Neurite-promoting substrate adhesion factors like LN
and FN seem to be required but are not sufficient for long-
term survival and stabilization of central neurons in
primary culture (Müller et al., 1989). In contrast to almost
pure neuronal cultures, neurons cocultured together with
astroglial cells may survive for prolonged periods even
under serumfree culture conditions, suggesting a
neurotrophic activity produced by the glial cells (Banker,
1980; Müller and Seifert, 1982). This view is further
supported by the detection of local enhancement of
neurotrophic activity presumably released by astroglia near
lesion sites in the injured adult rat brain (Nieto-Sampedro
et al., 1982; Manthorpe et al., 1983b). In fact, immature
astrocytes from rat brain grown in serumfree culture release
a neurotrophic activity that is diffusable in conditioned
medium and, when transferred to hippocampal or cortical
neurons which were seeded on PLL and LN-coated glass
coverslips, enhances neuronal survival significantly
compared to nonconditioned chemically defined hormone-
supplemented N2 (Bottenstein and Sato, 1979) medium (Fig.
5).

Preliminary biochemical characterization identified
the neurotrophic activity as a protein with an apparent
molecular weight >10kDa. Removal of this diffusable
neurotrophic support of ACM by transfer of the neuronal
culture into nonconditioned (nontoxic) control medium
resulted in neuronal cell death within 1-2 days suggesting
that astroglial trophic support may be permanently required,
at least in vitro, for "long-term" maintenance of these
brain neurons (unpublished observation).

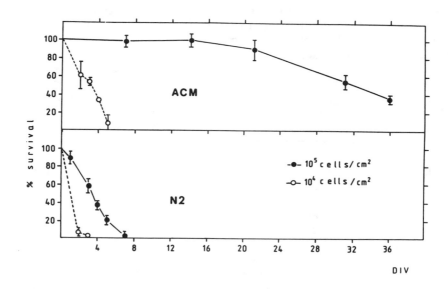

Figure 5. Effect of ACM and cell density on survival of hippocampal neurons in culture. Hippocampal neurons were seeded on LN-coated glass coverslips and grown in the presence of ACM (top) or nonconditioned N2 culture medium (bottom) at two cell densities (10^4 and 10^5 cells/cm²) and cell survival was assayed by MTT-assay as described (Matthiessen et al., 1989).

ROLE OF NEURONAL CELL CONTACT DENSITY FOR LONG-TERM SURVIVAL

Changes in cell density of serumfree neuronal cultures had significant effects on the degree of cell viability regardless whether the neurons were grown in serumfree nonconditioned N2 medium or under trophic glial support in ACM (Fig. 5). Increasing the cell density (e.g. from 10^4 to 10^5 hippocampal cells/cm²) markedly enhanced neuronal survival. However, further increase in cell density beyond 10^5 cells/cm² had no significant survival enhancing effect. Since neuronal cultures plated at low cell density may not survive for prolonged periods (>30 DIV) even in the presence of ACM but, instead, degenerate within one week (Fig. 5) a synergistic effect of astroglial neurotrophic support and cell contact density on neuronal survival is suggested.

It could further be demonstrated that the enhancement in neuronal survival in high density culture is not due to a concomitant rise in *astroglial* cells contaminating the neuronal culture but rather to an increase in *neuronal* density. Fig. 6 shows marked differences in neuronal survival when hippocampal cultures grown in ACM at cell densities of 10^4 and 2×10^4 cells/cm² were compared.

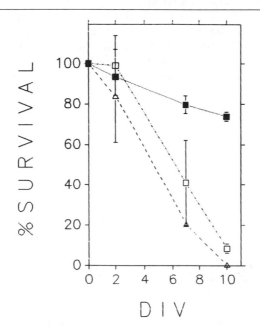

Figure 6. Effect of astroglial cell supplementation on survival of hippocampal neurons in culture. Hippocampal cultures highly enriched for neurons ($\geq 95\%$) were plated at (△) 10,000 cells/cm², (□) 10,000 cells/cm² plus 1,000 astroblasts/cm² and (■) 20,000 cells/cm². Mean ± S.D. (n=3).

It is interesting to note that further addition to the low density hippocampal culture (10^4 cells/cm²) of approximately 1,000 astroblasts/cm² (corresponding to 10% of the cultured cells) had very little effect on neuronal survival. This result strongly suggests that maintenance of neurons in a hippocampal culture of high cell density (e.g. 2×10^4 cells/cm²) is due to an increase in neuron-neuron rather than neuron-astroglia interactions. The nature of

this neuron-neuron stabilizing activity has yet to be
identified. This cellular interaction could either be
contact mediated or performed via diffusible molecules
acting e.g. in an autocrine fashion.

In contrast to low density hippocampal cultures (e.g.
10^4 cells/cm^2) neurons plated at high density developed into
tight neuritic networks expressing spontaneous bioelectrical
activity (Köller et al., 1990). Stabilization of the latter
cultures could thus be related to enhanced synaptic activity
and neuronal integration. On the other hand, recent evidence
from our laboratory suggested that neither chronic
inhibition of spike-evoked transmitter release nor
depolarization during development of hippocampal neurons in
high density culture had a significant influence on long-
term cell survival or axonal growth (unpublished
observation).

CONCLUSION

We have identified LN and FN as two prominent
constituents of astroglia released neurite-promoting
activity acting on primary neurons from embryonic rat brain.
LN is associated predominantly with heparan sulfate
proteoglycan in a high molecular weight complex. Recently it
could be demonstrated that astroglial LN appears to be
expressed in a modified molecular form lacking the A chain
entirely or in part (Matthiessen et al., 1989). Furthermore,
we have presented evidence for a neurotrophic protein or
proteins released by immature cerebral astrocytes in
serumfree defined culture which support(s) "long-term"
survival and stabilization of primary neurons derived from
embryonic rat brain. Evidence obtained with nerve cell
cultures suggested that the permanent presence of this
neurotrophic activity is necessary for maintenance and
stabilization of neuronal structure and function. Neurite-
promoting and neurotrophic astroglial proteins as well as
not yet identified neuron-neuron cell interactions seem to
be required but appear to be sufficient only in combination
for development and "long-term" survival of spontaneously
active neuronal networks.

ACKNOWLEDGEMENT

The excellent technical assistance of K. Dick is gratefully acknowledged. This work was supported in part by grants from the Deutsche Forschungsgemeinschaft (Mu 630/3-1,2).

REFERENCES

Adler R, Jerdan J, Hewitt AT (1985). Responses of cultured neural retinal cells to substratum-bound laminin and other extracellular matrix molecules. Dev Biol 206:100-114.

Banker GA (1980). Trophic interactions between astroglial cells and hippocampal neurons in culture. Science 209:809-810.

Beckh S, Müller HW, Seifert W (1987). Neurotrophic and neurite-promoting activities in astroglial conditioned medium. In: Glial-Neuronal Communication in Development and Regeneration. NATO ASI Series H: Cell Biology. Vol 2. HH Althaus and W Seifert, eds. Springer, Heidelberg, pp 385-406.

Bottenstein JE, Sato GH (1979). Growth of a rat neuroblastoma cell line in serum-free supplemented medium. Proc Natl Acad Sci USA 76:514-517.

Hall DE, Neugebauer KM, Reichardt LF (1987). Embryonic neural retinal cell response to extracellular matrix proteins: Developmental changes and effects of the cell substratum attachment antibody (CSAT). J Cell Biol 104:623-634.

Köller H, Siebler M, Schmalenbach C, Müller HW (1990). GABA and glutamate receptor development of cultured neurons from rat hippocampus, septal region, and neocortex. Synapse 5:59-64.

Liesi P, Dahl D, Vaheri A (1983). Laminin is produced by early rat astrocytes in primary culture. J Cell Biol 96:920-924.

Lindsay RM (1979). Adult rat brain astrocytes support survival of both NGF-dependent and NGF-insensitive neurons. Nature 282:80-82.

Manthorpe M, Engvall E, Ruoslahti E, Longo FM, Davis GE, Varon S (1983a). Laminin promotes neuritic regeneration from cultured peripheral and central neurons. J Cell Biol 97:1882-1890.

Manthorpe M, Nieto-Sampedro M, Skaper SD, Lewis ER, Barbin G, Longo FM, Cotman CW, Varon S (1983b). Neuronotrophic activity in brain wounds of the developing rat. Correlation with implant survival in the wound cavity. Brain Res 267:47-56.

Matthiessen P, Schmalenbach C, Müller HW (1989). Astroglia-released neurite growth-inducing activity for embryonic hippocampal neurons is associated with laminin bound in a sulfated complex and free fibronectin. Glia 2:177-188.

Müller HW, Seifert W (1982). A neurotrophic factor (NTF) released from primary glial cultures supports survival and fiber outgrowth of cultured hippocampal neurons. J Neurosci Res 8:195-204.

Müller HW, Schmalenbach C, Matthiessen HP (1989). Development and stabilization of neuronsl networks in culture: To the role of astroglial neurotrophic factors, cell contacts, and bioelectrical activity. In: Dynamics and Plasticity in Neuronal Systems. Proceedings of the 17th Göttingen Neurobiology Conference (N Elsner, W. Singer, eds), Thieme, Stuttgart, pp 11.

Nieto-Sampedro M, Lewis ER, Cotman CW, Manthorpe M, Skaper SD, Barbin G, Longo FM, Varon S (1982). Brain injury causes a time-dependent increase in neuronotrophic activity at the lesion site. Science 217:860-861.

Price J, Hynes RO (1985). Astrocytes in culture synthesize and secrete a variant form of fibronectin. J Neurosci 5:2205-2211.

Rogers SL, Letourneau PC, Palm SL, McCarthy J, Furcht LT (1983). Neurite extension by peripheral and central nervous system neurons in response to substratum-bound fibronectin and laminin. Dev Biol 98:212-220.

Selak I, Foidart JM, Moonen G (1985). Laminin promotes cerebellar granule cells migration in vitro and is synthesized by cultured astrocytes. Dev Neurosci 7:278-285.

Advances in Neural Regeneration
Research, pages 161–170
© 1990 Wiley-Liss, Inc.

ASTROCYTE REACTION IN INJURY AND REGENERATION

Sergey Fedoroff

Department of Anatomy, University of Saskatchewan,

Saskatoon, Saskatchewan S7N OWO

Astroglia are not a single well-defined cell type but rather a whole "family" of cells having diverse morphological phenotypes with regional specificity. The astroglia include radial glia (Rakic, 1984), fibrous and protoplasmic astrocytes (Privat and Ratabaul, 1986), ependymal cells (Bruni et al., 1985), Golgi-Bergmann cells (Wilkin and Levi, 1986), valate-protoplasmic astrocytes (Peters et al., 1976), pineal astrocytes (Papasozomenos, 1986) pituicytes (Wittkowski, 1986), Gomori-positive astrocytes (Srebro and Cichocki, 1971), perinodal astrocytes (Black and Waxman, 1988) and an unknown number of subpopulations of cells that may differ as to the types of receptors, ion channels, active transport and antigens they possess (Prochiantz and Mallat, 1988; Hansson, 1988, Cholewinski et al., 1988, Wilkin et al., 1990).

These cells can be grouped into a family because they have certain properties in common. All the cells are neuron supporting cells; all are in contact with either subpial external glia limitans, perivascular glial basement membrane or ventricular surfaces; they are coupled to each other by gap junctions or have contact with each other through adherent-type junctions. They all have, or had at some stage of their development, the potential to express glial fibrillary acidic protein (GFAP) in their intermediate filaments. Some, if not all, have small, regular, intramembranous particles, the orthogonal assemblies, in the cytoplasmic half of the membrane (Landis, 1986). Astroglia are present throughout the CNS although their density in various regions varies considerably. White matter has a higher density of astroglia than grey matter. In human cerebral cortex the glia/neuron ratio is 0.5 and in the dorso-medial thalamic nucleus it is 17.1 (Pope, 1978).

The first task of astroglia in development is to "fence" the CNS and they control the integrity of the blood-brain barrier throughout life. During embryonic development the establishment of normal functions of both neurons and astroglia seems to depend on specific interactions between the two cell types (Varon and Somjen, 1979; Hatten and Masson, 1986). Astroglia promote both the survival of neurons and neurite outgrowth (Banker, 1980, Lindsay,1979; Müller and Seifert, 1982; Noble et al., 1984; Rudge et al., 1985; Mattheissen et al., 1989) and may also influence the development of specific populations of neurons (Denis-Donini and Estenoz, 1988, Patel et al., 1988; Seaton et al., 1988; Patel et al., 1989). Conversely, neurons may influence the proliferation and maturation of astroglia (Hatten and Masson, 1986; Hayashi et al., 1988; Hunt et al., 1988). In culture, neurons develop more extensive dendritic trees when cultured on homotypic astroglia rather than heterotypic astroglia (Autillo-Touati et al., 1988). The immature astroglia are more permissive for neurite growth than astroglia from adult animals (Smith and Silver, 1988; Cohen et al., 1986; Tomaselli et al., 1988). In the chapter by R.H. Miller and G.M. Smith in this section, the maturation of astroglia and their state of permissiveness for neurite growth are discussed and in the chapter by S. David the acquisition of permissiveness for neurite growth at the site of lesion is dealt with.

During development astroglia do not react to injury or react only to a limited degree. Only in fairly advanced stages of embryonic development in man or postnatally in mice and rats do astrocytes respond to trauma and injury (Barrett et al., 1984; Grafe et al., 1983; Fedoroff and Doering, 1987) by swelling, hypertrophy with or without proliferation, formation of reactive astrocytes, and eventually, formation of glial scars (Reier and Houle, 1988). H.K. Kimelberg and his colleagues in a chapter in this section draw attention to the fact that the swelling of astrocytes alters membrane transport and they discuss the consequences. In another chapter M.B. Graeber and G.W. Kreutzberg give an account of the reaction of astroglia to injury and describe a mechanism by which astroglia and microglia strip the synaptic contacts from the regenerating neurons. In the chapter by F.J. Liuzzi, the way in which PNS-CNS interface astrocytes interact with the regenerating dorsal root axonal growth cones is discussed. This interaction helps to explain the role of astrocytes in CNS regeneration.

Astroglia have been referred to as the "liver of the brain" (Hamprecht, 1986) because they maintain the homeostasis of the neuronal environment. The functions of astroglia are many and various and are regulated by hormones, growth factors (see the section on growth factors, this volume) and cytokines (Benveniste, 1988). It has been suggested that all astroglia are coupled by gap junctions, forming an "astroglial functional syncytium" anchored to the pial and ventricular surfaces, blood vessels, and through the oligodendrocytes, to nerve fibers (Mugnaini, 1986; Kettenmann and Schachner 1985; Ransom and Carlini, 1986). It is quite possible that certain functional centers have their own astroglial synctium. The significance of a syncytium is that it can act as a spatial buffer of potassium ions (K^+ siphon), preventing accumulation of large amounts of K^+ in the intercellular spaces in areas where the neurons are highly active (Walz, 1989). In the chapter by J.M. Ritchie in this section, this aspect of astroglial function is discussed in relation to voltage-gated cation and anion channels.

The functions of astroglia are not limited by their coupling to each other; they also play a pivotal role in cell-cell communication in the CNS, mediated by humoral polypeptide factors (cytokines). By means of these factors astroglia interact with microglia, endothelium of the brain capillaries, oligodendroglia and lymphohemopoietic cells, T cells and macrophages. The cytokines released by neural cells resemble the cytokines of the hemopoietic system and include interleukin-1 (IL-1) (Fontana et al., 1982; Nieto-Sampedro and Berman, 1987), interleukin-6 (IL-6) (Frei et al., 1989), interferon α (IFNα) and interferon β (IFNβ) (Tedeschi et al., 1986; Salamat et al., 1988), tumor necrosis factor (TNF) (Robbins et al., 1987; Lieberman et al., 1989; Sawade et al., 1989), colony stimulating factor-1(CSF-1) (Hao et al., 1990), transforming growth factor (TGFα) (Loughlin et al., 1989) and a number of other factors which so far have not been studied sufficiently.

Astroglia are very plastic cells and easily respond to regulatory stimuli by assuming different functional states. The neurotrophic viruses (Frei et al., 1989; Suzumura et al., 1986), bacterial cell wall lipopolysaccharide (endotoxin) (Fontana et al., 1982; Lieberman et al., 1989), IFNγ (Fontana et al., 1986; Tedeschi et al., 1986) and probably a number of not yet identified factors released during brain injury or trauma at the site of lesion, can activate a number of genes in astrocytes resulting in the production of the respective protein products. Among the known activated genes are genes for nerve growth factor (NGF) (Frei et al., 1989; Furukawa et al., 1989), TNF (Lieberman et al., 1989), IFNα/β (Tedeschi et al., 1986; Salamat et al., 1988), IL-1 (Lieberman et al., 1989), and IL-6 (Frei et al., 1989). The cytokines secreted by activated astrocytes are all potent signal mediators, have target cells within and outside the nervous system and they mediate a number of physiological processes (Dinarello, 1988; Old, 1989).

Astrocytes interact with brain capillary endothelial cells by inducing the endothelial cells to adhere to each other by tight junctions, thus creating the blood brain barrier (Stewart and Wiley, 1981; Janzen and Raff, 1987). Secretion of TNF by activated astrocytes renders the endothelial cells of the brain capillaries adhesive to lymphohemopoietic cells thus facilitating their migration into the CNS (Simmons et al., 1988; Frohman et al., 1989). Similarly, astrocytes can be induced to release interferon alpha and beta (INFα/β) (Tedeschi et al., 1986). INF secreted by astrocytes and T lymphocytes can cause the expression of major histocompatability (MHC) class II antigens on subpopulations of astrocytes (Hirsch et al., 1983; Wong et al., 1984), thus acquiring the ability to present antigens to T lymphocytes in an MHC restricted fashion (Fontana et al., 1984). By secretion of CSF-1 the astroglia affect the survival and maturation of the microglia (Hao et al., 1990). By secreting IL-1 and PGE , astroglia have the potential to modulate inflammation and local as well as systemic immune response. Locally, astrocytes release IL-1 which induces the expression of the IL-2 receptor and secretion of IL-2 in T lymphocytes. In turn, IL-2 secreted by T lymphocytes stimulates proliferation and maturation of B lymphocytes (Dinarello, 1988). Secretion of prostaglandin (PGE) suppresses the proliferation and secretion of IL-2 (Goodwin and Webb, 1980; Merrill, 1989). Systemically, IL-1 can stimulate hypothalamic cells to secrete corticotrophic releasing factor (CRF) and through the hypothalamic-pituitary-adreno-corticosteroid neuroendocrine axis, indirectly suppress the immune response (Sundar et al., 1989; Weiss et al., 1989). Moreover, IL-1 by stimulating the sympathetic nervous system, which innervates the lymphoid organs, brings about a decrease in cellular immune responses (Sundar et al., 1989; Nance and Burns, 1989; Reder et al., 1989).

The complexity of the network of communications

between the glial cells in resting and activated states is difficult to fathom with the present state of knowledge. The regulatory stimuli that astrocytes receive can be of various intensities, synergistic or antagonistic to each other. In addition to signalling by cytokines, astroglial function is also affected by a number of growth factors, hormones and by neighboring neurons through release of neurotransmitters, neuropeptides and ions. Thus astrocytes are continuously signalling and receiving signals from various sources. It is within this complex framework that astrocyte function, behavior and their reaction in injury and regeneration must be viewed.

A challenge for the future is to learn how to manipulate the network of communication between the glia cells in such a way that they create conditions favorable for neurite regeneration. The chapters in this section on astrocyte reaction in injury and regeneration address a number of basic problems to do with neuronal regeneration, and facilitate understanding of the complexity of glial cell interactions.

REFERENCES

Autillo–Touati A, Chamak B, Araud J, Vuillet J, Seite R, Prochiantz A (1988). Region–specific neuro–astroglial interactions: Ultrastructural study of the in vitro expression of neuronal polarity. J Neurosci Res 19:326–342.
Banker GA (1980). Trophic interactions between astroglial cells and hippocampal neurons in culture. Science 209:809–810.
Balkwill FR, Burke F (1989). The cytokine network. Immunol Today 10:299–304.
Barrett CP, Donati EJ, Guth L (1984). Differences between adult and neonatal rats in their astroglial response to spinal injury. Exp Neurol 84:374–385.
Benveniste EN (1988). Lymphokines and monokines in the neuroendocrine system. Prog Allergy 43:84–120.
Black JA, Waxman SG (1988). The perinodal astrocyte. Glia 1:169–183.
Bruni JE, Del Bigio MR, Clattenburg RE (1985). Ependyma: normal and pathological. A review of literature. Brain Res Dev 9:1–19.
Cholewinski AJ, Hanley MR, Wilkin GP (1988). A phosphoinositide–linked peptide response in astrocytes: Evidence for regional heterogeneity. Neurochem Res 13:389–394.

Cohen J, Burne JF, Winter J, Bartlett P (1986). Retinal ganglion cells lose response to laminin with maturation. Nature 322:465–467.

Denis–Donini S, and M Estenoz (1988). Interneurons versus efferent neurons: Heterogeneity in their neurite outgrowth response to glia from several brain regions. Dev Biol 130:237–249.

Dinarello CA (1988). Biology of interleukin–1. FASEB J 2:108–115.

Fedoroff S, Doering LC (1987). Transplantation of mouse astrocyte precursor cells cultured in vitro into neonatal cerebellum. Ann NY Acad Sci 495:24–34.

Fontana A, Erb P, Pircher H, Zinkenagel R, Weber E, Fierz W (1986). Astrocytes as antigen–presenting cells. Part II: Unlike H–2K–dependent cytotoxic T cells, H–2Ia restricted T cells are only stimulated in the presence of interferon–γ. J Neuroimmunol 12:15–28.

Fontana A, Kristensen F, Dubs R, Gemsa D, Weber, E (1982). Production of prostaglandin E and an interleukin–1–like factor by cultured astrocytes and C6 glioma cells. J Immunol 129:2413–2419.

Fontana A, Weber E, Dayer JM (1984). Synthesis of interleukin 1/endogenous pyrogen in the brain of endotoxin–teated mice: step in fever induction. J Immunol 133:1696–1698.

Frei K, Malipiero UV, Leist PT, Zinkernagel, RM, Schwab ME, Fontana A (1989). On the cellular source and function of interleukin–6 produced in the central nervous system in viral diseases. Euro J Immunol 19:689–694.

Frohman EM, van den Noort S, Gupta S (1989). Astrocytes and intercerebral immune responses. Clin Immunol 9:1–9.

Furukawa Y, Tomioka N, Sato W, Satayoshi E, Hayashi K, Furukawa S (1989) Catecholamines increase nerve growth factor mRNA content in both mouse astroglial cells and fibroblast cells. FEBS Lett 247:463–467.

Goodwin JS, Webb DR (1980). Regulation of the immune response by prostaglandins. Clin Immunol Immunopthol 15:106–122.

Grafe MR (1983). Developmental factors affecting regeneration in the central nervous system: early but not late formed mitral cells reinnervate olfactory cortex after neonatal tract section. J Neurosci 3:617–630.

Hamprecht B (1986). Astroglia cells in culture: Receptors and cyclic nucleotides. S Fedoroff, A Vernadakis, (eds) "Astrocytes". New York, Academic Press, pp 77–106.

Hansson E, (1988). Astroglia from defined brain regions as studied with primary cultures. Prog Neurobiol 30:369–397.

Hao C, Guilbert LJ, Fedoroff S (1990). Production of CSF–1 by mouse astrocytes in vitro. J Neurosci Res (in press).

Hatten ME, Mason CA (1986). Neuron–astroglia interactions in vitro and in vivo. TINS 9:168–174.

Hayashi M, Hayashi R, Tanii H, Hashimoto K, Patel AJ (1988). The influence of nerve cells on the development of astrocytes. Dev Brain Res 41:37–42.

Hirsch MR, Wietzerbin J, Pierres M, Goridis C (1983). Expression of Ia antigens by cultured astrocytes treated with gamma–interferon. Neurosci Lett 41:199–204.

Hunt A, Hayashi M, Seaton P, Patel AJ (1988). Influence of nerve cells on the development of astrocytes. Biochem Soc Trans 16:295–296.

Janzen RL, Raff MC (1987). Astrocytes induce blood–brain barrier properties in endothelial cells. Nature 325:253–257.

Jedeschi B, Barrett JN, Keane RW (1986). Astrocytes produce interferon that enhances the expression of H–2 antigens on a subpopulation of brain cells. J Cell Biol 102:2244–2253.

Kettenmann H, Schachner M (1985). Pharmacological properties of GABA glutamate and aspartate induced depolarizations in cultured astrocytes. J Neurosci 5:3295–3301.

Landis DMD (1986). Membrane structure in astrocytes. S Fedoroff, A Vernadakis, (eds) "Astrocytes". New York, Academic Press, pp 61–76.

Lieberman AP, Pitha PM, Shin HS, Shin ML (1989). Production of tumor necrosis factor and other cytokines by astrocytes stimulated with lipopolysaccharide or a neurotropic virus. Proc Natl Acad Sci 86:6348–6352.

Lindsay RM (1979). Adult rat brain astrocytes support survival of both NGF–dependent and NGF–insensitive neurons. Nature 282:80–82.

Loughlin SE, Noriega JA, Lee G, Leslie FM, Annis CM, Fallon JH (1989). Development of transforming growth factor alpha immunoreactivity in cat brain. Soc Neurosci Abstr 15:710.

Mattheissen HP, Schmalenbach C, Müller HW (1989). Astroglia–released neurite growth–inducing activity for embryonic hippocampal neurons is associated with laminin bound in a sulfated complex and free fibronectin. Glia 2:177–188.

Merrill JE, (1989). Effect of lymphokines and monokines on glial cells in vitro and in vivo. Edward J Goetzel and Novera H Spector (eds). "Neuroimmune Networks: Physiology and Diseases". New York, Alan R Liss, pp 89–97.

Mugnaini E (1986). Cell junctions of astrocyte, ependyma, and related cells in the mammalian cerebral nervous system, with emphasis on the hypothesis of a generalized functional syncytium of supporting cells. Fedoroff S, Vernadakis A (eds): "Astrocytes", Vol 1. New York, Academic Press, pp 329–371.

Müller HW, Seifert W (1982). A neurotrophic factor (NTF) released from primary glial cultures supports survival and fiber outgrowth of cultured hippocampal neurons. J Neurosci Res 8:195–204.

Nance DM, Burns J (1989). Innervation of the spleen in the rat: absence of afferent innervation Soc Neurosci Abstr 15:713.

Nieto–Sampedro M, Berman MA (1987). Interleukin–1–like activity in rat brain: sources, targets and effects of injury. J Neurosci Res 17:14–219.

Noble M, Fok–Seang J, Cohen J (1984). Glia are a unique substrate for the in vitro growth of central nervous system neurons. J Neurosci 4:1892–1903.

Old LJ (1989). Tumor necrosis factor. Sci American 258:59–75.

Othen U, Lorez HP, Gadient R, Boeckh C (1989). Interleukin–1 injected into neostriatum of adult rat brain stimulates synthesis of nerve growth factor. Soc Neurosci Abstr 15:18.

Papasozomenos, S Ch (1986). Pineal astrocytes. S Fedoroff, A Vernadakis (eds). "Astrocytes", Vol 1, Orlando,, Academic Press. pp 209–223.

Patel AJ, Hunt A (1989). Regulation of production by primary cultures of rat forebrain astrocytes of a trophic factor important for the development of cholinergic neurons. Neurosci Lett 99:223–228.

Patel AJ, Hunt A, Seaton P (1988). The mechanism of cytosine arabinoside toxicity on quiescent astrocytes in vitro appears to be analogous to in vivo brain injury. Brain Research 450:378–381.

Peters A, Palay SL, deF Webster H (1976). The Fine Structure of the Nervous System: The Neurons and Supporting Cells. Philadelphia, WB Saunders Co pp 231–254.

Pope A (1978). Neuroglia: Quantitative aspects. Schoffeniels E, Franck G, Towers DB, Hertz L (eds): "Dynamic Properties of Glial Cells", Oxford, Pergamon Press, pp 13–20.

Privat A, Rataboul P (1986). Fibrous and protoplasmic astrocytes. S Fedoroff, A Vernadakis (eds), "Astrocytes" Vol 1, Orlando, Academic Press, pp 105–129.

Prochiantz A, Mallat M (1988). Astrocyte diversity. Ann NY Acad Sci 540:52–63.

Rakic P (1984). Emergence of neuronal and glial cell lineages in primate brain. IB Black, (ed) "Cellular and Molecular Biology of Neuronal Development." New York, Plenum Press, pp 29–50.

Ransom BR, Carlini WG (1986). Electrophysiological properties of astrocytes, Fedoroff S, Vernadakis A, (eds) "Astrocytes" Vol 2 Orlando, Academic Press, pp 1–49.

Redar AT, Karaszewski JW, Arnason GW (1989). Sympathetic nervous system involvement in immune responses of mice and in patients with multiple sclerosis. Goetzl EJ, Spector NH (eds) "Neuroimmune Networks: Physiology and Diseases". New York, Alan R. Liss, p 137–147.

Reier PJ, Houle JD (1988). The glial scar: Its bearing on axonal elongation and transplantation approaches to CNS repair. Waxman SG (ed) "Functional Recovery in Neurological Diseases", New York: Raven Press, pp 87–138.

Robbins DS, Shirazi Y, Drysdale B–E, Lieberman A, Shin HS, Shin, ML (1987). Production of cytotoxic factor for oligodendrocytes for stimulated astrocytes. J Immunol 139:2593–2597.

Rudge JS, Manthorpe M, Varon S (1985). The output of neurotrophic and neurite–promoting agents from rat brain astroglial cells: A microculture method of screening potential regulatory molecules. Dev Brain Res 19:161–172.

Salamat, SM, Tallent MW and Keane RW (1988). The role of astrocytes in immune responses within the central nervous system. Norenberg MD, Hertz L, Schousboe A (eds). "The Biochemical Pathlogy of Astrocytes" New York, Alan R. Liss, p 247–259.

Sawada M, Kondo N, Suzumura A, Marunouchi T (1989). Production of tumor necrosis factor–alpha by microglia and astrocytes in culture. Brain Research 491:394–397.

Seaton P, Hunt A, Patel AJ (1988). Production by astrocytes of a trophic factor for cholinergic neurons. Biochem Soc Trans 16:296–297.

Simmons D, Makgoba WM, Seed B (1988). ICAM, an adhesion ligand of LFA–1, is homologous to the neural cell adhesion molecule NCAM. Nature 331: 624–627.

Smith GM, Silver J (1988). Transplantation of immature and mature astrocytes and their effect on scar formation in the lesioned central nervous system. Prog Brain Research 78:353–361.

Srebro Z, Cichocki T (1971). A system of periventricular glia in brain characterized by large peroxisome-like organelles. Acta Histochem Bd 41:108–114.

Stewart PA, Wiley MJ (1981). Developing nervous tissue induces formation of blood-brain barrier characteristics in invading endothelial cells: A study using quail-chick transplantation chimeras. Dev Biol 84:184–192.

Sundar SK, Cierpial MA, Kilts CD, Weiss JM (1989). Brain interleukin-1 (IL-1) induced immune-suppression: mediation by CRF and sympathetic activation. Soc Neurosci Abstr 15:7.

Suzumura A, Lan E, Weiss SR, Silberberg DH (1986). Coronavirus infection induces H-2 antigen expression on oligodendrocytes and astrocytes. Science 232:991–993.

Tedeschi B, Barrett JN, Keane RW (1986). Astrocytes produce interferon that enhances the expression of H-2 antigens on a subpopulation of brain cells. J Cell Biol 102:2244–2253.

Tomaselli KJ, Neugebauer KM, Bixby JL, Lillien J, Reichardt LF (1988). N-Cadherin and integrins: two receptor systems that mediate neuronal process outgrowth on astrocytes. Neuron 1:33–43.

Varon SS, Somjen GG (1979). Neuron-glia interactions. Neurosci Res Program Bull 17:1–239.

Walz W (1989). Role of glial cells in the regulation of the brain ion neuroenvironment. Prog Neurobiol 33:309–333.

Weiss JM, Sundar SK, Cierpial MA, Ritchie J (1989). Brain interleukin-1 induced immunosuppression: dose response inhibition by alpha-MSH. Soc Neurosci Abstr 15:7.

Wilkin GP, Marriott DR, Cholewiuski AJ (1990). Astrocyte heterogeneity. TINS 13:43–46.

Wilkin GP, Levi G (1986). Cerebellar astrocytes. S Fedoroff, A Vernadakis (eds): "Astrocytes" Vol 1, Orlando, Academic Press, pp 245–268.

Wittkowski W (1986). S Fedoroff, A Vernadakis (eds): Pituicytes. "Astrocytes" Vol 1. Orlando, Academic Press pp 173–208.

Wong GHW, Bartlett PF, Clark-Levis I, Battye F, Schrader JW (1984). Inducible expression of H-2 and Ia antigens on brain cells. Nature 310:688–691.

**Advances in Neural Regeneration
Research, pages 171–183
© 1990 Wiley-Liss, Inc.**

CELL AND MOLECULAR INTERACTIONS THAT INFLUENCE
ASTROCYTE MEDIATED AXON OUTGROWTH

Robert H. Miller and George M. Smith

Center For Neuroscience
Case Western Reserve University
School of Medicine
Cleveland, Ohio 44106

The functional properties of astrocytes change during
maturation of the vertebrate central nervous system.
During development, immature astrocytes constitute a
major component of specific pathways that guide growing
axons toward their targets. Although the nature of these
pathways is unclear, they may provide mechanical guidance
by preformed channels in extracellular space between
adjacent cells (Singer et al., 1979) or chemical guidance
along diffusable (Cajal, 1927) or membrane-bound
gradients (Sperry, 1963). In the mature mammalian CNS,
extensive axonal outgrowth does not generally occur even
after lesions. Instead, the functions of mature
astrocytes have been proposed to provide structural
support, trophic factors and to regulate the ionic
environment (see Fedoroff and Vernadakis, 1986 for
review).

One dramatic demonstration of the different functional
properties of immature and mature astrocytes is in their
response to a lesion. Most injuries to the embryonic or
early neonatal mammalian CNS result in only limited
reactive gliosis, and rarely produce gliotic scarring or
extensive functional loss (Barrett et al., 1984; Grafe,
1983). However, in the mature CNS similar lesions
generally result in a severe functional deficit
characterized by axon loss or lack of growth, as well as
the formation of a pronounced glial scar. Glial scars
are comprised mostly of mature reactive astrocytes
(Barrett et al., 1984; Reier et al., 1983) and differ
from scars formed in non-neural tissue. In non-neural

tissue, fibroblasts secrete large amounts of
extracellular matrix material during scar formation. By
contrast, astrocytes, while they can participate in
intraparenchymal matrix formation, generally form scars
in the adult CNS through proliferation and the
combination of extension and hypertrophy of their
processes (Maxwell and Kruger, 1965; Miller et al.,
1986).

The limited axon growth seen following lesions to the
mature CNS is not an intrinsic property of mature CNS
axons but instead reflects the mature glial scar
environment which fails to support axonal growth
(Clemente and Windle, 1954; Reier et al., 1983). The
extent of scar formation in response to a specific lesion
can be reduced by transplanting pieces of fetal tissue
into the lesion cavity of mature animals, and this
reduction is generally accompained by an increase in
axonal growth (Kruger et al., 1986; Reier et al., 1986).
The reduction in scar formation and concomitant
enhancement of axon growth reflects a property of
immature astrocytes, since the transplantation of
immature astrocytes into the lesioned adult rat forebrain
also reduced scar formation (Smith et al., 1986) and
enhanced behavorial recovery after frontal cortex
ablations in adult rats (Kesslak et al., 1986).

The relative age of transplanted astrocytes is
important to reduce scar formation and subsequently
increase axon growth. For example, newborn rat brain
astrocytes cultured for 3-4 days invariably suppress
glial scar formation when transplanted into the adult
CNS, while astrocytes from P14 or older animals, or from
newborn rat brains which had been cultured for extended
periods, fail to repress scar formation when transplanted
into the adult CNS (Smith and Silver, 1988).
Furthermore, during regeneration of peripheral nerve
through implanted silicon chambers (Kalderon, 1988) or
after lesions of the corticospinal tract of neonatal rat
spinal cord (Schreyer and Jones, 1987) the introduction
of immature but not mature astrocytes supports axon
growth.

These observations suggest that changes in mammalian
astrocytes during maturation have a direct influence on
the cells' capacity to suppress glial scar formation and

promote axon growth. A number of factors may contribute
to the reduced capacity of mature astrocytes to support
axon growth. Molecules on the cell surface may change
during maturation such that mature astrocytes have
reduced expression of axon promoting molecules, or mature
astrocytes may express an axon outgrowth inhibiting
molecule such as those found on oligodendrocytes (Schwab
and Caroni, 1988). In addition, mature astrocytes may
structurally alter the neural environment by interacting
with other cell types to form a basal lamina that
inhibits axon growth (Kao et al., 1977) or by interacting
strongly with adjacent astrocytes to produce a physical
barrier to axon growth.

COMPARISON OF NEURITE OUTGROWTH OVER IMMATURE AND MATURE ASTROCYTES IN VITRO

The cellular complexity of mature glial scars and their
interaction with growing axons in vivo makes the analysis
of specific cellular function difficult. To examine the
capacity of a cell population to support axon outgrowth,
in vitro assay systems have been developed that simplify
this analysis. Neurite outgrowth in vitro is influenced
by a variety of different cellular and non-cellular
substrates (Letourneau, 1975; Noble, et al., 1984). In
addition, neurite outgrowth on cultured astrocytes is
mediated by neural cell surface molecules including N-
cadherin, laminin (Tomaselli et al., 1988), NCAM and L1
(Smith et al., 1989). The relative importance of these
molecules in mediating neurite outgrowth appears to
change with neuronal age (Cohen et al., 1986; Tomaselli
et al., 1988), but in general they appear to act in
combination such that antibody pertubation of a single
molecule only partially reduces neurite outgrowth
(Tomaselli et al., 1988; Smith et al., 1989).

Recently, the extent and molecular basis of neurite
outgrowth on immature and mature cultured astrocytes has
been compared (Smith et al., 1989). Neurite outgrowth
from embryonic rat cortical neurons on a confluent
monolayer of immature rat astrocytes was significantly
greater than the neurite outgrowth from a matched
population of neurons on a confluent monolayer of mature
astrocytes (Smith et al., 1989).

Differences in the capacity of immature and mature

astrocytes to promote neurite outgrowth are likely to be general phenomena. The relative difference in neurite outgrowth over immature and mature rat cortical astrocytes was not restricted to rat cortical neurons, but was also seen with neurons both from different CNS regions and from different species. For example, the relative extent of neurite outgrowth from E7 chick retinal neurons on immature and mature rat cortical astrocytes was similar to that seen with cortical rat neurons, even though total neurite outgrowth was more extensive. While NCAM appeared to be a major component mediating neurite outgrowth on immature astrocytes, its contribution on mature astrocytes was greatly reduced (Smith et al., 1989).

Although neurite outgrowth on cultures of immature astrocytes was significantly greater than that on mature astrocytes, the extent of neurite outgrowth on mature astrocytes in vitro was considerable. Extensive neurite outgrowth on mature astrocytes suggests that these cells retain some capacity to support axon outgrowth in vitro, and is in marked contrast to the lack of outgrowth seen through glial scars following most lesions to the mature CNS (Reier et al., 1983). One explanation for the differences in outgrowth in vivo and in vitro is that glial scars contain additional factors, absent from the cultures, which further contribute to inhibit axon growth.

INHIBITION OF AXON GROWTH IN THE LESIONED CNS

Cell types other than mature astrocytes are present in glial scars and may have the capacity to specifically inhibit axon growth. For example, oligodendrocytes and myelin from the mammalian CNS express specific proteins which under certain conditions strongly inhibit axon growth (Schwab and Caroni, 1988,). Most lesions to the mature CNS are likely to produce some myelin debris and this may contribute to the inhibition of axon growth. However, when grown in combination with astrocytes in vitro, oligodendrocytes appeared not to inhibit axon growth (Fawcett et al., 1987; Smith and Miller unpublished). In addition, many penetrating lesions produce not only gliosis but also a dense connective tissue scar and the formation of a basal lamina. This basal lamina has also been suggested to inhibit axon growth (Kao et al., 1977)

Not all gliotic responses in the mature CNS contain
significant amounts of myelin debris or connective tissue
scar, however, and considerable evidence suggests that
adult but not neonatal astrocytes inhibit axon growth in
the absence of other cell types. For example, following a
crush lesion to the dorsal root, neonatal rat axons
regenerate through the astrocyte-rich dorsal root
transitional zone and enter the spinal cord (Carlstedt et
al., 1987). However, following similar lesions in the
adult rat, regenerating axons are inhibited from entering
the adult spinal cord by astrocytes at the dorsal root
transitional zone (Liuzzi and Lasek, 1987). The
mechanism by which mature astrocytes effect this blockade
of axon growth is unknown, but has been proposed to
result from activation of physiological mechanisms within
the axon (Liuzzi and Lasek 1987). Furthermore, purified
mature but not immature astrocytes inhibit peripheral
axon growth when transplanted into peripheral nerves
using silicon chambers (Kalderon, 1988), suggesting that
the mature astrocytes have the capacity to inhibit axon
growth from a variety of neuronal cell types in the
absence of other cells.

CELL-CELL INTERACTIONS MAY REGULATE AXON GROWTH

One of the differences between neurite outgrowth in
culture and axonal regeneration in the mature CNS is the
architecture of the astrocyte environment. In vitro
neurites grow over the surface of a monolayer of glial
cells, and the rate of neurite outgrowth is influenced by
intrinsic neuronal properties (Lasek, 1988) as well as
the interaction of the growing axon directly with the
astrocyte substrate. Any interactions which occur
between adjacent astrocytes in the monolayer would be
unlikely to play a major part in influencing such axon
outgrowth.

By contrast, astrocytes in vivo form a three
dimensional environment through which axons grow. In
such an environment, the extent of axon growth will
depend not only on axon interactions with the astrocyte
substrate, but also indirectly on the interactions
between the surrounding astrocytes. In this case,
although mature astrocytes retain some capacity to

support axonal growth, if interactions between adjacent
mature astrocytes are significantly greater than between
adjacent immature astrocytes, axon growth may be further
inhibited. These conditions are described in Figure 1.

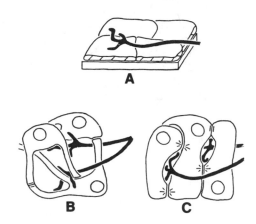

Figure 1. (A) Neurite outgrowth over cultured
astrocytes. Astrocyte/neuron interactions directly
influence axon growth. (B) Axon growth through an
immature astrocyte environment. Weak astrocytic
interactions produce a loosely packed astrocyte
environment through which axons can grow. (C) Axon
growth through a mature astrocyte environment. Strong
astrocytic interactions produce a tightly packed
astrocyte environment which may inhibit axon growth.

Changes in astrocyte/neuron and astrocyte/astrocyte
interactions occur during vertebrate CNS maturation.
During development, axons grow through extracellular
spaces between the processes of presumptive astrocytes in
a variety of locations including the developing optic
tract (Silver and Sidman, 1980), and spinal cord (Singer
et al., 1979). These extracellular spaces have been
suggested to provide specific "channels" in which growth
cones contact astrocyte cell surfaces and are directed
towards their targets. Similar channels have been
described in lesioned immature mammalian CNS (Dyson et
al., 1988) and regenerating newt spinal cord (Singer et
al., 1979). The presence of channels containing growth

cones in these specific locations may reflect relatively
weak astrocyte/astrocyte interactions while
astrocyte/neuron interactions are relatively strong at
this stage of development. Further, in regions where two
distinct axon tracts could potentially intermingle during
development, a compact arrangement of glia separates
them. In these regions extracellular spaces are small,
and the astrocyte plasma membranes are closely apposed to
each other, prehaps acting as a barrier to axon growth
between the two tracts (Silver et al., 1987).

The glial scar which forms following lesions to the
mature mammalian CNS has been proposed to form an
impenetrable barrier to axon growth (Clemente and Windle,
1954; Reier et al., 1983). In such regions of gliosis,
the plasma membranes of reactive astrocytes are closely
apposed to each other (Miller et al., 1986; Liuzzi and
Lasek, 1987), have an increased number of junctional
specializations (Nathaniel and Nathaniel, 1981) and there
are no large extracellular spaces. Growth cones fail to
grow through such a terrain; they either turn back or end
in synaptic-like terminals (Liuzzi and Lasek, 1987). The
inhibition of axon growth through a mature astrocyte
environment is consistent with an increase in astrocytic
interactions so that closely apposed astrocytes in the
mature glial scar form a barrier to further axon growth.

EXPERIMENTAL EVIDENCE OF CHANGES IN CELL-CELL
INTERACTIONS DURING CNS MATURATION

To compare interactions between neurons and astrocytes,
as well as between immature or mature astrocytes
themselves, short term adhesion and aggregation assays
were employed.

Cultures of immature and mature astrocytes were tested
for their capacity to bind probe cell populations
comprised of highly enriched embryonic rat cortical
neurons as well as immature or mature astrocytes. The
results are shown in Figure 2.

It is clear from these data that neurons ahere better
to immature than mature astrocytes, while
astrocyte/astrocyte adhesions increase with maturation.
To examine whether increased astrocyte adhesion during
maturation is accompanied by a morphological increase in

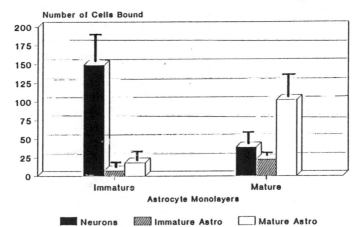

Figure 2. Comparision of cell adhesion to immature and
mature astrocyte monolayers. Immature astrocytes are more
adherent for neurons (solid bars) than mature astrocytes.
By contrast, mature astrocytes are more adherent for
mature astrocytes (open bars) than immature astrocytes are
for immature astrocytes (hatched bars)

cell/cell interactions, astrocyte aggregates were examined
by electron microscopy revealing a number of striking
differences. The cells in immature astrocyte aggregates
were loosely packed with large extracellular spaces
between them containing numerous processes from adjacent
astrocytes (Fig.3A). Most astrocytes were connected by
one or two gap junctions which frequently formed between
adjacent processes. By contrast, the cells in mature
astrocyte aggregates were comparatively closely packed,
with small extracellular spaces between them containing
few processes from adjacent cells (Fig.3B). Most adjacent
astrocytes were connected by numerous desmosomes (Fig.3B
and C) and well formed gap junctions (Fig.3D). These
observations suggest that the increased adhesion between
mature astrocytes seen in short term adhesion assays leads
to an increase in the extent of cell/cell apposition and
junction formation between adjacent mature astrocytes.
The increased cell-cell interaction and junction formation
between mature astrocyte may be an additional component

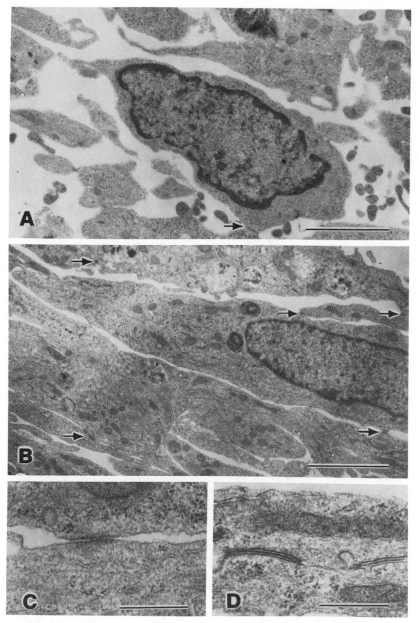

Figure 3. legend appears on page 180.

critical in the inhibition of axon growth through a three dimensional mature astrocyte environment such as that seen in regions of gliosis.

CONCLUSIONS

The extent of axon growth through a specific glial environment may be influenced directly through intrinsic neuronal properties and through interactions of the growing axon with its cellular substrate. In addition, growth may also be influenced indirectly through interactions between adjacent cells within the three dimensional milieu. During astrocyte maturation neurite outgrowth and astrocyte/neuron interactions are reduced while astrocyte/astrocyte interactions are increased. These findings raise the possibility that a critical component in inhibition of axon growth through the adult CNS is the extensive interaction between adjacent mature astrocytes.

It now becomes important to define the molecular basis of these different cell interactions. Because astrocyte/ neuron interactions decrease while astrocyte/astrocyte interactions increase during maturation, it seems likely that these cell-cell interactions are mediated through different cell surface components. Some major changes in the molecules mediating neurite outgrowth over immature and mature astrocytes have been defined (Smith et al., 1989). The identification of the molecular moieties involved in the increased astrocyte-astrocyte interaction seen in mature astrocytes and the generation of specific blocking antibodies should allow for a test of the hypothesis that increased astrocytic interactions contribute to the inhibition of axon growth through a

---

Figure 3. Electron micrographs from astrocyte aggregates. (A) Immature astrocytes have large extracellular spaces containing astrocyte processes and occasional gap junctions (arrow). (B) Mature astrocytes lack large extracellular spaces and have increased number of junctional specializations. (C) Desmosome-like junction in mature astrocyte aggregates. (D) Gap junction in mature astrocyte aggregates. Bar = 2.5um in A and B and 0.5um in C and D.

three dimensional astrocyte environment.

REFERENCES

Barrett CP, Donati EJ, Guth L (1984). Differences
  between adult and neonatal rats in their astroglial
  response to spinal injury. Exp Neurol 84:374-385.
Carlstedt T, Dalsgaard CJ, Molander C (1987). Regrowth
  of lesioned dorsal root fibers into the spinal cord of
  neonatal rats. Neurosci Lett 74: 14-18.
Cajal S Ramon y (1927). Studies in vertebrate
  neurogensis. Reprinted Springfield Il: Charles Thomas.
Clemente CD, Windle WF (1954). Regeneration of the
  severed nerves in the spinal cord of the adult cat.
  J Comp Neurol 101: 691- 731.
Cohen J, Burne JF, Winter J, Bartlett P (1986). Retinal
  ganglion cells lose response to laminin with maturation
  Nature 322: 465-467.
Dyson SE, Harvey AR, Trapp BD, Heath JW (1988).
  Ultrastructural and immunohistochemical analysis of
  axonal regrowth and myelination in membranes which form
  over lesion sites in the rat visual system. J
  Neurocytol 17:797-808.
Fawcett JW, Bakst I, Rokos J (1987). Interactions
  between glial cells and axons in vitro. Soc Neurosci
  Abs 13:1483.
Federoff S, Vernadakis A (1986). "Astrocytes" Vol.2.
  Cellular Neurobiology. Orlando: Academic Press.
Grafe MR (1983). Devlopmental factors affecting
  regeneration in the central nervous system: early but
  not late formed mitral cells reinnervate olfactory
  cortex after neonatal tract section. J Neurosci 3:617-
  630.
Kalderon N (1988). Differentiating astroglia in nervous
  tissue histogensis/regeneration: Studies in a model
  system of regenerating peripheral nerve. J Neurosci Res
  21:501-512.
Kao CC, Chang LW, Bloodworth JMB (1977). Axonal
  regeneration across transected mammalian spinal cords:
  An electron microscopic study of delayed microsurgical
  nerve grafting. Exp Neurol 54:591-615.
Kesslack JP, Nieto-Sampedro M, Globus J, Cotman CW
  (1986). Transplants of purified astrocytes promote
  behavioral recovery after frontal cortex ablation.
  Exp Neurol 92:377-390.
Kruger S, Sievers J, Hansen C, Sadler M, Berry M (1986).

Three morphologically distinct types of interface develop between adult host and fetal brain transplants: implications for scar formation in the adult central nervous system. J Comp Neurol 246:103-116.

Lasek RJ (1988). Studying the intrinsic determinants of neuronal form and function. Neurology and Neurobiology 37: 3-58.

Letourneau PC (1975). Possible role for cell-to-substrate adhesion in neuronal morphogensis. Dev Biol 44:77-91.

Liuzzi FJ, Lasek RJ (1987). Astrocytes block regeneration in mammals by activating the physiological stop pathway. Science 237: 642-645.

Maxwell DS, Kruger L (1965). The fine structure of astrocytes in the cerebral cortex and their response to focal injury produced by heavy ionizing particles. J Cell Biol 25:141-157.

Miller RH, David S, Patel R, Abney ER, Raff MC (1986). Is reactive gliosis a property of a distinct subpopulation of astrocytes? J Neurosci 6:22-29.

Natheniel EJH, Natheniel DR (1981). The reactive astrocyte. In Advances in Cellular Neurobiology. Academic Press Vol 2 pp.246-301.

Noble M, Fok-Seang J, Cohen J (1984). Glia are a unique substrate for the in vitro growth of central nervous system neurons. J Neurosci 4: 1892-1903.

Reier PJ, Bregman BS, Wujek JR (1986). Intraspinal transplantation of embryonic spinal cord tissue in neonatal and adult rats. J Comp Neurol 247: 275-296.

Reier PJ, Stensaas LJ, Guth L (1983). The astrocytic scar as an impediment to regeneration in the central nervous system. In Kao CC, Bunge RP and Reier PJ (eds): "Spinal cord reconstruction." New York: Raven Press, pp163-195.

Schreyer DJ, Jones EG (1987). Growth of corticospinal axons on prosthetic substrates introduced into the spinal cord of neonatal rats. Dev Brain Res 35:291-299.

Schwab ME, Caroni P (1988). Rat CNS myelin and a subtype of oligodendrocytes in culture represent a non-permisive substrate for neurite growth and fibroblast spreading. J Neurosci 8: 2381-2393.

Sperry RW, (1963). Chemoaffinity in the orderly growth of nerve fiber patterns and connections. Proc Nat Acad Sci USA 50: 703-710.

Silver J, Sidman RL (1980). A mechanism for the guidance and topographic patterning of retinal ganglion cell axons. J Comp Neurol 189:101-111.

Silver J, Poston M, Rutishauser U (1987). Axon pathway
boundaries in the developing brain. 1.Cellular and
molecular determinants that separate the optic and
olfactory projections. J Neurosci 7: 2264-2272.

Singer M, Nordlander RH, Egar P (1979). Axonal guidance
during embryogensis and regeneration in the spinal cord
of the newt: The blueprint hypothesis of neuronal
patterning. J Comp Neurol 185:1-22.

Smith GM, Miller RH, Silver J (1986). Changing role of
forebrain astrocytes during development, regenerative
failure and induced regeneration upon transplantation.
J Comp Neurol 251: 23-43.

Smith GM, Rutishauser U, Silver J, Miller RH (1989).
Astrocyte maturation in vitro alters the extent and
molecular basis of neurite outgrowth. Submitted Dev
Bio.

Smith GM, Silver J (1988). Transplantation of immature
and mature astrocytes and their effect on scar
formation in the lesioned central nervous system.
In Gash DM, Sladek JR (eds):"Progress in Brain
Research"v78, Elsevier, pp 353-361.

Tomaselli KJ, Neugebauer KM, Bixby JL, Lillien J,
Reichardt LF (1988). N- cadherin and integrins: two
receptor systems that mediate neuronal process
outgrowth on astrocytes. Neuron 1: 33-43.

Advances in Neural Regeneration
Research, pages 185–197
© 1990 Wiley-Liss, Inc.

DO REACTIVE ASTROCYTES INHIBIT REGENERATION ?

Samuel David

Centre for Research in Neuroscience,
McGill University and The Montreal
General Hospital Research Institute,
1650 Cedar Ave., Montreal, Quebec,
Canada, H3G 1A4

INTRODUCTION

Although injured neurons in the adult
mammalian central nervous system (CNS) fail to
regenerate though CNS tissue, peripheral nerve
grafting experiments have clearly demonstrated
that neurons in most regions of the adult
mammalian CNS can regenerate for long distances
under appropriate conditions (Ramon y Cajal, 1928;
Richardson et al., 1980; David and Aguayo, 1981;
Friedman and Aguayo, 1985; So and Aguayo, 1985;
Vidal-Sanz et al., 1988). These and other
transplantation studies such as embryonic CNS
tissue transplantation (Kromer et al., 1981;
Nornes et al., 1983; Bjorklund and Stenevi, 1984;
Bregman, 1988) and work on acallosal mice (Silver
and Ogawa, 1983; Smith et al., 1986) have helped
to emphasize the important role of CNS glia in
regulating axonal growth during development and
regeneration. The nature of these glial derived
influences are beginning to be understood.

In vitro studies suggest that at least three
types of extrinsic influences may contribute to
the success or failure of axon growth: (i) the
availability of appropriate growth factors
necessary for the survival of injured neurons

(Thoenin and Edgar, 1985; Barde, 1989); (ii) the presence of appropriate adhesion molecules on the cell surface or extracellular matrix, and functional receptors for these molecules (Carbonetto, 1984; Reichardt et al., 1989); and (iii) the presence or absence of inhibitory molecules that prevent neurite growth (Caroni and Schwab, 1988a, 1988b; Schwab and Caroni, 1988). Astrocytes and oligodendrocytes have both been cited as being responsible for inhibiting axonal regeneration.

In this review I will examine some of the evidence for the role of these two macroglial cell types in inhibiting axonal regeneration. The main focus however, will be to re-evaluate the role of reactive astrogliosis in the failure of axonal regeneration in the mammalian CNS.

INHIBITION BY OLIGODENDROCYTES AND CNS MYELIN

The long period of time required for the removal of myelin from the lesioned CNS, as well as the apparent regeneration of unmyelinated (monoaminergic) axons in the spinal cord (Bjorklund and Stenevi, 1979) and the hypothalamo-hypophyseal tract (Berry, 1979; Kiernan, 1979), led some investigators to suggest that the presence of myelin or myelin debris might play a role in the failure of CNS regeneration (Berry, 1979; Kiernan, 1979; Reier et al., 1983). However, the results of these morphological studies were open to other interpretations (see review by Reier et al., 1989) and they also did not provide direct evidence that CNS myelin inhibits regeneration. For these reasons, as well as the widely held view that astrocytes inhibit regeneration, this area of research remained dormant until recently.

Schwab and his colleagues have recently

shown that: (i) CNS myelin, unlike PNS myelin, is a very poor substrate for neurite growth and fibroblast spreading in vitro (Caroni and Schwab, 1988a); (ii) mature oligodendrocytes in cultures of rat optic nerve are a very poor substrate for neurite growth and fibroblast spreading (Schwab and Caroni, 1988); (iii) CNS white matter, but not grey matter is a non-permissive substrate for neurite growth in vitro (Savio and Schwab, 1989); (iv) the inhibitory effects are due to two minor proteins of 35 and 250 kDa, that are associated with CNS myelin (Caroni and Schwab, 1988a); and (v) monoclonal antibodies against these proteins can neutralize this inhibitory effect in vitro (Caroni and Schwab, 1988b) and also possibly in vivo (Savio et al., 1989). These studies provide good evidence that certain proteins associated with CNS myelin may have a marked inhibitory effect on neurite growth and axon regeneration.

INHIBITION BY ASTROCYTES

Despite the work that has been done on astrocytes, the role of reactive astrogliosis in inhibiting axonal regeneration still remains uncertain. There is evidence that astrocytes from the developing CNS provide a very good substrate for neurite growth in vitro (Noble et al., 1984; Fallon, 1985; Cohen et al., 1986; Reichardt et al., 1989). In contrast to this mature or reactive astrocytes in the mature mammalian CNS have long been suggested as having a negative influence on axonal regeneration. This conclusion has been based on a large number of studies, predominantly morphological (reviewed extensively by Reier et al., 1989; also see Liuzzi, in this volume).

Some of the studies using two experimental approaches will be reviewed here, because they provide some of the best evidence so far that astrocytes might inhibit regeneration. These two experimental approaches are: i) regeneration through the dorsal roots, either after crush injury or following anastomosis with other nerves (Carlstedt, 1983, 1985a, 1985b, 1988; Stensaas et al., 1987; Liuzzi and Lasek, 1987); ii) regeneration through adult and degenerated rat optic nerve segments grafted into the sciatic nerve of adult rats (Aguayo et al., 1978; Weinberg and Spencer, 1979; Reier et al., 1983; Anderson and Turmaine, 1986; Hall and Kent, 1987). In both types of experiments, when regenerating axons were examined several weeks after lesioning or grafting, the majority of the regenerating axons appeared to stop growing at the interface between the PNS and CNS, which was composed of reactive astrocytes and their processes.

Regeneration Through Dorsal Roots.

In these studies the majority of the dorsal root axons fail to regenerate into the CNS portion of the root and spinal cord after crush injury or anastomosis with autonomic nerves or ventral roots (see above for references). The majority of the axons that fail to regenerate appear to be confronted by the processes of reactive astrocytes at the interface between the PNS and CNS. However, these axons would be expected to encounter CNS myelin immediately after crossing into the CNS portion of the root, since in the uninjured animal they are myelinated by oligodendrocytes as soon as they traverse the PNS-CNS border (Berthold and Carlstedt, 1977). Also, Carlstedt (1988) has recently shown that dorsal root axons regenerate into the spinal cord in 2 day old post-natal rats, but not in 5 day old rats. At day 5 the dorsal root axons are myelinated, both in the PNS as well as in the CNS portion of the root (see figure 1 in Carlstedt, 1988). Therefore even though several weeks after crush lesion, the dorsal root axons in adult rats appear to abut astrocytes, and thus give the impression that they are being stopped by astrocytes, the failure of these axons to regenerate in this model could well be because the axons encounter CNS myelin with their associated inhibitory proteins (Caroni and Schwab, 1988a, 1988b) as soon as they cross the PNS-CNS interface. That reactive astrocytes may not be crucial in inhibiting regeneration is also supported by the finding that regeneration in the spinal cord is not enhanced in the absence of reactive gliosis (Guth et al., 1981).

Regeneration Through Segments of Optic Nerve.

When segments of normal adult rat optic nerve are grafted into the sciatic nerve of adult rats, the majority of the regenerating sciatic nerve axons fail to grow through the optic nerves (Aguayo, et al., 1978; Weinberg and Spencer, 1979; Reier et al., 1983; Anderson and Turmaine, 1986; Hall and Kent, 1987). When the grafts were examined several weeks after surgery, they consisted mainly of reactive astrocytes. However, in these experiments it is not possible to know whether regeneration was inhibited by astrocytes, oligodendrocytes or CNS myelin. This difficulty was obviated by the use of pre-degenerated optic nerve grafts which lacked myelin and consisted of an astrocytic scar (Reier et al., 1983; Hall and Kent, 1987). The majority of the axons in these experiments also failed to regenerate through the pre-degenerated optic nerve grafts. These results were therefore interpreted as indicating that reactive astrocytes in the adult mammalian CNS may inhibit axonal regeneration. However, we have recently shown that in this grafting model even embryonic rat optic nerve segments devoid of myelin are bypassed by the regenerating sciatic nerve axons (Giftochristos and David, 1988). The

simplest explanation for our results is that in
the presence of Schwann cells which are inevitably
present in this model, the regenerating peripheral
nerve axons choose to grow along Schwann cells
rather than central glia. Thus even embryonic
central glia, which would be expected to support
axon growth, are bypassed by the regenerating
peripheral nerve axons in preference to Schwann
cells. This model therefore, appears to have
limitations for testing the ability of CNS glia to
permit axonal regeneration.

Neurite growth in vitro on tissue sections of lesioned optic nerve.

Because of the uncertainty about the role of
reactive astrogliosis in the failure of axonal
regeneration, we decided to re-examine this using
an in vitro approach (David and Giftochristos,
1988b; David, 1989). We found that five days
after transecting the optic nerve in adult rats,
unfixed cryostat sections of the optic nerve have
greater adhesive properties near the site of
lesion, in that they permit better attachment of
PC-12 cells, than regions of the nerve away from
the lesion. Furthermore, PC-12 cells appeared to
adhere preferentially to areas that contain
astrocytes (David and Giftochristos, 1988b).
These astrocytes near the site of lesion are
larger, have more processes and stain more
intensely with antibodies against glial fibrillary
acidic protein, than astrocytes in the normal CNS.
They therefore have the characteristics of
reactive astrocytes (David, 1988). We have also
found that explants of embryonic chick dorsal root
ganglia (DRG) grow neurites easily over these
optic nerve sections near the site of transection,
whereas regions of the nerve away from the site of
transection, like the normal optic nerve, are
avoided by neurites from such explants (David,
1989; David et al., 1989). Thus within 5 days

after the induction of a lesion, the non-permissive nature of the adult CNS tissue is altered to a permissive state, but only near the site of lesion. This localized change in the non-permissive nature of the adult CNS tissue following lesions may account for axonal sprouting (Ramon y Cajal, 1928; also reviewed by Giftochristos and David, 1987), but lack of long distance axonal growth in the injured adult mammalian CNS. This localized change in the functional properties of CNS tissue near the site of lesion may be brought about by removal or neutralization of inhibitory influences (Caroni and Schwab, 1988a, 1988b), and/or the expression of growth promoting molecules (Reichardt, 1989; Nieto-Sampedro et al., 1983) by cells near the site of lesion.

Astrocytic "scars" generated 4-6 months after optic nerve transection in adult rats were also a surprisingly good substrate for neurite growth in our in vitro assay using explants of chick DRG's (David,1989; David et al., 1989). These experiments provide evidence that degenerated adult CNS white matter, consisting mainly of reactive astrocytes and lacking myelin, is able to support neurite growth in vitro, suggesting that the inhibitory influences present in the normal CNS are lost along this degenerated CNS pathway several months after lesioning. However, the inhibitory properties of the astrocyte-leptomeningeal interface at the edge of the wound is not fully known. The reasons why spontaneous regeneration does not occur in vivo along these degenerated pathways may be that by the time these inhibitory influences are lost, which may be several months, many of the injured neurons have died because of lack of trophic support, or they may no longer be in a growth mode.

CONCLUSIONS

Our in vitro studies suggest that CNS
lesions induce an immediate, but localized change
in the non-permissive nature of CNS white matter
to a permissive state near the lesion site. This
change may account for injury-induced axonal
sprouting in vivo. Studies with optic nerves that
were allowed to degenerate for 4-6 months indicate
that reactive astrogliosis does not inhibit
neurite growth in vitro.

ACKNOWLEDGEMENTS

This work was supported by grants from the
Canadian MRC and the Spinal Cord Research
Foundation.

REFERENCES

Aguayo, A.J., R. Dickson, J. Trecarten,
    M.Attiwell, G.M.Bray, and Richardson, P.M.
    (1978) Ensheathment and myelination of
    regenerating PNS fibers by transplanted optic
    nerve glia. Neurosci. Lett. 9:97-104.
Anderson, P.N. and M. Turmaine (1986) Axonal
    regeneration through living and freeze-dried CNS
    tissue. Neuropathol. Appl. Neurobiol. 12:389-
    399.
Barde, Y.A. (1989) Trophic factors and neuronal
    survival. Neuron 2:1-5.
Berry, M. Regeneration in the central nervous
    system. In Smith, W.T. & Cavanagh, J.B. (eds)
    Recent Advances in Neuropathology, no 1
    Edinburgh, Churchill Livingston, pp 67-111.
Berthold, C.H. and T.Carlstedt (1977) Observations
    on the morphology at the transition between the
    peripheral and the central nervous system in the
    cat.III Myelinated fibers in the S_1 dorsal root-
    lets. Acta Physiol. Scand. (Suppl) 446:43-60.

Bjorklund, A. and U. Stenevi (1979) Regeneration of monoaminergic and cholinergic neurons in the central nervous system. Physiol. Rev. 59:62-100.

Bjorklund, A. and U. Stenevi (1984) Intracerebral neural implants: Neuronal replacement and reconstruction of damaged circuitries. Ann. Rev. Neurosci. 7:279-308.

Bregman, B.S. (1988) Target-specific requirements of immature axotomized CNS neurons for survival and axonal elongation after injury. In Reier,P.J., Bunge, R.P & Seil,F.J.(eds) Current Issues in Neural Regeneration Research, Alan Liss, New York, pp 75-87.

Carbonetto, S. (1984) The extracellular matrix of the nervous system. Trends Neurosci. 7:382-387.

Carlstedt, T. (1983) Regrowth of anastomosed ventral root nerve fibers in the dorsal root of rats. Brain Res. 272:162-165.

Carlstedt, T. (1985a) Regenerating axons from nerve terminals at astrocytes. Brain Res. 347:188-191.

Carlstedt, T. (1985b) Regrowth of cholinergic and catecholaminergic neurons along a peripheral and central nervous pathway. Neurosci. 15:507-518.

Carlstedt, T. (1988) Reinnervation of the mammalian spinal cord after neonatal dorsal root crush. J. Neurocytol. 17:335-350.

Caroni, P. and M.E. Schwab (1988a) Two membrane protein fractions from rat central myelin with inhibitory properties for neurite growth and fibroblat spreading. J.Cell Biol. 106:1281-1288.

Caroni, P. and M.E. Schwab (1988b) Antibody against myelin-associated inhibitor of neurite growth neutralize non-permissive substrate properties of CNS white matter. Neuron 1:85-96.

Cohen, J., J.F. Burne, J. Winter and P. Bartlett. (1986) Retinal ganglion cells lose response to laminin with maturation. Nature 32: 465-467.

David, S. (1989) Astrocytes and axon growth in development and regeneration. J. Neurochem. 52:S32.

David, S.(1988) Reactive gliosis: Characterization

of injury-induced changes in astrocytes. In M.D. Norenberg, L.Hertz, A.Schousboe (eds) The Biochemical Pathology of Astrocytes, Alan R. Liss, New York, pp 123-134.

David, S. and A.J. Aguayo (1981) Axonal elongation into peripheral nervous system "bridges" after central nervous system injury. Science 214:931-933.

David, S. and N. Giftochristos (1988) Differences in the adhesive properties of astrocytes in the lesioned adult rat optic nerve. Neurosci. Abst. 14:1169.

David, S., C. Bouchard, O. Tasatas and N. Giftochristos (1989) Astrocytes in the lesioned mammalian central nervous system permit rather than inhibit regeneration. (submitted for publication).

Fallon, J.R. (1985) Preferential outgrowth of central nervous system neurites on astrocytes and Schwann cells as compared with nonglial cells in vitro. J. Cell Biol. 100:198-207.

Friedman, B. and A.J. Aguayo (1985) Injured neurons in the olfactory bulb of adult rat grow new axons along peripheral nerve grafts. J. Neurosci. 5:1616-1625.

Giftochristos, N. and S. David (1988a) Immature optic nerve glia do not promote axonal regeneration when transplanted into a peripheral nerve. Dev. Brain Res. 39:149-153.

Giftochristos, N. and S. David (1988b) Laminin and heparan sulphate proteoglycan in the lesioned adult mammalian central nervous system and their possible relationship to axonal sprouting. J. Neurocytol. 17:385-397.

Guth, L., C.P. Barrett, E.J. Donati, S.S Deshpande, E.X. Albuquerque (1981) Histopathological reactions and axonal regeneration in the transected spinal cord of hibernating squirrels. J. Comp. Neurol. 203:297-308.

Hall, S.M. and A.P. Kent (1987) The response of peripheral neurites to a grafted optic nerve.J.Neurocytol.   16:317-331.

Kiernan, J.A. (1979) Hypotheses concerned with axonal regeneration in the mammalian nervous system. Biol. Rev. 54: 153-197.

Kromer, L.F., A. Bjorklund and U. Stenevi (1981) Regeneration of the septohippocampal pathways in adult rats is promoted by utilizing embryonic hippocampal implants as bridges. Brain Res. 210:173-200.

Liuzzi, F.J. and R.J. Lasek (1987) Astrocytes block axonal regeneration in mammals by activating the physiological stop pathway. Science 237:642.

Nieto-Sampedro, M., E.R. Lewis, C.W. Cotman, M. Manthorpe, S.D. Skaper,G. Barbin, F.M. Longo and S. Varon (1982) Brain injury caused time-dependent increase in neurotrophic activity at the lesion site. Science 217:860-861.

Noble, M., J. Fok-Seang and J. Cohen (1984) Glia are a unique substrate for the in vitro growth of central nervous system neurons. J. Neurosci. 4:1892-1903.

Nornes, H., A. Bjorklund and U. Stenevi (1983) Reinnervation of the denervated adult spinal cord of rats by intraspinal transplants of embryonic brain stem neurons. Cell Tiss.Res. 230:15-35.

Ramon y Cajal, S. (1928) Degeneration and Regeneration of the Nervous System. (Translated by May, R.M.) Oxford University press, London.

Reichardt, L.S., J.L. Bixby, D.E. Hall, M.J. Ignatius, K.M. Neugebauer and K.J. Tomaselli (1989) Integrins and cell adhesion molecules: Neuronal receptors that regulate axon growth on extracellular matrix and cellsurfaces. Dev. Neurosci. 11:332-347.

Reier, P.J., L.J. Stensaas and L. Guth (1983) The astrocyte scar as an impediment to regeneration in the central nervous system. In C.C Kao, R.P.Bunge and P.J. Reier (eds), Spinal Cord Reconstruction. Raven Press, New York, pp 163-196.

Reier, P.J., Eng, L.F. and L. Jakeman (1989) Reactive astrocyte and axonal outgrowth in the injured CNS: Is gliosis really an impediment to regeneration? In F.J.Seil (ed), Neural Regeneration and Transplantation, Frontiers of Clinical Neuroscience, vol. 6, Alan R. Liss, New York, pp183-209.

Richardson, P.M., U. McGuinness and A.J. Aguayo (1980) Axons from CNS neurones regenerate into PNS grafts. Nature 284:264-265.

Savio, T. and M.E. Schwab (1989) Rat CNS white matter, but not gray matter, is non-permissive for neuronal cell adhesion and fiber outgrowth. J. Neurosci. 9:1126-1133.

Schwab, M.E. and P. Caroni (1988) Oligodendrocytes and CNS myelin are non-permissive substrate for neurite growth and fibroblast spreading in vitro. J. Neurosci. 8:2381-2393.

Silver, J. and M.Y. Ogawa (1983) Postnatally induced formation of the corpus callosum in acallosal mice on glia-coated cellulose bridges. Science 220: 1067-1069.

Smith, G.M., Miller, R.H. and J. Silver (1986) The changing role of forebrain astrocytes during development, regenerative failure, and induced regeneration upon transplantation. J. Comp. Neurol. 251:23-43.

So, K-F. and A.J. Aguayo (1985) Lengthy regrowth of cut axons from ganglion cells after peripheral nerve transplantation into the retina of adult rats. Brain Res. 328:349-354.

Stensaas, L.J., L.M. Partlow, P.R. Burgess and K.W. Horch (1987) Inhibition of regeneration: The ultrastructure of reactive astrocytes and abortive axon terminals in the transitional zone of the dorsal root. In F.J. Seil, E. Herbert, B.M. Carlson (eds) Neural Regeneration, Progress in Brain Research, vol.71, Elsevier, Amsterdam, pp 457-468.

Thoenin, H. and D. Edgar (1985) Neurotrophic factors. Science 229:238-242.

Vidal-Sanz, M., G.M. Bray, M.P. Villegas-Perez, S.

Thanos and A.J. Aguayo (1987) Axonal regeneration and synapse formation in the superior colliculus by retinal ganglion cells in the adult rat. J. Neurosci. 7:2894-2909.

Weinberg, E.L. and P.S. Spencer (1979) Studies on the control of myelinogenesis. 3. Signalling of oligodendrocyte myelination by regenerating peripheral axons. Brain Res. 162:273-279.

**Advances in Neural Regeneration
Research, pages 199–214
© 1990 Wiley-Liss, Inc.**

SWELLING-INDUCED MEMBRANE TRANSPORT CHANGES IN
ASTROCYTES

H. K. Kimelberg, S. Goderie, S. Pang[1], E.
O'Connor and H. Kettenmann[2]

Division of Neurosurgery and Program in
Neuroscience, Albany Medical College,
Albany, New York, U.S.A.; [1]Institute of
Biophysics, Academica Sinica, Beijing,
China; and [2]Institut fur Neurobiologie,
Universitat Heidelberg, Federal Republic
of Germany

INTRODUCTION
    Astrocytic swelling is an early event in a
number of pathological states including head injury,
ischemia, epilepsy and hepatic encephalopathy
(Kimelberg and Ransom, 1986). Whether such swelling
alters astrocytic properties, especially membrane
transport, has been relatively unexplored. As an
initial approach to this question we have studied
the membrane transport effects caused by swelling
primary astrocyte cultures in hypotonic media.
Astrocytes respond to exposure to hypotonic media
by rapidly swelling and then undergoing regulatory
volume decrease (RVD), a property shown by many
cell types which is caused by loss of intracellular
solutes, including amino acids and intracellular
ions such as KCl (Chamberlin and Strange, 1989;
Hoffman, 1987).
    In the light of current work, loss of ions under
such conditions may occur through a class of channels known as stretch-activated channels or SACs.
SACs can be experimentally activated in the surface
membrane of most cells by pressure applied through,
and measured by current changes within, a patch
pipette applied to the surface membranes of the

intact cells or, using the same methodology, in cells that have been swollen in hypotonic medium (Sachs, 1988).

There is a considerable body of work that shows that swelling of tissues and cells from both eury- haline invertebrates, where osmoregulation is a constant physiological challenge (Gilles et al., 1987), to mammalian cells, where it is likely to be restricted to pathological conditions (Verbalis and Drutarosky, 1988) or may occur during pregnancy in rats (Law, 1989), leads to release of amino acids and non-electrolytes such as urea and mannitol, as well as ions (Hoffman, 1987; Chamberlin and Strange, 1989). Such release, especially of taurine, is seen in primary astrocyte cultures during RVD (Pasantes- Morales and Schousboe, 1988; Kimelberg et al, 1989, 1990) and as a result of high $[K^+]_o$-induced swelling (Pasantes-Morales and Schousboe, 1989). If the excitatory amino acids glutamate and aspar- tate are released during astrocytic swelling in pathological states <u>in vivo</u>, this could lead to excitotoxicity and death of neurons (Choi, 1988).

METHODS

Primary astrocyte cultures (at least 95% pure as defined by immunocytochemistry for glial fibrillary protein) were prepared from 1 day old rat pups according to previously published methods (Frangakis and Kimelberg, 1984). They were grown in 12 well plastic trays for transport studies, or on glass cover slips for the electrophysiology studies. For uptake experiments cells were washed in a balanced salt solution consisting of (in mmoles): NaCl, 122; KCl, 3.3.; $CaCl_2$, 1.2; $MgSO_4$, 0.4; KH_2PO_4, 1.2; HEPES, 25, adjusted with NaOH to obtain a pH of 7.4; and glucose, 10. In Na^+-free solutions basic N- methyl-D-glucamine ($NMDG^+$) was added, and the pH was then adjusted to 7.4 with HCl. This solution was removed and the cells were then exposed to the same solution containing the appropriate radioactive plus unlabelled compounds. After the appropriate times the cells were then washed in a cold mannitol solution (Kimelberg and Frangakis, 1985). For efflux experiments, the cells were first loaded with the appropriate labeled compounds, washed in buffer and the released radioactivity measured (Kimelberg et al. 1990). Electrophysiology was by standard microelectrode techniques (Kimelberg and O'Connor, 1988).

RESULTS
Electrophysiology
    Shown in fig. 1 is the marked depolarization of astrocytes seen when rat primary astrocyte cultures are exposed to hypotonic solution. Two hypotonic conditions are shown; in the top trace in a) exposure to a solution from which 50mM NaCl was removed and in b) a solution from which 100 mM NaCl was removed. As can be seen there is a rapid initial depolarization followed by a gradual repolarization. A generalized RVD response for these cells (Kimelberg and Frangakis, 1985; Kimelberg and Goderie, 1988), which the membrane potential changes closely follow, is shown in c). Upon replacement of the hypotonic with isotonic solution it can be seen that the cells immediately return to their preswelling membrane potentials. This is because, although the cells have lost some K^+ (Kimelberg and Fragakis, 1985), they rapidly shrink upon reexposure to isotonic solution thereby maintaining $[K^+]_i$ and the membrane potential constant.

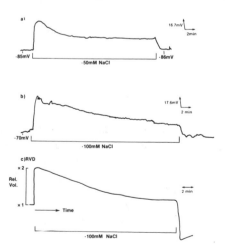

Fig. 1. Time course of depolarization of astrocytes when they were exposed for 30 min to balanced salt solutions from which 50 (a) or 100 (b) mM NaCl was removed. The perfusion solution was then changed back to the control solution. In (c) a generalized time course of volume changes occurring when astrocytes are exposed to a solution from which

100 mM has been removed (-100 mM NaCl) is shown for comparison. Recordings were corrected for liquid junction potential changes and the effects were not due to reduction of Na⁺ since the effects were not seen when sucrose replaced Na⁺ (from Kimelberg and O'Connor, 1988).

Similar membrane potential responses in response to hypotonic medium have also been reported by Ubl et al. (1988) for cultured opossum kidney cells and by Falke and Misler (1989) for Neuroblastoma cells.

Comparing cultured astrocytes and oligodendrocytes we found that oligodendrocytes showed several-fold smaller responses than astrocytes when exposed to the same hypotonic solution (Fig. 2).

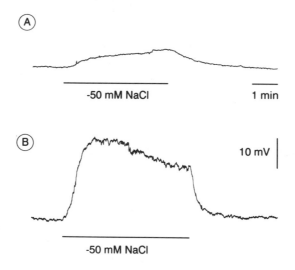

Fig. 2. Depolarization of a cultured mouse spinal cord oligodendrocyte (A) and rat cerebrocortical astrocyte (B) by exposure, as indicated by the bar, to solutions from which 50 mM NaCl was removed. The resting membrane potentials of the oligodendrocyte and astrocyte were -70 and -82 mV, respectively (from Kimelberg and Kettenmann, submitted).

We found that the smaller responses in oligodendrocytes could be simply explained as due to
dilution of $[K^+]_i$ by the cells' swelling as simple
osmometers. In contrast, in astrocytes only
approximately half of the swelling-induced
depolarization could be attributed to dilution of
$[K^+]_i$ (Kimelberg and O'Connor, 1988; Kimelberg and
Kettenmann, submitted). Since we have not studied
swelling in the oligodendrocytes we do not know if
they show a smaller degree of swelling due perhaps
to mechanical constraints, or whether there is an
absence of SACs or a low density which is
undetectable by measuring membrane potentials. A
recent preliminary study at the single channel
level has also shown the opening of K^+-selective
SACs in rat primary astrocyte cultures with
pressure applied through the cell – attached patch
pipette. A variety of different conductance
levels, but no ion selectivities, were reported
(Ding et al. 1989).

Viability of Cells on Swelling

The large membrane potential changes seen in
cells upon swelling in hypotonic medium raises the
question of whether the cells are undergoing a
nonspecific "lysis". One argument against non-
specific lysis is that the cells do not completely
depolarize as might be expected from a complete
breakdown of selective permeability, and the depolarization is rapidly reversible. Also the volume
changes are reversible since the cells show RVD
(Kimelberg and Frangakis, 1985; Kimelberg and Goderie, 1988; and see fig 1c).

We have also found that cells do not release
lactic dehydrogenase (unpublished observations)
and do not take up trypan blue when they are exposed
to this 960 dalton sulfonated compound during a 30
min exposure to minus 100 mM NaCl hypotonic
solution. The percentage of the cells that had
stained nuclei was 98 in the control (average of 2
samples of 50 cells each) and 95.8 ± 1.2 (mean of
3 samples of 50 cells, $\pm$ S.D.) in the swollen cells
respectively. Representative phase micrographs of
cells exposed to trypan blue are shown in fig. 3.
Also, we found that the subsequent growth rate of

50% confluent cultures was identical whether or not they had been exposed to minus 100 mM NaCl hypotonic solution for 30 minutes (unpublished observations).

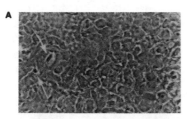
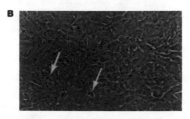
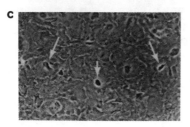

Fig. 3. Exposure of control and swollen cells to trypan blue. A) Serum containing growth medium was removed, the cells were washed with balanced salt solution (see Methods) and then exposed to 0.25% trypan blue in the same solution for 30 minutes at 37°. B) Cells previously exposed to isotonic solution for 30 minutes and then to hypotonic solution (minus 50 mM NaCl) for 1 minute plus 0.25% trypan blue. C) As in B) except cells were exposed to minus 100 mM hypotonic solution. White arrows show cells that stained for trypan blue. These were always $\geq$ 5% for all the conditions. Cells continued to exclude trypan blue for the entire 30 minute exposure to hypotonic solutions.

Swelling-Induced Ca^{2+} Uptake

One characteristic class of swelling activated channels are non-specific cation channels that allow divalent cations such as Ca^{2+} or Ba^{2+}, as well as Na^+ and K^+, to pass (Kullberg 1987; Sachs 1988; Falke and Misler, 1989). In fig. 4 we show that exposing astrocytes to media from which 50 mM (upper graph) or 100 mM (lower graph) NaCl had been removed leads to increased influx of Ca^{2+} as measur-

ed with $^{45}Ca^{2+}$. Since $^{45}Ca^{2+}$ was added with the
hypotonic or isotonic media at 0 time and the total
Ca^{2+} concentration was not changed, increased
uptake of Ca^{2+} is being seen. This could involve
increased surface binding of Ca^{2+} or increased
sequestration within intracellular organelles such
as mitochondria or endoplasmic reticulum (Meldolesi
et al.,1988). Since the normal free intracellular
Ca^{2+} has been found to be generally around $10^{-7}M$, the
steady state level of approximately 15 nmoles/mg
protein we measure with $^{45}Ca^{2+}$ gives 4.3 x $10^{-3}M$ for
a 3.5 ul intracellular volume per mg protein (Kimelberg and Frangakis, 1985). Thus only about 0.002%
of the total Ca^{2+} can be free, which is close to the
value suggested by Walz and Wilson (1986) based on
$^{45}Ca^{2+}$ uptake in mouse primary astrocyte cultures.
Since one can assume that the amount of surface
bound Ca^{2+} is likely to be relatively constant, then
the much greater uptake seen due to swelling astrocytes in hypotonic solutions is likely to represent
increased intracellular concentration and/or

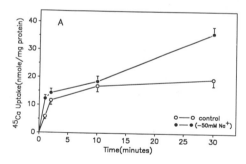

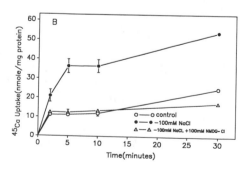

Fig. 4. Uptake of
$^{45}Ca^{2+}$ by astrocyte
cultures upon expo-
sure to minus 50
(A) or minus 100
(B) mM NaCl solut-
ions, as indicated
on   the   graphs.
$^{45}Ca^{2+}$ was added at
the same time as
the hypo-tonic or
isotonic media. In
(Δ) in B NaCl was
reduced by 100 mM
but isotonicity was
r e t a i n e d   b y
replacing it with
100 mM NMDG.Cl.

sequestration, with Ca^{2+} presumably entering via Ca^{2+} SACs. These effects are clearly dependent on swelling rather than the decrease in $[Na^+]_o$, since, as is shown in fig. 4B, maintaining isotonicity with N-methyl-Dglucamine (NMDG) results in no increased $^{45}Ca^{2+}$ influx. Whether this increased Ca^{2+} influx translates to an increase in free $[Ca^{2+}]_i$ with functional consequences such as the opening of other SACs, remains to be determined using fluorescent probes of intracellular Ca^{2+} and Ca^{2+} substitution studies.

<u>Swelling-Induced Release of Excitatory Amino Acids</u>

Fig. 5 shows that exposing astrocyte cultures that have been pre-loaded with $[^3H]$ labeled L-glutamate to hypotonic solutions (minus 50 mM NaCl) leads to massive efflux of this ^3H label. Interestingly, this efflux is blocked by a number of anion transport inhibitors such as furosemide and SITS, but not by the more specific $Na^+ + K^+ + 2Cl^-$ co-transport inhibitor, bumetanide (Warnock et al, 1983).

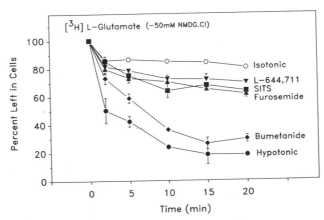

Fig. 5. Effect of different anion transport inhibitors on hypotonic media-induced efflux of $[^3H]$ L-glutamate into Na^+-free solutions ($\pm$ 50 mM NMDG.Cl) expressed as the percentage left in cells. Concentrations of inhibitors were 5 mM SITS and furosemide, and 1 mM L-644,711 and bumetanide.

One of these compounds, L644,711 (Cragoe et al. 1986), is a chloride co-transport inhibitor (Garay et al, 1986), and related compounds are potent chloride channel blockers (Landry et al, 1987). In fig. 6 we show a dose-response curve for inhibition by L644,711 of hypotonic media-induced release of the non-metabolizable [³H] D-aspartate from primary astrocyte cultures. The IC_{50} for inhibition is around 0.5mM.

Inhibition of release of excitatory amino-acids, such as glutamate and aspartate, from swollen astrocytes would be presumed to protect against potential neurotoxicity (Choi, 1988) due to release of these compounds from swollen astrocytes in pathological states in vivo, and indeed we have shown that L644,711 is markedly effective in reducing mortality in a closed head injury model (Cragoe et al, 1986; Kimelberg et al., 1987). These data are summarized in table 1.

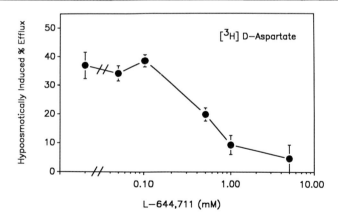

Fig. 6. Effect of increasing concentrations of L-644,711 on efflux of [³H] D-aspartate from rat primary astrocyte cultures due to exposure to hypotonic medium (removal of 50 mM NMDG.Cl in Na⁺ free medium).

DISCUSSION

A continuing theme in the papers in this section of this volume is that astroglia occupy a pivotal role in normal neuronal migration and process

Table 1

Effect of L-644,711 on the Mortality of Cats Subjected to an Acceleration-
Deceleration Plus Hypoxia Head Injury

Mode of Injection	Dose ug/kg	Treated Animals		Control Animals		Δ%
		Deaths/Total	% Mortality	Deaths/Total	% Mortality	
Intracisternal	0.57	7/15	47	9/18	50	3
	57	4/19**	21	11/28**	61	40
Intravenous	1000	12/25	48	14/25	56	8
	2500	5/21	24	8/19	42	18
	5000	1/19*	5	7/22*	33	27*
	10000	6/16**	38	15/19**	79	42**

Treated vs. controls level of significance: $^*p < 0.05$; $^{**}p < 0.025$ by Chi square test. Data for intravenously injected animals from Cragoe et al. (1986) and intracisternal from Kimelberg et al. (1987). Δ% = difference in % mortality.

extension during development. An intriguing implication is that under some conditions endogenous
astrocytes can be induced to recapitulate this
regenerative role after nervous system injury.
Alternatively, this could be accomplished by transplantation of young astrocytes grown in culture.

In this chapter we have emphasized a potential
mechanism for a pathological role for swollen astrocytes. Such swelling occurs as an early event in a
number of pathological states, including brain
ischemia and trauma (Kimelberg and Ransom, 1986).
In the present study we have sought to simulate
such swelling by simply exposing primary astrocyte
cultures to hypotonic medium. This technique has
been used for many years to study processes associated with volume regulatory decrease (RVD) in
a wide variety of animals (see Gilles et al.,
1987). Alternatively increasing external K^+ can be
used to induce astrocytic swelling in brain slices
and astrocyte cultures and extracellular K^+ is
known to increase to high levels of up to 80 mM in
vivo during ischemia (recently reviewed in Walz,
1989). However, increasing K^+ will introduce other
complication such as direct depolarization of the
plasma membrane, which could thus obscure purely
swelling related phenomena. The data presented in
this chapter show that hypotonic media-induced
swelling in cultured astrocytes is associated with
RVD, membrane depolarization and release of label
after loading with [^{3}H] D-aspartate or [^{3}H] L-
glutamate. The membrane depolarization seems to
follow the volume changes in that it is maximal
immediately after swelling in hypotonic media and
then repolarizes, paralleling the subsequent RVD
(see fig 1).

Release of organic compounds, as well as intracellular ions such as K^+ and Cl^-, are well established as the predominant mechanisms for RVD (Gilles
et al. 1987; Hoffman, 1987). Ionic release seems to
predominate in mammalian cells while in lower
vertebrates, and especially invertebrates, release
of amino acids, sulfonated amines such as taurine
and other compounds may predominate (Chamberlin and
Strange, 1989). Such processes are especially

well developed in euryhaline animals which are routinely exposed to water of varying salinity. For example, some annelids are exposed to water varying from 1 to 55 % saline (Gilles et al., 1987).

In relation to the mechanism of these swelling-induced transport changes, stretch-activated ion channels have recently been discovered using patch clamp single channel analysis (Guhary and Sachs, 1984). These stretch-activated channels (SACs) have now been found in a wide variety of cell types ranging from bacteria to mammalian cells (Kullberg, 1987). A recent preliminary study at the single channel level has shown the opening of SACs in astrocytes in primary cultures with pressure applied through the cell attached patch pipette (Ding et al. 1989). The SACs measured by cell attached patch clamp can also be activated in cells swollen in hypotonic media. In $\underline{Necturus}$ renal proximal cells stretch-activated K^+ channels are seen when the cells are swollen by around 60 % and these channels are identical to those activated by a suction of -6cm H_2O in the pipette (Sackin, 1989). Swelling of neuroblastoma cells in hypotonic medium has been shown to lead to rapid depolarization (Falke and Misler, 1989). Following the individual channels by whole-cell patch clamp showed that this behavior of the overall membrane potential correlated with an initial opening of a non-specific cation channel which would be responsible for the depolarization, followed by activation of K^+ selective channels which could be responsible for the repolarization we have seen in our studies. There was also a delayed opening of an anion channel, which could result in either a de- or repolarization depending on the anion equilibrium potential. This anion channel was permeant to anions at least of the size of acetate, and could be responsible for the increased efflux of glutamate and aspartate we see upon swelling astrocytes in hypotonic media. Thus the transport changes induced by swelling and underlying RVD in astrocytes and other cells presumable involves SACs for ions, but perhaps also swelling activated channels for amino acids and other osmoregulatory intracellular compounds.

Our finding of marked release of label after briefly loading the cells with [^{3}H] L-glutamate or [^{3}H] D-aspartate leads to the interesting possibility that swelling of astrocytes _in vivo_ may release excitotoxic compounds such as L-glutamate, which can then in turn cause neuronal injury due to excessive receptor activation (Choi, 1988). Thus any drugs that are found to inhibit such release, since astrocytes are likely to be a significant source of released L - glutamate in pathological states (Nicklas et al. 1987), may contribute to preventing neuronal injury and death in stroke or trauma. This hypothesis is supported by the finding that L644,711 causes significant improvement in recovery of cats from experimental closed head injury (Cragoe et al. 1986; Kimelberg et al. 1987).

ACKNOWLEDGMENTS

Unpublished work reported in this chapter was supported by NIH grant NS 23750 to H.K.K. We thank A. Davis for word processing.

REFERENCES

Chamberlin ME, Strange K (1989). Anisosmotic cell Volume regulation: A comparative view. Am J Physiol 257:C159-C173.

Choi DW (1988). Glutamate neurotoxicity and diseases of the nervous system. Neuron 1:623-634.

Cragoe Jr EJ, Woltersdorf Jr OW, Gould NP, Pietruszkiewicz AM, Ziegler C, Sakurai Y, Stokker GE, Anderson PS, Bourke RS, Kimelberg HK, Nelson LR, Barron KD, Rose JE, Szarowski D, Popp AJ, Waldman JP (1986). Agents for the treatment of brain edema. 2. [2,3,9,9a-tetrahydro-3-oxo-substituted-1H-fluoren-7-yl)oxy]alkanoic acids and some of their analogues. J Med Chem 29:825-841.

Ding JP, Bowman CL, Sokabe M, Sachs F (1989). Mechanical transduction in glial cells: SACS and SICS. Biophys J 55:244a.

Falke LC, Misler S (1989). Activity of ion channels during volume regulation by N1E115 neuroblastoma cells. Proc Natl Acad Sci USA 86:3919-3923.

Frangakis MV, Kimelberg HK (1984). Dissociation of neonatal rat brain by dispase for preparation of primary astrocyte cultures. Neurochem Res 9:1689-1698.

Garay RP, Hannaert PA, Nazaret C, Cragoe Jr EJ (1986). The significance of the relative effects of loop diuretics and anti-brain edema agents on the Na^+, K^+, Cl^- cotransport system and the $Cl^-/NaCO^-_3$ anion exchanger. Naunyn-Schmiedeberg's Arch Pharmacol 334:202-209.

Gilles R, Kleinzeller A, Bolis L (eds)(1987). "Current Topics in Membranes and Transport," Vol. 30, New York: Academic Press.

Guhary F, Sachs F (1984). Stretch-activated single ion channel currents in tissue-cultured embryonic chick. J Physiol (Lond) 352:685-701.

Hoffmann EK (1987). Volume regulation in cultured cells. In: Gilles R, Kleinzeller A, Bolis L (eds): "Current Topics in Membranes and Transport," Vol. 30, New York: Academic press, pp 125-180.

Kimelberg HK, Frangakis MV (1985). Furosemide- and bumetanide-sensitive ion transport and volume control in primary astrocyte cultures from rat brain. Brain Res 361:125-134.

Kimelberg HK, Kettenman H (submitted). Swelling-induced changes in electrophysiological properties of cultured astrocytes and oligo-dendrocytes. I. Effects on membrane potentials, input impedance and cell-cell coupling.

Kimelberg HK, Ransom BR (1986). Physiological aspects of astrocytic swelling. In: Fedoroff S, Vernadakis A (eds): "Astrocytes," Vol III, Orlando: Academic Press, pp 129-166.

Kimelberg HK, Goderie SK (1988). Volume regulation after swelling in primary astrocytes. In: Norenberg MD, Schousboe L, Hertz L (eds): "Biochemical Pathology of Astrocytes," New York: Alan R. Liss, pp 299-311.

Kimelberg HK, O'Connor ER (1988). Swelling-induced depolarization of astrocyte potentials. Glia 1:219-224.

Kimelberg HK, Cragoe Jr EJ, Nelson LR, Popp AJ, Szarowski D, Rose JW, Woltersdorf Jr OW, Pietruszkiewicz AM (1987). Improved recovery from a traumatic-hypoxic brain injury in cats by intracisternal injection of an anion transport inhibitor. Central Nervous System Trauma 4:3-14.

Kimelberg HK, Goderie S, Waniewski R (1989). Hypo-osmotic media-induced release of amino acids from astrocytes. Soc Neurosci Abstr 15: 353.

Kimelberg HK, Goderie SK, Higman S, Pang S, Waniewski RA (1990). Swelling-induced release of glutamate, aspartate and taurine from astrocyte cultures. J Neurosci, in press.

Kullberg R (1987). Stretch-activated ion channels in bacteria and animal cell membranes. Trends in Neurosci 10:38-39.

Landry DW, Reitman M, Cragoe Jr EJ, Al-Awqati Q (1987). Epithelial chloride channel. J Gen Physiol 90:779-798.

Law RO (1989). Effects of pregnancy on the contents of water, taurine, and total amino nitrogen in rat cerebral cortex. J. Neurochem 53:300-302.

Meldolesi J, Volpe P, Pozzan, T (1988). The intracellular distribution of calcium. Trends Neurosci 11:449-452.

Nicklas WJ, Zeevalk G, Hyndman A (1987). Inter-actions between neurons and glia in glutamate/glutamine compartmentation. Biochem Soc Trans 15:208-210.

Pasantes-Morales H, Schousboe A (1988). Volume regulation in astrocytes: A role for taurine as an osmoeffector. J Neurosci Res 20:505-509.

Pasantes-Morales H, Schousboe A (1989). Release of taurine from astrocytes during potassium-evoked swelling. Glia 2:45-50.

Sachs F (1988). Mechanical transduction in biological systems. CRC Critical Reviews in Biomedical Engineering 16:141-169.

Sackin H (1989). A stretch-activated K^+ channel sensitive to cell volume. Proc Natl Acad Sci USA 86:1731-1735.

Ubl J, Murer H, Kolb H.-A (1988). Ion channels activated by osmotic and mechanical stress in membranes of opossum kidney cells. J Membrane Biol 104:223-232.

Verbalis JG, Drutarosky MD (1988). Adaptation to chronic hypoosmolality in rats. Kidney Int 34:351-360.

Walz W (1989). Role of glial cells in the regulation of the brain ion microenvironment. Prog Neurobiol 33:309-333.

Walz W, Wilson DC (1986). Calcium entry into cultured mouse astrocytes. Neurosci Lett 67:301-306.

Warnock DG, Greger R, Dunham PB, Benjamin MA, Frizzell RA, Field M, Spring KR, Ives HE, Aronson PS, Seifter J (1983). Ion transport processes in apical membrane of epithelia. Fed Proc 43:2473-2487.

Advances in Neural Regeneration
Research, pages 215–224
© 1990 Wiley-Liss, Inc.

ASTROCYTIC REACTIONS ACCOMPANYING MOTOR NEURON REGENERATION

Manuel B. Graeber[1] and Georg W. Kreutzberg

Max-Planck-Institute for Psychiatry, 8033 Martinsried, F.R.G.

Introduction

Traumatic injury of a peripheral nerve is seldom followed by complete recovery of function. It is generally believed that local changes involving the peripheral nerve lesion site are the major cause underlying this clinical problem. This view is strongly supported by both clinical and experimental data on, for instance, the misguided outgrowth of axons or the formation of traumatic neuromas at sites of previous peripheral nerve injury. There is, however, comparably little known about whether the success of functional recovery after peripheral nerve trauma may also depend on changes which can be localized within the CNS itself.

After lesioning of their axon, motor neurons exhibit complex changes in their metabolism, morphology and electrophysiological properties. There is a decrease in enzymatic activities related to normal neuronal functioning, i.e. neurotransmission (Kreutzberg et al., 1984), but neuronal oxidative enzyme metabolism (Kreutzberg, 1963; Hamberger and Sjoestrand, 1966), growth factor receptor expression (Graeber et al., 1989a), and the production of proteins serving structural functions (Tetzlaff et al., 1988a) are increased. Abnormalities in the electrical properties of axotomized motor neurons are most conspicuous in their excitatory post-synaptic potentials (EPSP's) which are reduced in size and prolonged after axotomy (Eccles et al., 1958). These changes in electrophysiology are in good agreement (Kuno and Llinas, 1970b; Lux and Schubert, 1975; Munson et al., 1988) with the early morphological finding that synapses are physically separated from the surface of regenerating motor neurons (Blinzinger and Kreutzberg, 1968). Since then the "synaptic stripping" phenomenon has proven to be a very general feature of a neuron's response to axotomy (Kuno and Llinas, 1970b; Matthews and Nelson, 1975; Purves, 1975; for review see Cotman et al., 1981). However, the role of glial cells apparently involved in this process and the time course of their accompanying reactions have remained controversial (Torvik and

---

[1]Present address:Center for Neurological Diseases, Brigham and Women's Hospital and Harvard Medical School, Boston, U.S.A.

Skjoerten, 1971; Kerns and Hinsman, 1973; Sumner and Sutherland, 1973; Chen, 1978; Reisert et al., 1984). We have therefore reinvestigated the behavior of astrocytes and microglial cells which are located in the immediate neighborhood, i.e. the microenvironment, of regenerating motor neurons. In the experimental model employed, the facial nerve of rats is cut peripherally at the stylomastoid foramen while the brain parenchyma proper is left intact. The latter is of importance since axotomy causes a "sterile" lesion to the CNS which is devoid of recently blood derived inflammatory cells (Streit et al., 1988).

Early changes in the astrocytes

Probably through direct signaling from the injured nerve cells, astrocytes are stimulated to react following axotomy. As early as two days after operation there is a strong increase in immunoreactivity for the astrocyte specific glial fibrillary acidic protein (GFAP) in the facial nucleus of the affected side (Graeber and Kreutzberg, 1986). Post-embedding immunocytochemistry employing immunogold demonstrates at the ultrastructural level that the reactive astrocytes contain increased numbers of GFAP-positive glial filaments (Graeber and Kreutzberg, 1986), correlating well with their known hypertrophic appearance (Cammermeyer, 1955; Torvik and Skjoerten, 1971; Kerns and Hinsman, 1973). As a result, during the retrograde neuronal response GFAP-negative protoplasmic astrocytes transform into the GFAP-positive fibrous type. In contrast to direct CNS lesioning or retrograde degeneration where a glial scar develops (Streit and Kreutzberg, 1988), this change takes place without proliferation, acquisition of vimentin or increased histochemical oxidative enzyme activity in astrocytes (Hamberger and Sjoestrand, 1966; Graeber et al., 1988a,c). Using ^{35}S-methionine incorporation, two dimensional SDS-PAGE and in situ hybridization experiments, it has been further shown that following axotomy GFAP is newly synthesized by the reactive astrocytes (Tetzlaff et al., 1988b). This biochemical change precedes the increase in GFAP-immunoreactivity and can be detected 24 hours after axotomy. Interestingly, the time course and extent of reactive GFAP-expression are inversely related to the success of neuronal regeneration, indicating a direct relationship between the severity of neuronal injury and astrocytic activation. Thus, there is a stronger and more sustained increase in GFAP synthesis following facial nerve resection compared with simple crush lesioning (Tetzlaff et al., 1988b).

Other glial changes

Shortly after the astrocytic increase in GFAP there is a marked proliferation of local microglial cells (Cammermeyer, 1965; Sjoestrand,

1965; Kreutzberg, 1966), reaching a peak at day four after operation (Kreutzberg, 1968). Electron microscopic ^{3}H-thymidine autoradiography confirms that only microglial cells but not astrocytes undergo mitosis following rat facial nerve axotomy (Graeber et al., 1988c). The mitotic microglial cells initially appear in perineuronal positions where during the first post-operative week microglial pseudopods interpose between afferent axonal endings and the surface membranes of regenerating motor neurons (Blinzinger and Kreutzberg, 1968). After about 2 weeks the microglia leave their perineuronal positions and migrate into the neuropil (Kreutzberg, 1968).

Microglial cells are regarded to represent brain macrophage precursor cells which are intrinsic to the CNS (for recent review see Streit et al., 1988). This view is supported by the finding that microglial cells develop into brain macrophages when facial motor neurons are lethally injured and degenerate (Streit and Kreutzberg, 1988). However, there is no phagocytosis taking place during regeneration of facial motor neurons, though even in this situation microglial cells may newly express (Graeber et al., 1988a; Streit et al., 1989a,b) or increase (Graeber et al., 1988b) in antigens which are shared by monocytes/macrophages outside the CNS.

In contrast to astrocytes or microglia a response of oligodendrocytes to retrograde neuronal changes is virtually unknown (Torvik and Skjoerten, 1971; Barron et al., 1971). Apart from few morphological signs of activation accompanying late stages of regeneration (Graeber and Kreutzberg, unpublished observations), there are so far no data available on alterations of oligodendrocytic parameters following axotomy.

Delayed astrocyte reaction

When we followed the time course of the reactive GFAP expression accompanying motor neuron regeneration, we found that astrocytes, apart from newly synthesizing GFAP and reorganizing their cytoskeleton, also reshape their cell processes (Graeber and Kreutzberg, 1988). The astrocytes form very long cell extensions which cross the neuropil and come more and more close to the neuronal surfaces as regeneration proceeds. During the second to third week after axotomy these processes eventually take over the perineuronal positions of the microglia. Three weeks after the operation the cell bodies of the regenerating facial motor neurons are closely surrounded by GFAP-positive astrocytic profiles (Graeber and Kreutzberg, 1986). At the same time electron microscopy reveals that the astrocytes have developed sheet-like or lamellar processes which are layered in stacks around the regenerating nerve cells (Graeber and Kreutzberg, 1988). Such lamellar processes exhibit strong 5'-nucleotidase enzymatic activity in their plasma membrane and cover most neuronal surfaces with the apparent exception of small dendrites. As a result, very few intact synaptic contacts are preserved and the state of neuronal synaptic deafferentation initially associated with the microglial reaction is maintained for longer periods, i.e. months (Graeber and Kreutzberg, 1988). In spite of this isolation, peripheral reinnervation of the musculature recommences about four weeks after cut lesioning. Thus, normal syaptic input seems not to be needed by the motor neuron for regrowing its axon and reinnervation of the musculature. We have, however, observed perineuronal astrocytic lamellar stacks later than three months and up to 300 days after cut lesioning experiments when their presence seems to parallel a discrete but long-lasting deficit in the performance of complex fine motor movements of whiskers on the affected side (Graeber and Kreutzberg, unpublished observations).

Role of microglia and astrocytes in the synaptic stripping process

An active role of microglia in the synaptic stripping process has been suggested by several authors (Blinzinger and Kreutzberg, 1968; Kerns and Hinsman, 1973; Sumner and Sutherland, 1973; Kreutzberg and Barron, 1978). The basis for this hypothesis is that during early stages of the axonal reaction regenerating motor neurons may be almost completely encircled by microglial cell processes which are often directly attached to the neuronal surface membrane. However, as stated in the original publication (Blinzinger and Kreutzberg, 1968), it is more frequently observed that exceedingly thin, sheet-like astrocytic cytoplasmic processes separate the microglia from the regenerating nerve cells. Some authors have therefore concluded that an extensive separation of boutons by microglia does not take place (Chen, 1978) and that the microglial contribution to the regeneration process is probably negligible (Reisert et al., 1984). Yet, these interpretations neglect that even in unoperated motor neurons all surface areas which are devoid of synapses are normally covered by astrocytic cell processes (Poritsky, 1969). Thus, since the perineuronal microglial population rapidly expands following axotomy, the presence of single astrocytic cytoplasmic sheets interposed between microglial and neuronal membranes can be sufficiently explained by the space occupying behavior of the microglia and does not necessarily imply an active role of the astrocytes at this stage of synaptic reorganization. Our data on GFAP- and vimentin-expression (Graeber and Kreutzberg, 1986; Tetzlaff et al., 1988b; Graeber et al., 1988a) further strongly suggest that cytoskeletal changes which are likely to precede the reshaping of cell processes (Graeber and Kreutzberg, 1988) peak at least two weeks earlier in microglia than in astrocytes. In fact, there is a good correlation between the time course of changes in the cytoskeleton of glial cells and the new appearance of perineuronal microglial and lamellar astrocytic cell processes at their respective time points, i.e. during the first and third week after operation (Blinzinger and Kreutzberg, 1968; Torvik and Skjoerten, 1971; Kerns and Hinsman, 1973; Sumner and Sutherland, 1973; Graeber and Kreutzberg, 1988). Finally, evidence for an involvement of microglial cells in the synaptic stripping process of motor neurons is derived from studies with the cytostatic drug, adriamycin, showing that chromatolytic motor neurons do not lose their afferent synaptic contacts when the microglial reaction is inhibited (Graeber et al., 1989b).

A reshaping of astrocytic cell processes and a new appearance of astrocytic lamellae accompanying motor neuron regeneration has been previously observed (Barron et al., 1971; Torvik and Soereide, 1972; Sumner and Sutherland, 1973; Chen, 1978; Reisert et al., 1984). However, while astrocytic lamellar processes in regenerating rat hypoglossal nuclei return to normal status within three months (Sumner and Sutherland, 1973; Reisert et al., 1984), no such recovery has been reported for cat spinal (Chen, 1978) and rat facial motor nuclei (Graeber and Kreutzberg, 1988). Concomitant to the persistence of astrocytic lamellar stacks in these systems the number of synapses at most neurons does not return to normal by 90 days after injury (Chen, 1978; Graeber and Kreutzberg, 1988). Rather, this change may have a long-lasting character (Fig. 1).

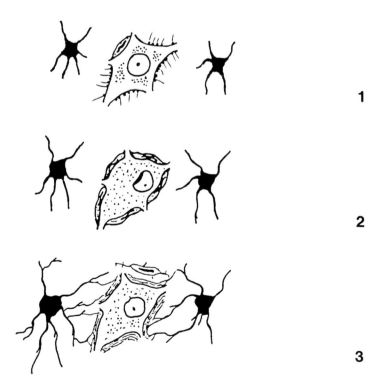

Fig. 1 Schematic drawing summarizing the glial reactions accompanying motor neuron regeneration. 1. During normal state, 2. One week after axotomy, 3. Three months after axotomy.

Functional implications

Axotomy alters most electrical properties of a motor neuron (for review see Munson et al., 1988). Some of these changes, e.g. the slower rising and smaller potential of monosynaptic EPSP's (Eccles et al., 1958), directly relate to the early synaptic stripping process (Kuno and Llinas, 1970b; Lux and Schubert, 1975; Munson et al., 1988). Other alterations in neuronal properties include the occurrence of spike-like dendritic depolarizations or partial spikes (Eccles et al., 1958; Kuno and Llinas, 1970a) which are Na^+-dependent (Sernagor et al., 1986). It has been speculated that the physical separation of synapses by glial cells provides a favorable setting for the molecular changes underlying this phenomenon, i.e. the insertion of new Na+ channels in the soma and dendritic membranes of regenerating motor neurons (Sernagor et al., 1986).

Whereas the synaptic efficacy of group I afferent fibers recovers even without functional reconnection of motor neuron and muscle (Munson et al., 1988), the restorative potential of other synaptic contacts may be less well developed. Eccles et al. (1958), for instance, found some evidence for abnormal connexions in two of three cat spinal cords that had longer periods of chromatolysis, and in some central neurons the physiological changes may be even irreversible (Faber, 1984). In addition, our findings strongly suggest that astrocytes may interfere with the restoration of normal synaptic contacts on regenerating motor neurons. This view is in good agreement with recent studies demonstrating that astrocytes may be actively involved in the reduction of synaptic density (Meshul et al., 1987; Meshul and Seil, 1988). In the rat facial nucleus the astrocytic involvement is most prominent during late stages of regeneration where the overall arrangement of synaptic contacts remains abnormal for several hundred days after cut lesioning. Therefore, although the exact synaptic organization of normal and regenerating facial motor nuclei is as yet ill-defined, it may be envisioned that complex aspects of normal neuronal functioning, e.g. the performance of fine motor movements, are especially concerned. Finally, a formation of astrocytic lamellar processes with wrapping of dendrites has been also observed following hemisection of rat spinal cord (Bernstein et al., 1975). It seems thus not unlikely that the post-traumatic formation of astrocytic lamellar processes may be of general importance for CNS functional repair.

There are so far no data available on functional interactions between glial cells during motor neuron regeneration. However, it is tempting to speculate on the astrocyte-microglial relationship following axotomy. Microglial cells which undergo a "neurofugal" migration only during regeneration but not degeneration of motor neurons clearly have a strong cytotoxic potential (for review see Streit et al., 1988). From a teleological point of view the astrocytic lamellar reaction may thus serve a two-fold function in both isolating and *at the same time* protecting the motor neuron during regeneration.

Conclusions

Axotomy leads to a substantial loss of afferent synaptic contacts from the surface of regenerating motor neurons. Microglial cells are likely to be involved in this process. Long-term, astrocytes interfere with the restoration of synaptic integrity but may also protect the injured neurons against cytotoxic microglial cells. Since astrocytic lamellar processes maintain a synaptic deafferentation of regenerating motor neurons for longer periods, i.e. several months, functional consequences may particularly involve the restoration of fine motor movements. We suggest an astrocytic lamellar reaction to be considered when functional recovery after peripheral nerve trauma is prolonged although peripheral reinnervation of the musculature has been achieved.

References

Barron KD, Chiang TY, Daniels AC, Doolin PF (1971) Subcellular accompaniments of axon reaction in cervical motoneurons of the cat. In: Zimmerman HM (ed) Progress in Neuropathology, Vol. 1, Grune & Stratton, New York, pp 255-280

Bernstein JJ, Wells MR, Bernstein M (1975) Dendrites and neuroglia following hemisection of rat spinal cord: effects of puromycin. In: Kreutzberg GW (ed) Physiology and Pathology of Dendrites, Advances in Neurology, Vol. 12, Raven Press, New York, pp 439-451

Blinzinger K, Kreutzberg G (1968) Displacement of synaptic terminals from regenerating motoneurons by microglial cells. Z. Zellforsch. 85: 145-157

Cammermeyer J (1955) Astroglial changes during retrograde atrophy of nucleus facialis in mice. J. Comp. Neurol. 102: 133-150

Cammermeyer J (1965) Juxtavascular karyokinesis and microglia cell proliferation during retrograde reaction in the mouse facial nucleus. Ergeb. Anat. Entwicklgs. Ges. 38: 1-22

Chen DH (1978) Qualitative and quantitative study of synaptic displacement in chromatolyzed motoneurons of the cat. J. Comp. Neurol. 177: 635-664

Cotman CW, Nieto-Sampedro M, Harris EW (1981) Synapse replacement in the nervous system of adult vertebrates. Physiol. Rev. 61: 684-784

Eccles JC, Libet B, Young RR (1958) The behaviour of chromatolysed motoneurones studied by intracellular recording. J. Physiol. 143: 11-40

Faber DS (1984) Reorganization of neuronal membrane properties following axotomy. Exp. Brain Res., Suppl. 9: 225-239

Graeber MB, Kreutzberg GW (1986) Astrocytes increase in glial fibrillary acidic protein during retrograde changes of facial motor neurons. J. Neurocytol. 15: 363-373

Graeber MB, Kreutzberg GW (1988) Delayed astrocyte reaction following facial nerve axotomy. J. Neurocytol. 17: 209-220

Graeber MB, Streit WJ, Kreutzberg GW (1988a) The microglial cytoskeleton: vimentin is localized within activated cells in situ. J. Neurocytol. 17: 573-580

Graeber MB, Streit WJ, Kreutzberg GW (1988b) Axotomy of the rat facial nerve leads to increased CR3 complement receptor expression by activated microglial cells. J. Neurosci. Res. 21: 18-24

Graeber MB, Tetzlaff W, Streit WJ, Kreutzberg GW (1988c) Microglial cells but not astrocytes undergo mitosis following rat facial nerve axotomy. Neurosci. Lett. 85: 317-321

Graeber MB, Raivich G, Kreutzberg GW (1989a) Increase of transferrin receptors and iron uptake in regenerating motor neurons. J. Neurosci. Res., in press

Graeber MB, Streit WJ, Kreutzberg GW (1989b) Formation of microglia-derived brain macrophages is blocked by adriamycin. Acta Neuropathol. (Berl.), in press

Hamberger A, Sjoestrand J (1966) Respiratory enzyme activities in neurons and glial cells of the hypoglossal nucleus during nerve regeneration. Acta Physiol. Scand. 67: 76-88

Kerns JM, Hinsman EJ (1973) Neuroglial response to sciatic neurectomy. II. Electron microscopy. J. Comp. Neurol. 151: 255-280

Kreutzberg GW (1963) Changes of coenzyme (TPN) diaphorase and TPN-linked dehydrogenase during axonal reaction of the nerve cell. Nature 199: 393-394

Kreutzberg GW (1966) Autoradiographische Untersuchung über die Beteiligung von Gliazellen an der axonalen Reaktion im Facialiskern der Ratte. Acta Neuropathol. (Berl.) 7: 149-161

Kreutzberg GW (1968) Über perineuronale Mikrogliazellen (Autoradiographische Untersuchungen). Acta Neuropathol. (Berl.), Suppl. 4: 141-145

Kreutzberg GW, Barron KD (1978) 5'-Nucleotidase of microglial cells in the facial nucleus during axonal reaction. J. Neurocytol. 7: 601-610

Kreutzberg, G.W., Tetzlaff, W., and Toth, L. (1984) Cytochemical changes of cholinesterases in motor neurons during regeneration. In: Brzin, M., Barnard, E.A., and Sket, D. (eds.) Cholinesterases - Fundamental and Applied Aspects, de Gruyter, Berlin, pp. 273-288

Kuno M, Llinas R (1970a) Enhancement of synaptic transmission by dendritic potentials in chromatolysed motoneurones of the cat. J. Physiol. (Lond.) 210: 807-821

Kuno M, Llinas R (1970b) Alterations of synaptic action in chromatolysed motoneurones of the cat. J. Physiol. (Lond.) 210: 823-838

Lux HD, Schubert P (1975) Some aspects of the electroanatomy of dendrites. In: Kreutzberg GW (ed) Advances in Neurology, Vol. 12, Raven Press, New York, pp. 29-44

Matthews MR, Nelson VH (1975) Detachment of structurally intact nerve endings from chromatolytic neurones of rat superior cervical ganglion during the depression of synaptic transmission induced by post-ganglionic axotomy. J. Physiol. (Lond.) 245: 91-135

Meshul CK, Seil FJ, Herndon RM (1987) Astrocytes play a role in regulation of synaptic density. Brain Res. 402: 139-145

Meshul CK, Seil FJ (1988) Transplanted astrocytes reduce synaptic density in the neuropil of cerebellar cultures. Brain Res. 441: 23-32

Munson JB, Foehring RC, Sypert GW (1988) Target-dependence of spinal motoneurons. In: Reier PJ, Bunge RP, Seil FJ (eds) Current Issues in Neural Regeneration Research, Alan R. Liss, New York, pp. 55-64

Poritsky R (1969) Two and three dimensional ultrastructure of boutons and glial cells on the motoneuronal surface in the cat spinal cord. J. Comp. Neurol. 135: 423-452

Purves D (1975) Functional and structural changes in mammalian sympathetic neurones following interruption of their axons. J. Physiol. (Lond.) 252: 429-463

Reisert I, Wildemann G, Grab D, Pilgrim Ch (1984) The glial reaction in the course of axon regeneration: a stereological study of the rat hypoglossal nucleus. J. Comp. Neurol. 229: 121-128

Sernagor E, Yarom Y, Werman R (1986) Sodium-dependent regenerative responses in dendrites of axotomized motoneurons in the cat. Proc. Natl. Acad. Sci. USA 83: 7966-7970

Sjoestrand, J. (1965) Proliferative changes in glial cells during nerve regeneration. Z. Zellforsch. 68: 481-493

Streit WJ, Kreutzberg GW (1988) Response of endogenous glial cells to motor neuron degeneration induced by toxic ricin. J. Comp. Neurol. 268: 248-263

Streit WJ, Graeber MB, Kreutzberg GW (1988) Functional plasticity of microglia: a review. Glia 1: 301-307

Streit WJ, Graeber MB, Kreutzberg GW (1989a) Peripheral nerve lesion produces increased levels of major histocompatibility complex antigens in the central nervous system. J. Neuroimmunol. 21: 117-123

Streit WJ, Graeber MB, Kreutzberg GW (1989b) Expression of Ia antigen on perivascular and microglial cells after sublethal and lethal motor neuron injury. Exp. Neurol., in press

Sumner BEH, Sutherland FI (1973) Quantitative electron microscopy on the injured hypoglossal nucleus in the rat. J. Neurocytol. 2: 315-328

Tetzlaff W, Bisby MA, Kreutzberg GW (1988a) Changes in cytoskeletal proteins in the rat facial nucleus following axotomy. J. Neurosci. 8: 3181-3189

Tetzlaff W, Graeber MB, Bisby MA, Kreutzberg GW (1988b) Increased glial fibrillary acidic protein synthesis in astrocytes during retrograde reaction of the rat facial nucleus. Glia 1: 90-95

Torvik A, Skjoerten F (1971) Electron microscopic observations on nerve cell regeneration and degeneration after axon lesions. II. Changes in the glial cells. Acta Neuropathol. (Berl.) 17: 265-282

Torvik A, Soereide AJ (1972) Nerve cell regeneration after axon lesions in newborn rabbits. J. Neuropathol. Exp. Neurol. 31: 683-695

**Advances in Neural Regeneration
Research, pages 225–236
© 1990 Wiley-Liss, Inc.**

REGULATION OF AXONAL REGENERATION THROUGH THE DORSAL ROOT
TRANSITIONAL ZONE IN ADULT MAMMALS

Francis J. Liuzzi

Department of Anatomy and Neurobiology
and Department of Neurosurgery, Eastern Virginia
Medical School, Norfolk, Virginia 23501

INTRODUCTION

When dorsal root axons are severed by crushing or
cutting the dorsal roots in adult mammals, the axons grow
unimpeded within the PNS environment of the root. Yet, as
Ramon y Cajal (1928) noted, when the growing axon tips
encounter the CNS environment of the dorsal root
transitional zone (DRTZ), they do one of three things.
Horseradish peroxidase (HRP) anterograde injury-filling of
regenerating dorsal root axons in adult rats reveals a
small number of axons that continue through the DRTZ, grow,
arborize and apparently synapse within the dorsal gray
matter (Liuzzi and Lasek, 1987b). Similarly, anterograde
injury-filling of regenerating dorsal roots shows that some
regenerating dorsal root axons, upon reaching the DRTZ,
turn and grow back into the PNS environment of the dorsal
root (Liuzzi, unpublished observation; Reier and Houle,
1988). The majority of regenerating dorsal root axons,
however, stop at the junction between the PNS environment
of the root and the CNS environment of the spinal cord
(Stensaas, et al., 1987; Liuzzi and Lasek, 1986, 1987a;
Carlstedt, 1989). In this PNS-CNS interface region, the
growth cones of regenerating axons are transformed into
stable, stationary axon endings among the astrocytic
processes and somata which characterize the CNS side of the
DRTZ following dorsal root injury. The ultrastructural
morphologies of the axo-glial endings in the DRTZ are
similar in many ways to presynaptic terminals (Carlstedt,
1985; Stensaas, et al., 1987 and Liuzzi and Lasek, 1986,
1987a). They are relatively small, contain numerous small
spherical vesicles, a few dense-cored vesicles, a number of
mitochondria and are essentially devoid of neurofilaments
and microtubules (Liuzzi and Lasek, 1986,1987a).

HYPOTHESES ADVANCED TO EXPLAIN THE FAILURE OF AXONS TO BREACH THE DORSAL ROOT TRANSITIONAL ZONE

Since the time of Ramon y Cajal's reports on dorsal root axonal regeneration in mammals (1928), there have been a number of different hypotheses advanced to explain the failure of regenerating axons to penetrate the DRTZ and to grow into the spinal cord.

The first and perhaps most widely held hypothesis views the gliosis in the region as an impenetrable physical barrier to axonal growth. Indeed, the ultrastructural appearance of the CNS side of the DRTZ following dorsal root injury reveals a stereotypical glial scar composed of hypertrophic astrocytic somata and their tightly interwoven processes packed with intermediate filaments.

Although this hypothesis is appealing for its simplicity, it fails to consider the ability of a small number of regenerating axons to breach the DRTZ from the root and of central axons to regenerate out of the spinal cord into a denervated dorsal root (Carlstedt, 1989; Kodama, et al., 1989). More importantly, the hypothesis fails to encompass the immutable fact that astrocytes are living, dynamic cells with a broad range of behaviors. An ever-increasing literature shows that astrocytic behaviors include, but are not limited to, the expression of a myriad of neurotransmitter receptors (Hansson, et al., 1986), the ability to produce, under certain circumstances, extracellular matrix molecules (ECMs) such as laminin (Liesi, et al., 1983; Liesi, et al., 1984b) and type IV collagen (Wujek, et al., 1989), as well as the ability to interact with the immune system, as shown by their ability to produce interferon (Tedeschi, et al., 1986).

A more recently proposed hypothesis to explain the failure of regenerating dorsal root axons to grow through the DRTZ has been advanced by Bignami, Chi and Dahl (1984). They examined the DRTZ after root injury immunohistochemically with antisera to neurofilament protein, glial fibrillary acidic protein (GFAP) and laminin. Staining with a neurofilament antisera revealed a similar finding to that obtained from anterograde injury-filling of regenerating dorsal roots with HRP. It showed that a few regenerating axons traversed the DRTZ (Bignami, et al., 1985). More importantly, Bignami and his colleagues (1985) showed that laminin staining was confined to the PNS side of the DRTZ suggesting, contrary to what has been shown for some reactive astrocytes (Liesi, et al., 1984b and Giftochristos and David, 1988), that reactive astrocytes in the region do not express detectable levels of this ECM after dorsal root injury. These authors conclude that the absence of laminin on the CNS side of the DRTZ is responsible for the failure of regenerating axons to traverse the region.

It is important to note, however, that while laminin has been strongly implicated as a substrate for axonal growth *in vitro* (Liesi, et al., 1984a; Manthorpe, et al., 1983) and, as a component of the basal lamina, in the peripheral nervous system (Ide, et al., 1983) there is data to suggest that its absence in the DRTZ of adult mammals may not be sufficient to explain failed axonal regeneration through the region. Indeed, *in vitro* studies have shown that neurites grow effectively on astrocyte monolayers, even in the presence of antibodies that have been shown to block laminin-associated neuritic extension (Tomaselli, et al., 1986; David, 1988). These tissue culture data indicate that the robust neuritic extension observed on astrocytic monolayers is mediated by astrocytic surface molecules other than laminin (David, 1988). Recently, in support of the *in vitro* findings, Giftochristos and David (1988) have provided *in vivo* data showing that axonal sprouts in severed adult rat optic nerves are associated with laminin-negative, but not with laminin-positive astrocytes, again suggesting that the presence of laminin is not essential for axonal growth on astrocytic membranes, even in the case of the adult mammalian CNS.

THE PHYSIOLOGICAL STOP PATHWAY HYPOTHESIS: AN INTERACTION BETWEEN TRANSITIONAL ZONE ASTROCYTES AND NEURONAL GROWTH CONES

A number of years ago, Liuzzi and Lasek (1986; 1987a,b) began to explore the mechanisms by which regenerating axons are stopped at the adult rat DRTZ. Coincident with those studies, they were continuing studies begun by Lasek and Black (1977) which were directed at the question of "How do axons stop growing?". Earlier studies in Lasek's laboratory (Hoffman and Lasek, 1975; Lasek and Hoffman, 1976) had shown that slowly transported axonal cytoskeletal proteins, particularly the neurofilament triplet proteins, are not degraded as they move down the axons toward their terminals. Yet, upon reaching the presynaptic terminals, these proteins are rapidly degraded. Based on these earlier findings, Lasek and Black (1977) proposed that the breakdown of neurofilament proteins in the axon terminals was dependent upon the activation of axonal proteases by the interactions of the axon terminals with their target cells. To test their hypothesis, they made ligation neuromas in guinea pig hypoglossal nerves and studied the slow axonal transport of cytoskeletal proteins into axon terminals in the absence of target cells. They found, using ^{3}H-lysine injections into the hypoglossal nucleus followed by gel electrophoresis and fluorography of consecutive hypoglossal nerve segments, that slowly transported proteins moved into the neuroma and that the neurofilament triplet proteins had a particularly long residence time in that region.

Liuzzi and Lasek repeated those experiments and used electron microscopy to examine axon endings in hypoglossal neuromas. The ultra-structural analyses confirmed the biochemical data and showed not only massive accumulations of neurofilaments in the axon endings within the neuromas, but also large accumulations of membranous organelles within those endings (Liuzzi and Lasek, unpublished observations; Figure 1).

At the same time that Liuzzi and Lasek were studying the ultrastructural characteristics of axon terminals in ligation neuromas, their ultrastructural examinations of regenerated dorsal root axon endings in the DRTZ revealed morphologies dramatically different from those observed in the case of physically blocked axons within the neuromas. Interestingly, they observed, as Carlstedt (1985a) had reported earlier from his ultrastructural observations of motor axon terminals in the DRTZ after ventral-to-dorsal root anastomoses, that the regenerated dorsal root axonal endings had many of the morphological characteristics of synaptic terminals (Liuzzi and Lasek, 1986, 1987a). They were relatively small compared to the distended endings in the neuroma. And, more importantly, they were not characterized by accumulations of membranous organelles and were devoid of microtubules as well as neurofilaments.

It was obvious that if the astrocytes of the DRTZ were acting merely as a physical barrier, then the morphologies of the dorsal root axonal endings in the region should more closely resemble the physically blocked axon endings observed in the ligation neuroma. The similarity of the dorsal root axo-glial endings to presynaptic terminals, particularly the absence of neurofilaments in those endings, suggested that the proteolytic mechanisms, which are normally activated when an axon contacts an appropriate target, were activated when the growing axon tips contacted astrocytic processes within the DRTZ. Moreover, the fact that motoneuron axon endings swelled with neurofilaments and membranous organelles when physically blocked in hypoglossal neuromas (Liuzzi and Lasek, unpublished observations), yet similar axons formed synaptoid terminals when they contacted astrocytes in the DRTZ following ventral-to-dorsal root anastomoses (Carlstedt, 1985a), suggested that the phenomenon was not

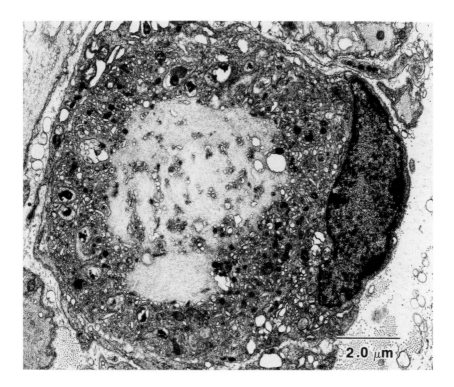

Figure 1. Electron micrograph of a physically blocked motoneuron axonal ending within a hypoglossal neuroma three weeks after ligating the hypoglossal nerve in an adult guinea pig. The ending is immensely swollen by accumulated neurofilaments and membranous elements.

specific to primary afferent axons and lent further credence to the idea that there was a physiological interaction occurring between axon and astrocyte in this region. In addition, not only are the axon endings of different types of axons affected similarly by the DRTZ astrocytes, but Carlstedt (1985b) has reported evidence that the phenotypic expression of the astrocytes, particularly the amount of intermediate filaments within them, is determined by the type of axons that contact them. When he coapted the hypogastric nerve made up of catacholaminergic axons to a cut dorsal root, he found astrocytes with fewer glial filaments as compared to those observed when cholinergic, motor axons, or dorsal root axons regenerated into the DRTZ (Carlstedt, 1985b).

Following the initial observations of axon endings in ligation neuromas where axons are physically blocked in the absence of targets and axo-glial endings in the DRTZ following crush, Liuzzi and Lasek (1986; 1987a) proposed the hypothesis that astrocytes block axonal regeneration through the DRTZ by activating the physiological stop pathway.

The physiological stop pathway is normally activated when axons contact appropriate targets and is made up of a sequence of events which change a motile growth cone into a stationary stable axon terminal. The early events of the physiological stop pathway are unknown but probably involve axo-glial membrane interactions that result in the cessation of filopodial extension and exploration by the growth cone.

At least two of the later events in the stop pathway appear to be protease-dependent (Liuzzi, in press). One of these events had already been suggested by the work of Lasek and Black (1977) when they proposed that proteases extant in the axon were activated within presynaptic terminals by contact with target cells, and that this proteolytic activation was responsible for the disassembly of neurofilaments. The idea of protease activation in synaptic terminals as a mechanism for the removal of cytoskeletal elements, particularly neurofilaments, was further substantiated by Roots' (1983) observation that intratectal injections of leupeptin, a protease inhibitor, caused an accumulation of neurofilaments within presynaptic terminals of fish tecta, much as reduced temperatures had, by inhibiting enzyme activity in those endings.

Evidence for protease activation in a second component of the physiological stop pathway was recently provided by Sahenk and Lasek (1988). It has been suggested by Bisby (1987) that proteolysis is involved in the removal of membranous elements from normal axon terminals by the conversion of anterogradely transported membranous elements to retrogradely transported elements. Sahenk and Lasek (1988) confirmed Bisby's notion by showing that local application of protease inhibitors to axonal endings disrupted anterograde-to-retrograde conversion resulting in a decreased retrograde transport of proteins from the terminals and an accumulation of membranous organelles within the axon tips.

When the physiological stop pathway is not activated, then, as in the case of physical blockade in a ligation neuroma where target cells are absent, neurofilaments and membranous elements accumulate in the axon endings. To definitively test the hypothesis that DRTZ astrocytes are not acting merely as a physical barrier to axonal growth, but rather are activating the physiological stop pathway, Liuzzi and Lasek (1986; 1987a) compared the ultrastructural morphologies of dorsal root axonal endings in ligation neuromas of the L5 dorsal root to axo-glial endings at the DRTZ. Just as motoneuron axons stopped in a hypoglossal neuroma swell with neurofilaments and membranous organelles, those dorsal root axons physically blocked in the dorsal root swell with neurofilaments and membranous organelles (Figure 2). By contrast, the axo-glial endings in the DRTZ are relatively small and, as stated above, have morphologies reminiscent of synaptic terminals (Liuzzi and Lasek, 1987; Liuzzi, in press; Figure 3). These findings

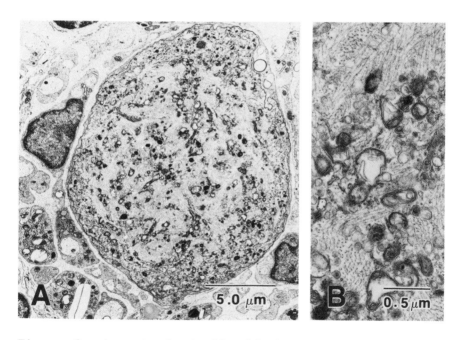

Figure 2. **A.** A physically blocked dorsal root axonal ending. This ending which did not contact astrocytes of the DRTZ is distended by the continuous flow of neurofilaments and membranous organelles into the ending and the inaction of the proteolytic mechanisms needed to disassemble and remove them. **B.** Higher magnification of an area within the ending. (from Liuzzi and Lasek, 1987a, copyright 1987 by the AAAS)

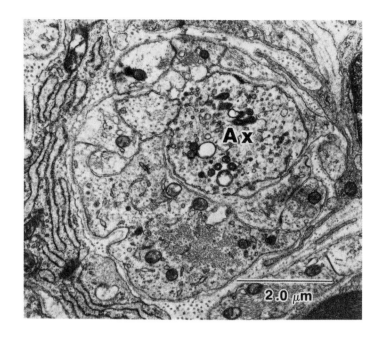

Figure 3. An axo-glial ending (Ax) in the DRTZ three weeks after dorsal root crush. In contrast to the swollen ending in Figure 2, this ending, which is surrounded by astrocytic processes, is small and completely devoid of neurofilaments. In addition, it contains a few mitochondria and small vesicles. (from Liuzzi and Lasek, 1987a, copyright 1987 by the AAAS)

convincingly demonstrate that inhibition of axonal growth through the DRTZ must involve more than a simple physical blockade by astrocytes in the region.

Recently, Liuzzi (in press) conducted experiments to further test the physiological stop pathway hypothesis. Lumbar dorsal roots were crushed as in the previous experiments, except that two to four weeks after the dorsal root crushes, leupeptin, a protease inhibitor, was infused for one week into the region of the DRTZ by a lumbar intrathecal catheter attached to an Alzet 2001 mini-osmotic pump. Control animals received crushes alone or crushes followed by saline infusions.

Control axo-glial ending morphologies were essentially the same as observed in the earlier study (Liuzzi and Lasek, 1987). By contrast, axo-glial endings exposed to the protease inhibitor were distended with both neurofilaments as well as membranous organelles (Figure 4). These observations further support the idea that the physiological stop pathway is activated at the DRTZ.

SUMMARY

A novel hypothesis has recently been proposed to explain the failure of regenerating dorsal root axons to grow through the DRTZ, a PNS-CNS interface. This hypothesis and the data supporting it suggest that astro-

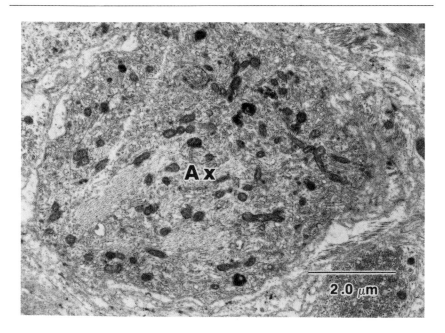

Figure 4. Swollen axo-glial ending (Ax) in the DRTZ following one week of intrathecal leupeptin infusion. This ending, like the physically blocked endings of the hypoglossal nerve and dorsal root, is distended by accumulated neurofilaments and membranous organelles.

cytes within the DRTZ are not merely a physical barrier to axonal elongation. Rather, it appears that astrocytes exploit a physiological pathway extant within the tips of growing axons which is normally activated by target cells. The activation of the physiological stop pathway transforms the motile axonal growth cone into a stable stationary axon ending wherein cytoskeletal and membranous elements, which are continually being transported down the axon, are either disassembled or converted for removal from the axon tip and return to the neuronal soma.

ACKNOWLEDGEMENTS

The author would like to thank Dr. Bruce Tedeschi for critically reading the manuscript. In addition, he would like to thank Sandy Kohler and Terri Munson for their technical assistance. This work was supported by a grant from the NIH (NS24309) and a grant from the Spinal Cord Research Foundation.

REFERENCES

Bisby MA (1987). Does recycling have functioning other than disposal? In Bisby MA and Smith RS (eds): "Axoplasmic Transport," New York: Alan R. Liss, pp.365-383.

Bignami A, Chi NH, Dahl D (1984). Regenerating dorsal roots and the nerve entry zone: an immunofluorescence study with neurofilament and laminin antisera. Exp Neurol 85:426-436.

Carlstedt T (1985a). Regenerating axons form terminals at astrocytes. Brain Res 347:188-191.

Carlstedt T (1985b). Regrowth of cholinergic and catecholaminergic neurons along a peripheral and central nervous pathway. Neurosci 15:507-528.

Carlstedt T, Cullheim S, Risling M, Ulfhake B (1989). Nerve fibre regeneration across the PNS-CNS interface at the root-spinal cord junction. Brain Res Bull 22:93-102.

David S (1988). Neurite outgrowth from mammalian CNS neurons on astrocytes in vitro may not be mediated primarily by laminin. J Neurocytol 17:131-144.

Giftochristos N, David S (1988). Laminin and heparan sulphate proteoglycan in the lesioned adult mammalian central nervous system and their possible relationship to axonal sprouting. J Neurocytol 17:385-397.

Hansson E, Nilsson A, Eriksson P, Nilsson M, Sellstrom A (1986). Heterogeneity among astrocytes, evaluated by biochemical parameters. In Grisar T, Franck G, Hertz L, Norton WT, Sensenbrenner M, Woodbury DM (eds): "Dynamic properties of glia cells II. Cellular and molecular aspects," New York: Pergammon Press, pp 235-243.

Hoffman PN, Lasek RJ (1975). The slow component of axonal transport. Identification of major structural polypeptides of the axon and their generality among mammalian neurons. J Cell Bio 66:351-366.

Ide C, Tohyama K, Yokota R, Nitatori T, Onodera S (1983). Schwann cell basal lamina and nerve regeneration. Brain Res 288:61-75.

Kodama RT, Smith KJ, Liuzzi FJ (1989). Does the regeneration of central axons into adenervated peripheral nerve require CNS trauma? Anat Rec 223:62A.

Lasek RJ, Black MM (1977). How do axons stop growing? Some clues from the metabolism of proteins in the slow component of axonal transport. In Roberts S, Lajtha A, Gispen WH (eds): "Mechanisms, Regulation and Special Functions of Protein Synthesis in the Brain," Amsterdam: Elsevier/North-Holland Biomedical Press, pp 161-169.

Lasek RJ, Hoffman PN (1976). The neuronal cytoskeleton, axonal transport and axonal growth. In Goldman R, Pollard T, Rosenbaum J (eds): "Cell Motility", Cold Springs Harbor: Cold Spring Harbor Laboratory, pp 1021-1049.

Liesi P, Dahl D, Vaheri, A (1984a). Neurons cultured from developing rat brain attach and spread preferentially to laminin. J Neurosci Res 11:241-251.

Liesi P, Kaakkola S, Dahl D, Vaheri A (1984b). Laminin is induced in adult brain astrocytes by stereotaxic lesioning. EMBO J 3:683-686.

Liuzzi FJ (in press). Proteolysis is a critical step in the physiological stop pathway: Mechanisms involved in the blockade of axonal regeneration by mammalian astrocytes. Brain Res.

Liuzzi FJ, Lasek RJ (1986). Astrocytes at the dorsal root, root-cord interface activate degradative mechanisms in the terminals of regenerated dorsal root axons. Soc Neurosci Abstr 12:697.

Liuzzi FJ, Lasek RJ (1987a). Astrocytes block axonal regeneration in mammals by activating the physiological stop pathway. Science 237:642-645.

Liuzzi FJ, Lasek RJ (1987b). Some dorsal root axons regenerate into the adult rat spinal cord. An HRP study. Soc Neurosci Abstr 13:395.

Manthorpe M, Engvall E, Ruoslahti E, Longo FM, Davis GE, Varon S (1983). Laminin promotes neuritic regeneration from cultured peripheral and central neurons. J Cell Bio 97:1882-1890.

Ramon y Cajal S (1928). "Degeneration and regeneration of the nervous system." London: Oxford University Press, pp 531-557.

Reier PJ, Houle JD (1988). The glial scar: its bearing on axonal elongation and transplantation approaches to CNS repair. In Waxman SG (ed): "Functional recovery in neurological disease," New York: Raven Press, pp 87-138.

Roots BI (1983). Neurofilament accumulation induced in synapses by leupeptin. Science 221:971-972.

Sahenk Z, Lasek RJ (1988). Inhibition of proteolysis blocks anterograde-retrograde conversion of axonally transported vesicles. Brain Res 460:199-203.

Stensaas LJ, Partlow LM, Burgess PR, Horch KW (1987). Inhibition of regeneration: the ultrastructure of reactive astrocytes and abortive axon terminals in the transitional zone of the dorsal root. In Seil FJ, Herbert E, Carlson BM (eds): "Progress in Brain Research," vol. 71, New York: Elsevier, pp 457-468.

Tomaselli KJ, Reichert LF, Bixby JL (1986). Distinct molecular neuronal process outgrowth on non-neuronal cell surfaces and extracellular matrices. J Cell Bio 103:2659-2672.

Wujek JR, Haleem-Smith H, Freese E, Yamada Y (1989). Cultured mammalian astrocytes synthesize collagen type IV: Evidence that astrocytes may participate in basement membrane formation at CNS boundaries. Soc Neurosci Abstr 15:510.

**Advances in Neural Regeneration
Research, pages 237–252**

VOLTAGE-GATED CATION and ANION CHANNELS in the SATELLITE CELLS OF THE MAMMALIAN NERVOUS SYSTEM

J. Murdoch Ritchie

*Department of Pharmacology, Yale University School of
Medicine, New Haven, CT 06510*

Introduction

The earliest indication that the satellite cells of the nervous system express voltage-gated, Hodgkin-Huxley type sodium channels came from experiments on mammalian myelinated peripheral nerve (although this was not appreciated at the time). Using radiolabeled saxitoxin as a marker for sodium channels Ritchie et al. (1981) showed that in rabbit sciatic nerve that had been demyelinated *in vivo* with lysolethicin and then allowed to remyelinate, the saxitoxin-binding capacity after an initial fall rose to a value 2-3 times that of the control nerve as remyelination proceeded. At the time, this maintained increase in saxitoxin-binding capacity was attributed solely to the fact that in remyelinated nerve the number of nodes per unit length of fiber characteristically increases greatly. A similar finding was subsequently made (Ritchie, 1982) in crushed rabbit nerve when, after Wallerian degeneration had occurred, the axons were allowed to regenerate. After first decreasing to about half its original value, the saxitoxin binding rapidly increased to a maintained value that was 2-3 times that of the control contralateral nerve (Fig. 1A). Again, the increase in sodium channel content (determined from the maximal saturable binding of labeled saxitoxin) was taken to reflect the known increase in the number of nodes per unit length that occurs in regeneration (it being assumed that the number of sodium channels per node remains roughly constant).

This conclusion from the regeneration and remyelination experiments, though highly plausible, was soon brought into question by the corresponding findings in degenerated nerve trunks (Ritchie & Rang, 1983). In these experiments a length of sciatic nerve was isolated *in vivo* by section high and low in the thigh, great care being taken to prevent axonal regeneration. When these experiments were carried out on rat nerve (Fig. 1B,

interupted line) the expected result was obtained, namely that the saxitoxin binding capacity rapidly decreased after nerve section as Wallerian

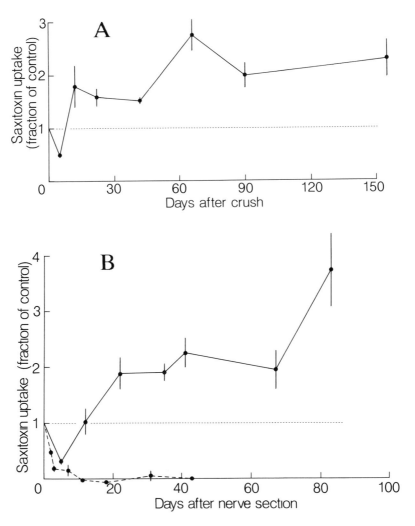

Figure 1. (A) The binding of saxitoxin to regenerating rabbit sciatic
nerve. The saturable saxitoxin uptake after a crush with fine watchmak-
er's forceps is expressed as a fraction of that in control contralateral nerve.
The bars show ± 1SEM. Each point is the mean of 4-7 (total 42) experiments. (B) The corresponding uptake by degenerating rat and rabbit
sciatic nerve after section in the thigh region. Each point is the mean of
results from 3-12 (total 39) rabbit, and 2-4 (total 15) rat sciatic nerves.

degeneration occurred; and it soon reached a value that was indistinguishable from zero . In the rabbit, however, the saxitoxin binding capacity of the degenerating nerve trunk, which fell to less than half in the first few days, returned to its original value by ten days; and thereafter it reached, and maintained for more than three months, a value about twice as much. Ritchie & Rang (1983) concluded that this increased binding in sectioned degenerated rabbit sciatic nerve must be to non-neuronal sites. They suggested that these sites were, in fact, situated on the surface membrane of the Schwann cells, which had greatly proliferated in number as axonal degeneration had progressed. Part of the evidence for this conclusion was that diphtheria toxin, which seems to kill Schwann cells relatively specifically without significantly affecting axons (at least in low concentrations), virtually abolished the saxitoxin-binding capacity of sciatic nerves that had been cut 30-60 days previously.

We soon confirmed that these saxitoxin binding sites were indeed sodium channels in electrophysiological experiments on cultured Schwann cells with the patch clamp method (Hamill et al., 1981). These electrophysiological experiments (Chiu et al., 1984; Shrager et al.,1985) showed that rabbit cultured Schwann cells do indeed express plasmalemmal voltage-gated sodium channels. Soon afterwards, we showed that such voltage-gated sodium channels were also present in rat cultured astrocytes (Bevan et al., 1985) . Furthermore, it was shown that the satellite cells of both the peripheral and central nervous systems express not just voltage-gated sodium channels but also voltage-gated potassium (Chiu et al., 1984; Shrager et al., 1985; Howe & Ritchie, 1988) and chloride (Gray & Ritchie, 1986; Howe & Ritchie, 1988) channels.

Sodium Channels

Figure 2 shows "whole-cell" records of the ionic current in both a rabbit cultured Schwann cell (A) and a rat cultured astrocyte (B). The particular Schwann cell in Fig. 2A was cultured from sciatic nerves of 1- or 2-day old rabbits. The sciatic nerve, it should be noted, is predominantly myelinated in the adult. Essentially identical results have been obtained from Schwann cells derived from neonatal vagus nerves (which are predominantly non-myelinated in the adult) and from adult sciatic and vagus nerves (Howe & Ritchie, 1990). The Schwann cells were prepared as in Shrager et al. (1985). The astrocytes were prepared according to the method described by McCarthy & de Vellis (1980) from rat cerebral cortex of 1- or 2-day old rats; more than 90% were type 1 astrocytes and were GFAP-positive, the remaining cells being fibroblast-like.

In both kinds of satellite cell, an early inward sodium current is clearly seen in Figure 2. In the particular Schwann cell illustrated, little or no delayed outward current is present, although potassium currents (as large as 12 nA) are usually seen. In the astrocyte illustrated, the outward current is particularly prominent.

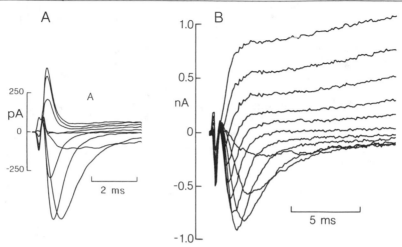

Figure 2. Ionic currents (leak subtracted) in whole-cell recordings from a rabbit cultured Schwann cell (*A*) and a rat cultured astrocyte (*B*). Cells were held at -70 mV, pulsed for 100 ms to -100 mV to remove sodium channel inactivation, and then taken in 10 or 20 mV steps to a series of potentials between -60 and +100 mV (*A*) or between -50 and +50 mV (*B*).

The sodium current in both kinds of satellite cell is in general similar to that recorded from the rabbit node of Ranvier (Chiu *et al.*, 1979). Thus, as Fig. 3*A* shows, the mid-point of the *h*-infinity curve is at a membrane potential of about -80 mV; and as can be seen from the peak current-voltage (*I/V*) curve in Fig. 3*B*, the inward current, which is first detectable when the cell is depolarized to -60 mV, reverses at a value very close to the predicted reversal potential for a perfectly Na$^+$-selective channel (which with the solutions used in this experiment was +69 mV).

The satellite cell and axolemmal sodium currents, however, are not identical. First, although the general shape of each *I/V* curve is similar, the mid-point of the first phase of both the Schwann cell and cortical astrocyte *I/V* curves is shifted about 25-30 mV in the depolarizing direction relative to that of the axolemma (Shrager *et al.*, 1985; Bevan *et al.*, 1985). A similar shift in the *I/V* curve also occurs in some optic nerve astrocytes, but in the *opposite* direction. Thus, Barres *et al.* (1989) have recently shown that the *I/V* curves of type 1 optic nerve astrocytes are displaced by about 10 mV in the *hyper*polarizing direction relative to the *I/V* curves of their associated retinal ganglion cells. Whether this represents an intrinsic difference between neuronal and satellite cell sodium channels, or whether this merely reflects a difference in the environment of the sodium channel in the different kinds of cell, remains unclear at the moment. It is pertinent that the position of the I/V curves of the ganglion cells is in fact identical to that of type 2 astrocytes i.e. there is no glial-neuronal shift (Barres *et al.*, 1989).

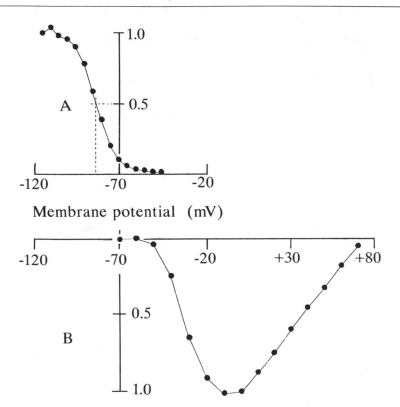

Figure 3. The normalized h-infinity (*A*) and peak current-voltage relation (*B*) for a rat cultured astrocyte.

The second difference is in the saxitoxin (and tetrodotoxin) sensitivity of astrocytes. Saxitoxin binding experiments reveal that both Schwann cells and astrocytes exhibit a high affinity binding site with an equilibrium dissociation constant of about 2 nM (Bevan *et al.*, 1985). In Schwann cells, electrophysiological patch clamp experiments reveal a similar high-affinity receptor for saxitoxin in the sodium channel (Howe & Ritchie, 1990). However, in astrocytes, very much larger concentrations of both saxitoxin and tetrodotoxin are required to affect conduction: thus, about 30 nM saxitoxin or 500 nM tetrodotoxin is required to half-block the whole-cell sodium current in cortical rat astrocytes (Bevan *et al.*, 1985). These astrocytes thus express two sensitivities to saxitoxin. There is a high affinity site revealed in the binding experiments, and a much lower affinity site revealed in the electrophysiological experiments. Whether this means there are two different kinds of sodium channel, or whether there is a single sodium channel that can exist in two states, is unclear at the moment. It should be noted that type 1 astrocytes from the rat optic nerve do exhibit high affinity block by tetrodotoxin (Barres *et al.*, 1989).

What is the function of satellite cell sodium channels?

The normal resting potential of cultured Schwann cells is quite low, being about -30 to -40 mV (Chiu *et al.*, 1984; Shrager *et al.*, 1985; Howe & Ritchie, 1990), at which potential all sodium channels would be inactivated (see Fig. 3). A similar small resting potential was found in the cortical astrocytes studied by Bevan *et al.* (1985), although some optic nerve astrocytes have resting potentials of -70 to -90 mV (see Barres *et al.*, 1989). Schwann cells obtained from explanted rabbit sciatic nerves similarly exhibit low resting potentials: according to Fig. 3 of Chiu & Wilson (1989) the average resting potential in Schwann cells from freshly explanted rabbit sciatic nerve is about -20 mV; and it rises to a peak value of about -50 mV at 8 days - still well into the region of complete inactivation. It seems unlikely, therefore, that these channels play any direct role in electrophysiological function either of Schwann cell or of at least some astrocytes.

One possible explanation for the presence of Schwann cell sodium channels is that they provide a local source of sodium channels for the axolemma of the neurons they ensheath (see Gray & Ritchie, 1986). This might be an important factor if the lifetime of the axolemmal sodium channels were as short as it is in the cultured Schwann cells. As can be seen in Fig. 4, the full expression of saxitoxin binding in a primary culture of Schwann cells takes about 6 days to reach a plateau after the culture is first set up. The initial absence of saxitoxin binding capacity seems to be a result of the dissociation procedure, which involves exposure of the Schwann cells to large concentrations of proteolytic enzyme and collagenase. The saxitoxin binding capacity is destroyed by this procedure; and it recovers relatively slowly only as synthesis of new sodium channels progresses (Ritchie, 1988). If, once the sodium channel expression has reached its plateau, the culture is now re-exposed to the proteolytic enzyme, the saxitoxin binding capacity is again destroyed; and it recovers along the same time course as before. The time constant of recovery is about 3 days. Conversely, exposure of the cells to to tunicamycin, an inhibitor of glycosylation, leads to a progressive exponential fall in saxitoxin binding capacity, again with a time constant of about 3 days.

These experiments with protease and tunicamycin both lead to the conclusion that the Schwann cell sodium channels have an average life-time of about 3 days (based on the assumption that the steady state density of Schwann cell sodium channels is maintained by a constant synthesis of channels in the face of a rate of loss from the membrane proportional to the amount of channel already present). Such a rapid turnover would clearly impose a large metabolic load on a neuron if all the channels in the axon had to be made in its cell body. It has been calculated (Ritchie, 1988) that a small neuron might be required to replace 8% of its total cell protein mass daily just as sodium channels - a replacement that would present a not inconsiderable metabolic load. In remyelinating and regenerating

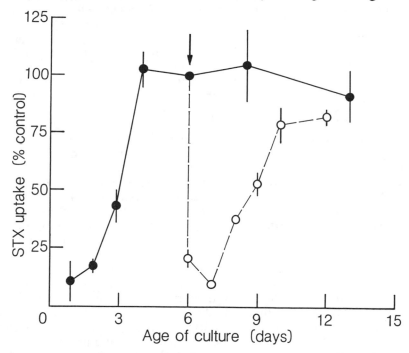

Figure 4. The uptake of labeled saxitoxin by rabbit cultured Schwann cells at various times after setting up the primary cell culture. At each time point, triplicate determinations of the saturable uptake at 2.4 nM were made of each on at least 3 different preparations. Each uptake was expressed as a fraction of the value at 6 days and the mean values obtained (the bars represent $\pm$ 1 SEM). At 6 days, one batch was re-exposed to the proteolytic enzyme used for dissociation (broken line) and the recovery of saxitoxin binding followed.

myelinated nerve, where there are many more nodes per unit length of nerve, and presumably more sodium channels (see Ritchie *et al.*, 1981; Ritchie, 1982), the load would be even more extreme. Nevertheless, although this hypothesis is very intriguing and has some circumstantial morphological and biochemical support (see Gray & Ritchie, 1985), *direct* evidence in its favor is lacking at the moment.

Extraneuronal sodium channels are present both normally and pathophysiologically

Extraneuronal sodium channels are clearly present in abnormal or pathophysiological circumstances. Thus, they were first demonstrated in Wallerian degeneration in rabbit peripheral nerve trunks (Ritchie & Rang, 1983) and subsequently in primary cultures of Schwann cells (Chiu *et al.*, 1984; Shrager *et al.*, 1985). Such extraneuronal sodium channels, however, must also be present in normal nerve, because the amount that can be attributed solely to binding to the nodal axolemma is far too small to account for more than a fraction of the total binding of 19.9 fmole/mg (Ritchie & Rogart, 1977). Chiu & Schwarz (1987) from electrophysiological experiments give a value of 24,000 sodium channels per node for a rabbit sciatic axon of diameter 18-20 μm, whose nodal area would be about 35 μm^2 (Rydmark & Berthold, 1983); Neumcke & Stämpfli (1982) give a similar number of 21,000 for rat node. The nodal channel density is thus about 750/μm^2. Gating current measurements in corresponding rabbit sciatic nodes give an upper limit of 82,000 channels per node (Chiu & Ritchie, 1981). Even if the density were as high as 2,000/μm^2 (so allowing for electrically silent or inactivated channels), binding to the nodal axolemma would only be about 2.7 fmole/mg. Given that fibroblasts do not bind saxitoxin at all (Gray *et al.*, 1986), that binding to the non-myelinated fibers (including their associated non-myelinating Schwann cells) in the sciatic nerve is about 2.8 fmole/mg (Ritchie & Rogart, 1977), and that the binding to the internodal axolemma, with a density of less than 25/μm^2 (Ritchie & Rogart, 1977; Chiu & Schwartz, 1988), cannot be more (and may indeed be considerably less) than 4.8 fmole/mg, it becomes clear that about half of the observed total binding of 19.9 fmole/mg must have been to Schwann cells of normal *myelinated* axons. Even in the Schwann cells of normal rat sciatic nerve, where in cell culture (Shrager *et al.*, 1985) and in Wallerian degeneration *in vivo* (Ritchie & Rang, 1983) there is relatively little expression of plasmalemmal Schwann cell sodium channels, such channels must be also abundant because the saturable uptake of saxitoxin by rat sciatic nerve is even greater than in rabbit nerve. Indeed, rat sciatic nerve has a saxitoxin-binding capacity of nearly triple that in rabbit sciatic nerve, which would be even more difficult to account for solely in terms of neuronal binding (Ritchie, 1984). Just why expression of these sodium channels in the rat is absent, or perhaps down-regulated, in pathophysiological situations is not clear at the moment.

In summary, the balance sheet in normal rabbit myelinated nerve trunks seems to be that, as far as *numbers* are concerned, the bulk of the sodium channels (about 50%) are extraneuronal and are associated with myelinating Schwann cells. Less than 25% of the channels are associated with the internodal axolemma; about 15% are associated with the non-myelinated fibers and their ensheathing non-myelinating Schwann cells; and the remaining small percentage is associated with the nodal axolemma. The plasmalemmal *densities*, however, are in quite a different order; and there is a considerable inhomogeneity present. The nodal channel density is at least $750/\mu m^2$; the Schwann plasmalemmal density is about $30/\mu m^2$ (Shrager et al., 1985); the internodal axolemmal density is less than $25/\mu m^2$ (Ritchie & Rogart, 1977; Chiu & Schwarz, 1987); and fibroblasts do not bind saxitoxin in measurable amounts (Gray et al., 1986).

One puzzling feature of the extranodal sodium channels is the large variation in size of the sodium currents that is found from one cell to the next. Although practically all cultured Schwann cells express sodium currents, the amplitude varies by 2 orders of magnitude -- from tens of pA to values as large as 1-2 nA. This lability in current amplitude (see also Chiu et al., 1984) is observed too with astrocytic sodium currents (Bevan et al., 1985; Barres et al., 1989). It is interesting that this large *individual* variation in the size of the sodium current occurs in the face of a relatively constant *population* expression of sodium channels: cultures of rabbit Schwann cells bind saxitoxin to the extent of 200-400 fmole/mg protein with comparatively little variation.

Potassium channels

Cultured rat astrocytes and cultured rabbit Schwann cells both express a delayed voltage-dependent outward current. As is the case with the voltage-dependent sodium currents, the amplitude of this current varies greatly from one individual cell to the next. In some cells it is quite small (as, for example, in the Schwann cell in Fig. 2A) whereas in others it is much larger (for example, in the astrocyte in Fig. 2B) and may be as high as 12 nA. Because satellite cells also express plasmalemmal chloride channels, the potassium currents are usually studied in the absence of extracellular chloride (the main anion in the bathing solution being gluconate).

At least two types of potassium channel are present in cultured Schwann cells (Howe & Ritchie, 1988). While both kinds are equally sensitive to channel block by TEA, the two populations are not equally sensitive to block by 4-aminopyridine (i.e. there is a 4-AP-sensitive and a relatively 4-AP-insensitive population of channels). Figure 5, for exam-

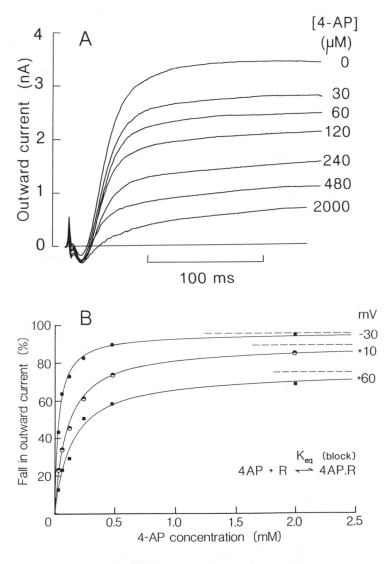

Figure 5. (*A*) Ionic currents (leak subtracted) in a Schwann cell pulsed from a holding potential of -70 mV to a test potential of +10 mV in the presence of various concentrations of 4-AP; concentrations in μM are indicated at the side of each record. (*B*) The decrease in outward current expressed as a percentage of the current in 4-AP free solution at that potential (and two others) is plotted as a function of 4-AP concentration. The curves are least-squares fits to rectangular hyperbolae.

ple, shows the ionic currents in a Schwann cell pulsed from a holding potential of -70 mV to a test potential of +10 mV in the presence of various concentrations of 4-AP. As can be seen, the potassium current (which is first detectable at a potential of about -50 mV) progressively decreases as the 4-AP concentration is progressively increased. But the degree of block of the potassium current clearly approaches a limiting value. This value can be estimated by plotting the fall in outward current as a function of 4-AP concentration (Fig. 5B), and then fitting the data to a rectangular hyperbola. As can be seen, about 15% of the current evoked by depolarization to +10 mV is relatively insensitive to 4-AP. The 4-AP insensitive fraction is relatively smaller at -30 mV; and it is relatively much larger at +60 mV.

Howe & Ritchie (1988) also pointed out that there is a small third component of outward current which is largely insensitive to both 4-AP and to TEA and has no clear correspondence with any axolemmal potassium channel described so far. Whether or not these three kinds of channel correspond with the three described by DuBois (1981) for frog nodes of Ranvier on the basis of their kinetic behavior is at present unclear.

Functional significance of satellite cell potassium channels

One suggestion for the function of at least one of these groups of potassium channels in astrocytes and Schwann cells is that it is involved in Schwann cell proliferation. As early as 1967, Lubin had suggested that intracellular potassium is important in protein synthesis; and, indeed, subsequent work has shown that voltage-dependent potassium channels are involved in cell division in T lymphocytes (DeCoursey et al., 1984) and rabbit fibroblasts (Gray et al., 1986). It is interesting, therefore, that Chiu & Wilson (1989) have recently shown in experiments on sectioned rabbit sciatic nerve that the increase in thymidine incorporation that accompanies the proliferation of Schwann cells during Wallerian degeneration is completely inhibited by small concentrations of TEA. When the TEA is removed, thymidine incorporation resumes. Potassium channels, thus, are involved in some way in Schwann cell proliferation: when they are blocked cell proliferation does not occur.

This, however, may not be the only function of satellite cell potassium channels. It seems clear that at least some of the glial astrocytic cells in the central nervous system are involved in the spatial buffering of potassium ions. A problem arises in the central nervous system because active neurons release potassium into a relatively restricted extracellular space. The result is a rise in extracellular potassium concentration, which if not dealt with would lead to a block of neuronal function. As is well known from the work of Kuffler and his colleagues (e.g. Kuffler et al., 1956) two properties of the glial cells enable them to buffer this rise in extracellular potassium concentration. The first is that the astrocytes are electrically coupled together to form a large glial syncytium. The second is they have a high potassium permeability. The result is that there is a potential difference between active regions with high extracellular potassium concentrations and more remote, neuronally inactive, parts of the syncytium. This potential difference causes a current to flow that drives potassium into the glial cell syncytium in the region of high extracellular concentration and out of the glial cells more remotely. The net effect is a transfer of potassium from a region where the extracellular potassium concentration is high to one where it is low. Much of this buffering would occur through potassium channels that are already open at rest. Indeed, Newman has pointed out that the inward rectifier potassium channels in single glial cells of the retina that he elegantly studies are particularly well adapted to this function of transferring potassium away from the region of electrically active retinal ganglion cells into the vitreous humor. The retinal glial cell achieves this by a strikingly non-uniform distribution of potassium conductance along its length, which allows for the influx of potassium ions in the region of the retinal ganglion cells, but restricts the efflux principally, in the different species studied (Newman, 1987), to an area of high conductance abutting either the vitreous humor or retinal blood vessels. The voltage-dependent channels described above would be recruited only with intense neuronal activity, which might lead to dangerously high extracellular potassium concentrations -- high concentrations which would in turn open the potassium channels.

Chloride channels

In the first experiments describing voltage-gated sodium and potassium channels in rat cultured astrocytes it was noted that only about 70% of the outward current was sensitive to TEA (Bevan *et al.*, 1985). This outward current also persisted when the main cation in the pipette was cesium, which would have been expected to block completely outward potassium current (Fig. 6A). This persisting current, which is seen more clearly in Fig. 6B on a longer time base, is the result of an inward movement of chloride ions. Thus, when the chloride of the bathing medium is replaced by the larger organic anion gluconate, there is a rapid abolition of this outward current (Fig. 6C), which is quickly restored on replacing gluconate with chloride again. As might be expected from a chloride current, this outward current is blocked by the disulfonate stilbene inhibitors of chloride transport, DIDS and SITS.

This channel is somewhat more permeable to the bromide ion than to chloride ion. It is reasonably permeable to methylsulfate, sulfate and isethionate, it is sparingly soluble to acetate, and it is hardly at all permeable to glutamate, aspartate, or gluconate (Gray & Ritchie, 1986).

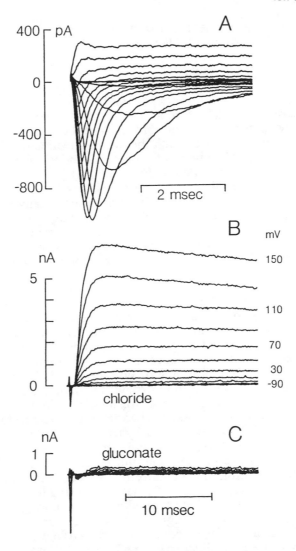

Figure 6. (*A*) Ionic currents (leak subtracted) in whole-cell recordings from a rat cultured astrocyte. The pipette solution contained 150 mM CsCl. The cell was held at -70 mV, pulsed for 100 ms to -100 mV to remove sodium channel inactivation and then taken in 10 mV steps to a series of potentials between -70 and +120 mV. (*B*) Records of the outward currents (whole-cell recording) from a rat cultured astrocyte (with N-methyl-(+)-glucamine gluconate in the pipette). The cell was held at -70 mV, pulsed to -100 mV for 100 msec, and then brought to the potentials indicated. (*C*) The same family of records as in (*B*) obtained shortly after the sodium chloride of the bathing medium had been replaced by sodium gluconate.

A similar chloride channel has now been shown to be present in rabbit Schwann cells (Howe & Ritchie, 1988).

Function of chloride channels

The astrocyte chloride current can first be detected with depolarizations to membrane potentials of about -50 mV; and it continues to increase at more positive potentials. Under physiological conditions, chloride is the ion carrying the current through the anion-selective conductance, so that from the physiological point of view this conductance can probably be considered to be a chloride conductance. Although many chloride channels have been described in other tissues, few resemble the voltage-gated conductance in Schwann cells and astrocytes. Many (for example, ligand-activated channels) show little or no voltage-dependence; and others, which do show a strong voltage-dependence, are quite different in character, being open near 0 mV and closing rapidly on changing the potential by more than 20 mV in either direction (see Gray & Ritchie, 1986 for references).

As to the function of the astrocytic chloride channels Bevan et al. (1985) pointed out that voltage-gated chloride channels could provide a useful adjunct to the potassium buffering mechanism described above that is often ascribed to astrocytes, particularly under extreme conditions where high external potassium concentrations would substantially depolarize the astrocyte. The presence of voltage-gated chloride channels would permit chloride to enter the astrocytes with potassium released by locally active neurons. The presence of the chloride channels has the advantage of allowing the potassium that has been released by the active neurons to be stored locally in the nearby astrocyte as potassium chloride rather than being dumped remotely, as in the hypothesis generally proposed (e.g. Coles & Orkand, 1983; Gardner-Medwin, 1983). This in turn means that the potassium may be more readily accessible to the neuron when it attempts to recapture its lost potassium during the recovery process. Such a mechanism could work in addition to a more general transfer of potassium from regions of high to low concentration. Clearly, the Schwann cell chloride channels could similarly aid in clearing potassium from the periaxonal extracellular space of peripheral axons.

ACKNOWLEDGEMENTS

This work was supported in part by grants NS08304 and NS12327 from the USPHS and by a grant RG1162 from the National Multiple Sclerosis Society.

REFERENCES

Barres BA, Chun LLY, Corey DP (1989). Glial and neuronal forms of the voltage-dependent sodium channel: characteristics and cell-type distribution. Neuron 2:1375-1388.

Bevan S, Chiu SY, Gray PTA, Ritchie JM (1985). The presence of voltage-gated sodium, potassium and chloride channels in rat cultured astrocytes. Proc R Soc Lond B 225:299-313.

Chiu SY, Ritchie JM (1981). Ionic and gating currents in mammalian myelinated nerve. In Waxman SG, Ritchie JM (eds): "Demyelinating Diseases." New York: Raven, pp 313-328.

Chiu SY, Ritchie JM, Rogart RB, Stagg D (1979). A quantitative description of membrane currents in rabbit myelinated nerve. J Physiol (Lond) 292:149-166.

Chiu SY, Schwarz W (1987). Sodium and potassium currents in acutely demyelinated internodes of rabbit sciatic nerves. J Physiol (Lond) 391:631-649.

Chiu SY, Shrager P, Ritchie JM (1984). Neuronal-type Na^+ and K^+ channels in rabbit cultured Schwann cells. Nature 311:156-157.

Chiu SY, Wilson GF (1989). The role of potassium channels in Schwann cell proliferation in Wallerian degeneration of explant rabbit sciatic nerves. J Physiol (Lond) 408:199-222.

Coles JA, Orkand RK (1983). Chloride enters receptors and glia in response to light or raised external potassium in the retina slices of the bee drone, *Apis mellifera.* J Physiol (Lond) 357:11P.

DeCoursey TE, Chandy KG, Gupta S, Cahalan MD (1984). Voltage-gated K channels in human T lymphocytes: a role in mitogenesis? Nature 307:465-468.

DuBois JM (1981). Evidence for the existence of three types of potassium channel in the frog Ranvier node membrane. J Physiol (Lond) 318:297-316.

Gardner-Medwin AR (1983a). A study of the mechanisms by which potassium moves through brain in the rat tissue. J Physiol (Lond) 355:353-374.

Gray PTA, Chiu SY, Bevan S, Ritchie JM (1986). Ion channels in rabbit cultured fibroblasts. Proc R Soc Lond B 227:1-16.

Gray PTA, Ritchie JM (1985). Ion channels in Schwann and glial cells. Trends in Neurosci 8:411-415.

Gray PTA, Ritchie JM (1986). A voltage-gated chloride conductance in rat cultured astrocytes. Proc R Soc Lond B 228:267-288.

Hamill OP, Marty A, Sakmann B, Sigworth FJ (1981). Improved patch-clamp techniques for high-resolution current recording for cells and cell-free membrane patches. Eur J Physiol 391:85-100.

Howe JR, Ritchie JM (1988). Two types of potassium current in rabbit cultured Schwann cells. Proc R Soc Lond B 235:119-127.

Howe JR, Ritchie JM (1990). Sodium currents in Schwann cells from myelinated and non-myelinated nerves of neonatal and adult rabbits. J Physiol (Lond) In the Press.

Kuffler SW, Nicholls JG, Martin AR (1984). "From Neuron to Brain." Sunderland MA: Sinauer.

Kuffler SW, Nicholls JG, Orkand (1966). Physiological properties of glial cells in the central nervous system of amphibia. J Neurophysiol 29:768-787.

Lubin M (1967). Intracellular potassium and macromolecular synthesis in mammalian cells. Nature 213:451-453.

McCarthy K, de Vellis J (1980). Preparation of separate astroglial and oligodendroglial cell cultures from rat cerebral tissue. J Cell Biol 85:890-902.

Neumcke B, Stämpfli R (1982). Sodium currents and sodium-current fluctuations in rat myelinated nerve fibres. J Physiol (Lond) 329:163-184.

Newman EA (1987). Distribution of potassium conductance in mammalian Müller (glial) cells: a comparative study. J Neurosci 7:2423-2432.

Orkand RK (1982). Signalling between neuronal and glial cells. In Sears TA (ed): "Neuronal-glial Cell Interrelationships." Heidelberg: Springer-Verlag, pp 147-158.

Ritchie JM (1982). Sodium and potassium channels in regenerating and developing mammalian myelinated nerves. Proc R Soc Lond B 215:277-287.

Ritchie JM (1984). Distribution of sodium and potassium channels in mammalian myelinated nerve. In Serratrice *et al.* (eds): "Neuromuscular Diseases". New York: Raven, pp 247-252.

Ritchie JM (1988). Sodium-channel turnover in rabbit cultured Schwann cells. Proc R Soc Lond B 33:423-430.

Ritchie JM, Rogart RB (1977). Density of sodium channels in mammalian myelinated nerve fibers and nature of the axonal membrane under the myelin sheath. Proc Nat Acad Sci USA 74:211-215.

Ritchie JM, Rang HP (1983). Extraneuronal saxitoxin binding sites in rabbit myelinated nerve. Proc Natl Acad Sci USA 80:2803-2807.

Ritchie JM, Rang HP, Pellegrino R (1981). Sodium and potassium channels in demyelinated and remyelinated mammalian nerve. Nature 294:257-259.

Rydmark M, Berthold C-H (1983). Electron microscopic serial section analysis of nodes of Ranvier in lumbar spinal roots of the cat: a morphometric study of nodal compartments of fibres of different sizes. J Neurocytol 12:537-565.

Shrager P, Chiu SY, Ritchie JM (1985). Voltage-dependent sodium and potassium channels in mammalian cultured Schwann cells.

Advances in Neural Regeneration
Research, pages 253–255
© 1990 Wiley-Liss, Inc.

MOLECULAR MECHANISMS RELEVANT TO REGENERATION

Jeremy P. Brockes

Ludwig Institute for Cancer Research
91 Riding House Street, London WIP 8BT
England

The four contributions to this section on molecular mechanisms relevant to regeneration cover a diverse set of topics. Nonetheless they can all be accomodated within the developmental history of the neuron. That is, its birth from precursor cells in the neuroepithelium, its adoption of a mature phenotype, and its participation in regeneration after the appropriate stimuli. A major effort in regeneration research has been, and continues to be, the identification of those environmental influences, such as soluble factors, extracellular matrix, or proximity to other cells, that can influence the neuron. It is understandable that much of this work treats the neuron as a black box, but the present contributions are indicative of our increasing understanding of the intracellular machinery. They are concerned with molecules such as signal transduction proteins, transcription factors and cytoskeletal proteins that mediate basic processes in the developing and regenerating nerve cell.

It has been very difficult to analyze in vertebrates how an undifferentiated precursor is triggered to become a neuron. Recent investigations of neurogenesis in the *Drosphila* eye have used a combined genetic and molecular approach to identify molecules involved in this fundamental process. Such investigations have already uncovered the role of a membrane associated tyrosine kinase in mediating formation of the R7 photoreceptor. The *Drosphila* eye is a nonclonal system of development that may be a powerful model for vertebrate development, particularly in terms of basic molecular mechanisms.

A second, previously refractory problem that is now yielding to molecular analysis is that of positional specification in the developing vertebrate CNS. Here again, studies on *Drosphila* have provided the tools to isolate vertebrate transcription factors containing the homeobox or zinc finger motifs. The pattern of expression of these molecules has already had a considerable impact on our understanding of the metameric organization of the developing CNS, particularly in the hindbrain.

The effects of stress and injury on neurons, as well as the response to trophic factors, are all mediated by signal transduction proteins that include some of the previously identified proto-oncogenes. It is most important to try and elucidate the mechanisms involved in these processes that can change the internal state of the nerve cell. A fundamental aspect of mobilizing the neuron for process extension is the expression of genes for cytoskeletal proteins. The availability of cloned probes for these genes has allowed us to appreciate the subtlety of their regulation in both development and regeneration.

In order to help the reader appreciate some of the parallels between the various topics in this section, I should like to mention two general issues that are common to them. One is the relationship between development and regeneration, an old question that is receiving new impetus from the molecular studies. Are there fundamental differences of mechanism resulting from the need to establish regenerative events within the constraints of a mature rather than a developing nerve cell? Do stress and injury responses play a role in mediating this requirement? To what extent is positional specificataion "remembered" in regeneration, and will it be necessary to reevoke expression of developmental transcription factors?

The second general issue arises from the fact that most of the components under consideration are used in other, nonneural cells, and we can derive added insights from appreciating this. For example, the proto-oncogenes such as tyrosine kinases, fos or ras are most familiar in the context of control or proliferation. In the postmitotic neuron they are apparently used to mediate processes such as repair, cellular commitment, and process extension. What are the mechanistic parallels to be drawn from a consideration of these molecules in the different contexts? The expression of homeobox genes in the developing CNS has provided the clearest example of their position dependent expression in vertebrates. Nonetheless they are also expressed in other embryonic fields such as the limb and one wonders if there are mechanistic similarities, and precisely what aspects of the neuronal phenotype are determined by their expression. Recent work has uncovered even more parallels with *Drosphila* in terms of the large scale organization of the gene clusters and their patterns of expression.

These mechanisms are relevant to regeneration not just in the basic sense of our understanding of the process. We can look forward to a time when we can take advantage of this understanding to allow manipulation of these events to promote regeneration.

**Advances in Neural Regeneration
Research, pages 257–275
© 1990 Wiley-Liss, Inc.**

CHANGES IN CYTOSKELETAL GENE EXPRESSION DURING AXONAL
REGROWTH IN MAMMALIAN NEURONS

Monica M. Oblinger and Johnson Wong

Department of Cell Biology & Anatomy,
Chicago Medical School, North Chicago, IL
60064

INTRODUCTION

In the peripheral nervous system, axonal regeneration
after disconnection of the axon from its cell body by a
crush lesion follows an orderly pattern that ultimately
results in the reconstitution of function. It is clear that
the cytoskeletal polymers, microfilaments, microtubules, and
NFs, play important roles in all phases of the regrowth of
axons. During the first phase of regrowth, sprouting, fine
caliber sprouts emerge from the parent stump of axon that
remains attached to the cell body and begin to grow distally
(Fig. 1). During this stage, actin microfilaments are
essential for growth cone motility. Next, the active
elongation phase of growth ensues. The insertion of
microtubules to stabilize the elongating daughter axons is
critical to this phase. Finally, provided that an
appropriate target is contacted and an appropriate
connection is made, the new axons enter the last phase of
regeneration, maturation. This final stage involves the
radial growth of the new axons by the recruitment of
increased numbers of neurofilaments (NFs) into the axons
(Lasek et al., 1983), as well as the remyelination of axons
by Schwann cells. Thus, during all stages of regeneration,
the cytoskeleton provides the basis for motility, structure
and stabilization of the new axons. Recent studies have
documented major changes in the biosynthesis of various
cytoskeletal components during axonal regeneration and
helped to define the molecular mechanisms by which the
cytoskeleton influences axonal growth. In the following
section, we review the general scheme by which the axonal
cytoskeleton is generated and examine how axotomy impinges
on this scheme.

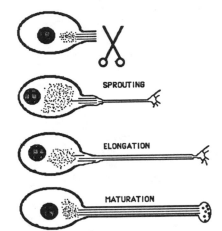

SPROUTING

ELONGATION

MATURATION

FIGURE 1. Schematic diagram showing the major steps in axonal regeneration that involve the neuronal cytoskeleton.

THE AXONAL CYTOSKELETON IS GENERATED BY A HIGHLY VECTORIAL PROCESS WHICH IS ALTERED BY AXONAL INJURY

The vectorial process that supplies the axonal cytoskeleton begins in the neuronal cell body with the transcription of cytoskeletal genes and ends at the axon tip with the degradation of the cytoskeletal polymers (Fig. 2). Since transcription is the first step in the flow of genetic information, changes at this level could have major effects downstream on the composition of the axonal cytoskeleton. At present, nothing is known about the effects of axon injury on the transcription of cytoskeletal genes. However, a fair amount has been learned about the next level in the vectorial process, the mRNA level. The level of various cytoskeletal protein mRNAs in cells is set by both transcription rate and degradation. Without distinguishing between these two factors, *in situ* hybridization methods have provided a sensitive assay for measuring changes in steady state levels of various mRNA species. Recent studies of rat dorsal root ganglion (DRG) neurons have shown that peripheral axotomy induces changes in the level of NF, tubulin and actin mRNAs (Hoffman et al., 1987; Wong and Oblinger, 1987; Hoffman and Cleveland, 1988, Oblinger et al., 1989a). The consensus is that NF mRNA levels decrease and tubulin and actin mRNA levels rise during the initial weeks after axotomy.

Translation of cytoskeletal proteins is the next major step in the vectorial process that generates the axonal cytoskeleton (Fig. 2). Studies in DRG and other types of neurons have shown that the synthesis of NF proteins is significantly reduced in the first few weeks after axotomy (Oblinger and Lasek, 1985, 1988; Greenberg and Lasek, 1988). During the same interval, actin synthesis increases and tubulin synthesis either increases or doesn't change, depending on experimental conditions (Greenberg and Lasek, 1988, Oblinger and Lasek, 1985, 1988). It is likely that these changes in protein synthesis are driven by changes in the levels of translationally active mRNAs. Most of the newly synthesized cytoskeletal proteins are destined for export into the axon, and thus, the level of biosynthesis is a critical determinant of the number of NFs, microtubules and microfilaments in axons.

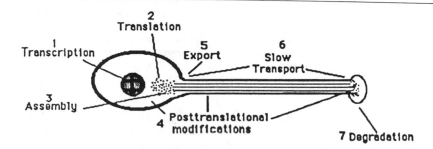

FIGURE 2. Schematic diagram illustrating the central dogma about the biogenesis of the neuronal cytoskeleton. The scheme begins with the utilization of genetic information in the nucleus and progresses numerically to the degradation step at the axon terminal.

Several intermediate steps lie between translation and axonal transport of the cytoskeletal elements, but these are less well understood. Assembly of cytoskeletal proteins into polymer is clearly an important step since cytoskeletal proteins do not appear to be transported in the monomer form (reviewed in Lasek, 1988). While assembly of cytoskeletal proteins is tightly temporally linked to translation in normal neurons (Black et al., 1986), nothing is presently known about this process in injured neurons. Also, the mechanisms by which the cytoskeleton is exported from the soma into the axon are poorly understood. Several studies have suggested that the export of NFs from the soma may be affected by axotomy since NFs accumulate in the soma of some axotomized neurons (Goldstein et al., 1987). More complex mechanisms such as selective export/routing of NFs into the 2 axonal branches of DRG cells after axotomy have also been described (Oblinger and Lasek, 1985, 1988). The signal(s)

that target cytoskeletal or associated proteins for export
to the axon (or other neuronal compartments) remain to be
identified and then studied during axonal regrowth.

The final pathway for expression of the cytoskeletal
genes is axonal transport (Fig. 2). NFs and microtubules
are conveyed through axons by slow axonal transport (Lasek
and Hoffman, 1976). After axotomy, reduced levels of NF
protein and increased levels and rates of tubulin transport
in intact axonal regions of injured neurons have been
reported (Hoffman and Lasek, 1980; Oblinger and Lasek,
1988). Changes in the rate as well as the amount of NF
transport are known to have morphological consequences. For
example, a reduced level of NFs entering the axonal
transport system after distal axotomy results in a reduction
in axon caliber which proceeds somatofugally at the rate of
slow transport (Hoffman et al., 1987). After axotomy, slow
axonal transport also functions to move the cytoskeletal
polymers from the parent axons into and through the
regenerating sprouts (McQuarrie and Lasek, 1988; Oblinger et
al., 1989a).

From the preceding discussion, it is clear that there
are numerous levels at which factors generated by an axotomy
could act to alter the flow of genetic information which
ultimately generates the cytoskeleton. In the following
sections we will discuss some of our recent findings on
axotomy-induced changes in cytoskeletal biosynthesis and
discuss how we envision that these alterations feed-forward
on the actual process of regeneration.

REGULATION OF NF TRIPLET GENES DURING REGENERATION

Recently, we and others documented a down regulation
of NF-L, one of the three NF genes, in adult rat DRG neurons
after axotomy (Wong and Oblinger, 1987; Hoffman et al.,
1987; Oblinger et al., 1989a). As a result, we became
interested in the question of whether or not all of the NF
genes were coordinately regulated during regeneration.
During initial neural development, the three NF proteins are
not expressed coordinately. The low (NF-L, ~68kDa) and
middle (NF-M, ~145kDa) molecular weight subunits appear
temporally before the high molecular weight (NF-H, ~200kDa)
protein (Willard and Simon, 1983). This pattern of NF
protein expression appears to be driven by a similar pattern
of change in NF mRNA expression during development (Julien
et al., 1986).

We used quantitative *in situ* hybridization methods to

compare changes in the levels of each of the NF mRNAs in
adult L5 DRG neurons from 1d to 8 weeks after sciatic nerve
crush (Wong and Oblinger, 1989). Histological sections of
DRGs were hybridized with ^{35}S-labeled cDNA probes specific
for the various NF mRNA species (NF-L, Lewis and Cowan,
1985; NF-M, Julien et al., 1986; NF-H, Robinson et al.,
1986) and analyzed as described (Wong and Oblinger, 1987).
The results indicated that, generally, the 3 NF mRNAs
undergo similar patterns of change after axotomy (Fig. 3).
That is, all 3 mRNA species are reduced during the initial
weeks after injury, and all 3 mRNAs recover to
nearly normal levels of expression at later times (Fig. 3).
There are also differences, the most notable being that NF-H
mRNA levels downregulate more slowly than NF-L and NF-M.
Overall, however, the NF gene family appears to be regulated
in a coordinate manner during regeneration.

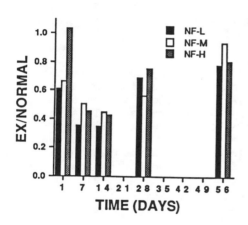

FIGURE 3. Time course
of changes in NF triplet
mRNA levels after axotomy as
determined by quantitative
in situ hybridization with
[35]S-labeled cDNA probes
specific for each of the
different NF mRNAs. From
autoradiograms, the mean
density of silver grains
over large-sized (>1000 μm^2)
L5 DRG neurons at each of
the indicated days after
sciatic nerve crush was
determined and expressed as
a fraction of the normal
value.

In many axotomy experiments the uninjured
contralateral neurons serve as the comparison for axotomized
neurons. However, a variety of changes in contralateral
neurons have been reported after peripheral nerve injury
(Watson, 1968; Lieberman, 1971; Pearson et al., 1988).
Recently, we have observed major changes in the expression
of NF mRNAs in contralateral, uninjured DRG neurons after
axotomy (Wong & Oblinger, 1990). Using quantitative *in situ*
hybridization methods, a robust downregulation in NF-L mRNA
levels in uninjured contralateral DRG neurons has been found
after both central (Fig. 4) and peripheral branch axotomy
(not shown). The reductions in NF-L mRNA levels in the
contralateral neurons, while not as substantial as in
axotomized neurons, are still quite dramatic (Fig. 4).

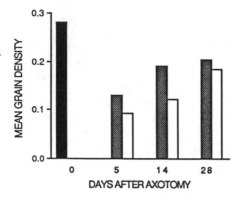

FIGURE 4. Changes in NF-L mRNA levels in axotomized (open bars) and contralateral control (stippled bars) L5 DRG neurons after dorsal root crush. Solid bar indicates the mRNA level found in normal, untreated, control neurons. Mean grain densities over large-sized neurons were determined from autoradiograms generated by *in situ* hybridization with a ^{35}S-labeled cDNA probe.

In large myelinated axons, axonal caliber is determined largely by the number and density of NFs (Lasek et al., 1983; Hoffman et al., 1988). A reduction in NF number in proximal regions of injured axons can result from downregulated levels of NF mRNA expression (Hoffman et al., 1987). Thus, our findings of reduced NF mRNA levels in contralateral DRG neurons after axotomy suggest that the diameter of contralateral sensory axons might be altered after axotomy. Interestingly, reductions in the size of axons in the contralateral sciatic nerve as well as the ipsilateral nerve after unilateral crush injury were documented much earlier this century (Fig. 5; Greenman, 1913). Our current findings on mRNA changes demonstrate the underlying molecular basis for the reported changes in the caliber of contralateral (Greenman, 1913) as well as the axotomized (Hoffman et al., 1987; Greenman, 1913) DRG axons.

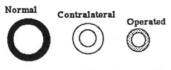

Average areas of largest nerve fibers
(proximal to lesion site)

FIGURE 5. Schematic diagram illustrating the changes in the caliber of sciatic nerve axons after distal crush. Note that contralateral as well as injured axons decrease in size. Redrawn from Figure 3 in Greenman et al., 1913.

Why do changes occur in contralateral neurons after axotomy? One possibility is that the changes are a result of compensatory sprouting of contralateral axons. Originally proposed as a "work hypertrophy" effect by Watson

(1968), the idea is that an increased work load on the contralateral limb which occurs after denervation of the other limb stimulates axonal sprouting (to innervate a larger or more active target). For motor fibers, sprouting of uninjured motor fibers on the contralateral side of the animal after axotomy has been documented (Ring et al., 1983). If sprouting of sensory fibers also occurs, the molecular changes in NF expression observed in contralateral neurons may simply accompany such axonal growth. The time course of possible sprouting events for contralateral sensory fibers has yet to be examined.

How are the NF genes regulated? While the answers to this question are not known, it has been suggested that factor(s) derived from target cell interactions are important to NF gene expression (Hoffman et al., 1988). The possibilities for such a factor are exogenous molecules (released by the target) that are taken up at the axon tip and retrogradely transported to the neuron cell body, or molecules produced in the cell body that are transported to the end of the axon where they are modified and subsequently returned to the cell body. We favor the second possibility due to results of our recent studies of DRG neurons after dorsal root (central branch) lesions (Wong and Oblinger, 1990). Crushed dorsal root axons of rats do not "successfully regenerate" in the sense of reestablishing functional connections with appropriate target neurons in the CNS. However, when we examined the time course and magnitude of change in NF-L mRNA levels after central axotomy using quantitative *in situ* hybridization methods, we found that the changes are nearly identical to those seen after peripheral branch axotomy (Wong and Oblinger, 1990; also see Figs. 3 & 4 above). That is, during the initial 2 weeks after axotomy the level of NF-L mRNA is reduced; at later times, recovery towards control values occurs.

Regenerating central branch DRG axons are known to make aberrant synaptic-like endings on astrocytes at the CNS entry zone (Liuzzi and Lasek, 1987). It has been proposed that mature astrocytes induce the formation of such terminal structures by providing a functional "stop" signal to growing axons (Liuzzi and Lasek, 1987). The aberrant endings made by regenerating dorsal root axons on astrocytes at the CNS entry zone can apparently degrade cytoskeleton since electron microscopic examination has demonstrated that these endings are devoid of NFs and microtubules (Liuzzi and Lasek, 1987). In normal neurons, NF proteins are degraded in the axon terminal by calcium activated neutral proteases called calpains (Lasek et al., 1983). It is possible that NF degradation products generated at functional axon endings by calpains and transported retrogradely back to the cell body are important in regulating NF gene expression in a positive direction. If this is the case, then after axotomy, when the cell is deprived of such products, NF gene expression would be downregulated, and after reconnection and formation of a functional axon tip (with respect to degradation), NF gene expression would recover.

While undoubtedly overly simplistic, this model can account for the central branch axotomy results discussed above. The aberrant axoglial endings which are active in NF degradation would enable recovery of normal levels of NF mRNA expression in the DRG neurons in spite of the fact that the dorsal root axons had not regrown to their original target neurons. The model is also useful when considering the events of normal neural development. Radial growth of axons during development has generally been found to ensue once target connection is made. In that case, functional terminals begin to degrade NFs and this could promote increased expression of NF genes, thereby enabling maturation to occur. Clearly, tests of this hypothesis are needed but it is encouraging that a recent study reported that the use of leupeptin, a calpain inhibitor, to block NF degradation (with resulting NF accumulation in axonal terminals) resulted in a significant reduction in NF mRNA levels in retinal neurons (Smith et al., 1988).

It is apparent that NFs are important in maturation and radial growth of axons during development and regeneration. However, why are NFs downregulated during the initial stages of axonal regeneration? It is possible that NF expression is downregulated because the large numbers of NFs present in mature parent axons are an impediment to effective axonal sprouting and elongation, events which are more dependent on the efficient delivery of microfilament and microtubules. This issue will be discussed further in later sections of this review. Recent findings have shown that not all neuronal intermediate filaments (IF) are downregulated during regeneration. The following section discusses the changes that occur after axotomy in the expression of a newly discovered IF.

PERIPHERIN, A NOVEL TYPE III NEURONAL INTERMEDIATE FILAMENT, IS UPREGULATED DURING REGENERATION.

DRG neurons are among a subset of neurons in the adult nervous system that express a 57kDa, neuron-specific intermediate filament (IF) protein (Portier et al., 1984; Parysek and Goldman, 1988; Parysek et al., 1988, Brody et

al., 1989). Due to its presence in the PNS and apparent
absence in the CNS, this 57kDa IF protein was termed
"peripherin" (Portier et al., 1984). Peripherin is present
in small neurons of the DRG, sympathetic ganglia, most
cranial nerves and ventral motor neurons in the adult rat
(Portier et al., 1984; Leonard et al., 1988; Parysek and
Goldman, 1988; Brody et al., 1989). Recently, it has been
found that a small number of nuclear groups in the adult rat
CNS also express peripherin (Leonard et al., 1988; Parysek
and Goldman, 1988; Brody et al., 1989). The predicted amino
acid sequence of peripherin indicates that it is a member of
the type III IF class which also includes vimentin, desmin
and glial fibrillary acidic protein (Leonard et al., 1988;
Parysek et al., 1988) rather than the type IV IF class which
includes the NF triplet.

We recently provided evidence for the upregulation of
peripherin during axonal regeneration on several levels
(Oblinger et al., 1989b; Wong and Oblinger, 1989). Table 1
summarizes the information we currently have about
peripherin expression in axotomized DRG neurons. By
quantitative *in situ* hybridization methods, the peripherin
mRNA level in large DRG neurons is increased 14d after
sciatic nerve crush, a time at which NF mRNA expression is
maximally decreased. A more extensive examination of the
time course of peripherin mRNA changes by quantitative *in
situ* hybridization has revealed that peripherin mRNA levels
in large-sized DRG neurons increase within 1 day and remain
elevated for 8 wks after peripheral axotomy (Wong and
Oblinger, 1989). Interestingly, RNA blots fail to show this
change. The reason for this may be that peripherin
expression in the small neurons of the DRG (which contain
the majority of the peripherin message in the adult rat)
decreases slightly after axotomy while the large cell
expression of the mRNA increases (Table 1, Oblinger et al.,
1989b). Pulse-labeling studies have demonstrated that
peripherin synthesis in axotomized DRG neurons is increased
14d after sciatic nerve crush (Table 1). Immunocytochemical
examination of axotomized DRG neurons has revealed increased
levels of immunodetectable peripherin after axotomy (Table
1). Finally, the amount of peripherin entering regenerating
axonal sprouts by slow axonal transport has been found to
increase significantly if a conditioning lesion is used to
upregulate peripherin synthesis in DRG neurons 2 wks prior
to a second axotomy (Table 1). Thus, a number of lines of
evidence indicate that peripherin is regulated in a
direction opposite to that of the NF proteins after axotomy.

The finding that peripherin expression is upregulated
after axotomy of DRG neurons supports the idea that this

protein has an important function during active axonal elongation. In the DRG, it is of particular interest that the major increase in peripherin expression occurs in the large neurons of the DRG (which do not normally express much of this protein in the adult). Our preliminary findings indicate that large DRG cells express significant levels of peripherin at earlier developmental stages. Whether or not peripherin is present in the same or different IFs as the NF proteins remains to be determined in future studies. However, in either event, altered amounts of peripherin relative to the NF proteins in the cytoskeleton of regenerating axonal sprouts may alter the properties of the axonal cytoskeleton. Our findings suggest that such a change may be beneficial to the axonal regrowth process.

Table 1.   Peripherin Expression in DRG
            Neurons at 14d Post-axotomy

Peripherin mRNA level
        - Quantitative *in*   (↑)[1]
          situ hybridization
        - RNA blot analyses   (no change)[2]
Peripherin synthesis   (↑)
Immunodetectable levels   (↑)[3]
Transport in axonal sprouts   (↑)
    after priming lesion
----

[1] Large cells only; small neurons show a slight
   reduction in peripherin mRNA levels.
[2] Total DRG RNA was examined.
[3] Both large and small neurons.
(Data from Oblinger et al., 1989b)

TUBULIN EXPRESSION IS GENERALLY INCREASED DURING AXONAL REGROWTH

Several studies have demonstrated that tubulin gene expression is generally increased after axotomy (Hoffman et al., 1987; Oblinger et al., 1989a). However, not all tubulin genes appear to be influenced to the same extent by axotomy. For example, the expression of the class II ß-tubulin mRNA is greatly increased after axotomy (6-fold) while the class I and IV ß-tubulin mRNAs increase to a much lesser extent (Hoffman and Cleveland, 1988). Interestingly, the class II ß-tubulin gene is also normally expressed at much higher levels in the immature brain than in the adult (Bond et al., 1984). The class III (neuron-specific) ß-tubulin gene has not yet been evaluated in axotomized neurons. The expression of an α-tubulin mRNA which is the major species expressed during embryonic neuronal development also increases after axotomy (Miller et al., 1989). However, another α-tubulin mRNA species that is known to be constitutively expressed does not increase during regeneration (Miller et al., 1989).

It is commonly assumed that changes in the expression of tubulin genes are somehow be related to the progress of axonal regeneration and also to the success or failure of axonal reconnection with appropriate targets. Microtubules are known to be essential for sprout elongation and the increased expression of tubulin might facilitate sprout elongation by upregulating the overall supply of microtubules. Alternatively, the changes in tubulin expression after injury might serve to alter the composition of neuronal microtubules since the expression of certain tubulin isotypes appears to be selectively increased over others. Presumably, once reconnection of axons with appropriate targets occurs, tubulin expression would return to normal. If the target provided a factor/signal to the neuron which resulted in recovery of the normal homeostatic pattern of tubulin gene expression, we might predict that failure of a regenerating axon to reconnect with normal targets would continue to drive high levels of tubulin expression in the neuron. With continued failure to reconnect, other factors might shut down tubulin gene expression to below normal levels. In fact, our recent studies of DRG neurons after central axotomy show that failure to reconnect with original targets does not maintain high levels of tubulin mRNA expression (Wong and Oblinger, 1990). Instead, after an initial increase in tubulin mRNA levels in DRG cells, tubulin gene expression falls well below (~50% below) normal levels.

Because microtubules have a number of important functions in a variety of cell types, the identification of the actual factors and molecular details of tubulin gene regulation is an important avenue of research. It has long been known that the level of tubulin monomer in cells is an important factor in tubulin gene expression (Cleveland et al., 1981). As the concentration of monomer in cells decreases, tubulin synthesis as well as mRNA levels increase and vice-versa. It is not known whether or not axotomy affects the polymer/monomer ratio for tubulin in neurons. However, it is very likely that additional factors are also involved in the regulation of tubulin gene expression during what is often a long time course of axonal regeneration.

CHANGES IN CYTOSKELETAL GENE EXPRESSION AFFECT THE
COMPOSITION, MORPHOLOGY AND GROWTH PROPERTIES OF
REGENERATING SPROUTS

Studies of the conditioning lesion phenomenon
originally suggested that cell body changes, particularly
those involving production of the cytoskeleton, contribute
to a more efficient regenerative process (reviewed in
McQuarrie, 1983). Regenerating axons of neurons that had
been primed or conditioned by a distal axotomy a few weeks
earlier grow at a faster rate after a subsequent lesion than
do axons regrowing from a naive neuron after only a single
axotomy. We have verified this phenomenon in the rat DRG
system (Fig. 6). A conditioning lesion of the sciatic nerve
accelerates the elongation rate of the fastest growing DRG
axons by about 25% and also increases the rate of growth of
the slower growing population of DRG axons (Oblinger and
Lasek, 1984).

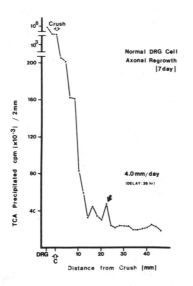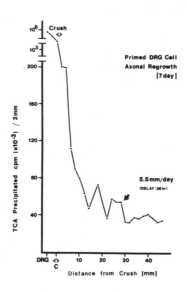

FIGURE 6. Assessment of regeneneration of primed and normal DRG axons
using the fast axonal transport method (Oblinger and Lasek, 1984). The
furthest distance from the proximal test crush site (C with arrow) at
which significant protein radioactivity was found 12 hrs after labeling
the L5 DRG with ^{35}S-methionine defines the outgrowth distance. Note
that this point is more distal in the primed condition at 7d after test
crush. A crush of the distal sciatic nerve 2 weeks prior to the test
crush served as the priming lesion. Estimated growth rates, using a
previously defined initial delay of 36h for the onset of sprouting, are
indicated.

Is it possible to relate the augmented growth rate of DRG axons after a conditioning axotomy to the series of molecular changes that have been discussed above? In our attempt to do so, we reasoned that if the molecular changes in cytoskeletal gene expression in the cell body have a direct role in the conditioning lesion phenomenon, they must reach the level of the axon and thus be detectable at that level. In the simplest version, we hypothesized that regenerating axonal sprouts elaborated by conditioned neurons must differ from those elaborated by unprimed neurons with respect to their cytoskeletons. To test this hypothesis, we examined the protein composition of the axonally transported cytoskeleton in regrowing axonal sprouts formed by primed and unprimed DRG cells using a novel modification of the axonal transport paradigm (Oblinger et al., 1989a).

In this paradigm, ongoing protein synthesis in the ganglion is labeled immediately before peripheral DRG axons are crushed at a site very close (several mm) to the DRG (Fig. 7). As the regenerating axons grow out, they incorporate newly synthesized radiolabeled proteins that are exported from the cell body. At later times, the labeled cytoskeletal proteins that have been axonally transported into the sprouts can be studied by gel electrophoresis/ fluorography. By doing a priming lesion of the distal sciatic nerve 2 weeks before the protein labeling/proximal nerve crush procedure, primed DRG neurons having altered synthesis patterns can be used to generate sprouts. The composition of such sprouts can then be compared with that of sprouts from unprimed DRG neurons.

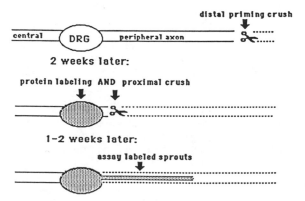

FIGURE 7. Schematic diagram of the paradigm used to examine cytoskeletal protein transport in regenerating sprouts. For the unprimed condition the distal priming crush is omitted.

An advantage of this paradigm for studies of cytoskeletal proteins is that cell body changes are quickly

transferred to the new axons because the injury site is
located very close to the cell body. This is an important
consideration since the rate of slow transport (1 mm/day) is
quite slow and, in the case of distal injuries, the products
of altered synthesis patterns in the cell body would require
many days/weeks to reach the axotomy site. Using this new
paradigm, we recently found that axonal sprouts of primed
DRG cells contain significantly less labeled NF protein and
more tubulin than do sprouts made by unprimed DRG neurons
(Oblinger et al., 1989a). The regrowing sprouts of
conditioned neurons also transport significantly greater
amounts of peripherin than do those of unprimed neurons
(Oblinger et al., 1989b). Figure 8 illustrates these
biochemical differences.

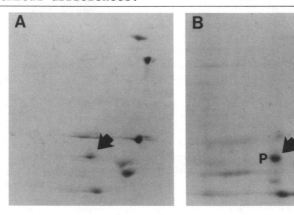

FIGURE 8. Fluorographs of 2D gel-separated proteins in a 10 mm piece of
regenerating nerve (just distal to the crush) 7d after labeling the L5
DRGs with ^{35}S-methionine and crushing the peripheral L5 nerve 2 mm from
the DRG. (A) unprimed DRG system, (B) primed system; a conditioning
lesion of the distal sciatic nerve preceded the labeling/proximal crush
by 2 weeks. L,M, H indicate the NF triplet, T indicates tubulin and P
with the arrow indicates peripherin.

The observed differences in the proteins transported
in regrowing sprouts under the two conditions leads one to a
simple prediction: that the morphology of sprouts
elaborated by primed and unprimed DRG neurons differs. To
directly examine this, quantitative morphometric analyses of
electron microscopic (EM) sections of regenerating axons in
the two conditions were done. The ultrastructure of axonal
sprouts from unprimed and primed DRG neurons was indeed
found to be strikingly different. Regenerating axons of
primed neurons contain few identifiable NFs and many more

microtubules than do those of unprimed DRG neurons (Fig. 9).
Quantitative analysis has revealed that the regenerating
axonal sprouts of primed DRG cells have a smaller average
cross-sectional area than do those of unprimed neurons
(Oblinger et al., 1989a).

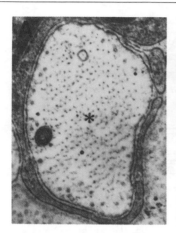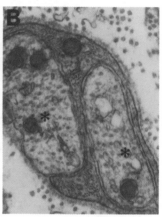

FIGURE 9. Electron micrographs showing the ultrastructure of axonal
sprouts from (A) unprimed and (B) primed DRG neurons. Thin sections
were obtained 9 mm from the proximal test crush site at 12d. Several
axons are indicated by asterisks. Note that the sprouts in the primed
condition have fewer NFs and more microtubules than do those in the
unprimed condition.

These findings provide support for the hypothesis that
sprouts from conditioned neurons differ from those
elaborated by unprimed neurons with respect to their
cytoskeleton. The augmented growth rate of conditioned
neurons can be correlated with a reduction in NFs and an
increase in microtubules in the sprouts. The idea of a
relationship between growth rate and the composition of the
cytoskeleton has also received support from developmental
studies. For example, during development, the axonal growth
rate is significantly faster than in the adult, the rate of
slow transport is faster, and slow transport conveys far
less NF protein than in the adult (Willard and Simon, 1983,
Hoffman et al., 1988). Thus, the model that has emerged is
that axonal sprouts which have a relatively NF-rich
cytoskeleton do not elongate as efficiently as those that
have fewer NFs and relatively more microtubules (Fig. 10).
If an adult neuron is to undergo regeneration, a
downregulated level of NF gene expression coupled with an
increased expression of appropriate tubulin genes appears to

be beneficial to the growth process. In the PNS, conditioning lesions are thus one way of recapturing the neuron's own
effective developmental strategy for growing its axon.

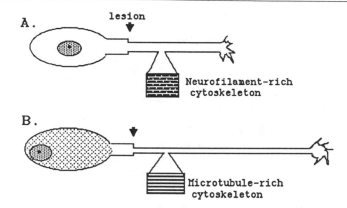

FIGURE 10. Schematic diagram summarizing the effect of a conditioning
lesion on axonal regeneration. Normally, a DRG cell stimulated to
regenerate by a proximal crush will elaborate sprouts that contain a
fair number of NFs (A). However, DRG neurons which have been primed by
a prior injury (B) and have downregulated NF expression and upregulated
tubulin expression will elaborate microtubule-rich sprouts that are
thinner and grow faster.

    How do we envision that down regulation of NFs affects
growth rate? Axonal growth rate is dependent on many
factors, from environmental conditions to intrinsic
mechanisms such as polymer elongation and translocation
(Lasek, 1988). The relationship between structural element
supply by slow transport and the rate of elongation maybe
fairly strict. Sliding of cytoskeletal polymers relative to
each other has been proposed as the motile model for slow
transport (Lasek, 1986). In that model, NFs are the "drag"
on the system since they are the slowest moving, most
numerous and, if crosslinked, the bulkiest of the elements
in the cytoskeleton. A reduction in NF number might
facilitate the sliding of other cytoskeletal elements. In
this way, a reduction in NF number could ultimately result
in a faster rate of supply of microtubules and other
elements needed to support the advance of regenerating
sprouts. Even when a lesion is more distally placed, the
supply of structural elements could be accelerated thru any
proximal sections of parent axons that have already changed
composition due to a downregulated level of NF expression.
In the future, it will be of interest to further test these

ideas using other methods of affecting NF number in the axon. This might be possible through pharmacological treatment or, eventually, by manipulations of regulatory regions of NF genes.

REFERENCES

Black, MM, Keyser, P and Sobel, E (1986). Interval between the synthesis and assembly of cytoskeletal proteins in cultured neurons. J Neurosci 6:1004-1012.

Bond, JF, Robinson, GS and Farmer, SR (1984). Differential expression of two neural cell-specific β-tubulin mRNAs during rat brain development. Mol Cell Biol 4:1313-1319.

Brody, BA, Ley, CA and Parysek, LM (1989). Selective distribution of the 57kd neural intermediate filament protein in the rat CNS. J Neurosci 9:2391-2401.

Cleveland, DW, Lopata, MA, Sherline, P and Kirschner, MW (1981). Unpolymerized tubulin modulates the level of tubulin mRNAs. Cell 25:537-546.

Goldstein, ME, Cooper, HS, Bruce, J, Carden, MJ, Lee, VM-Y and Schlaepfer, WW (1987). Phosphorylation of neurofilament proteins and chromatolysis following transection of rat sciatic nerve. J Neurosci 7:1586-1594.

Greenberg, SE and Lasek, RJ (1988). Neurofilament protein synthesis in DRG neurons decreases more after peripheral axotomy than central axotomy. J Neurosci, 8:1739-1746.

Greenman, MJ (1913). Studies on the regeneration of the peroneal nerve of the albino rat: number and sectional areas of fibers: area relation of axis to sheath. J Comp Neurol 23:479-513.

Hoffman, PN and Cleveland, DW (1988). Neurofilament and tubulin expression recapitulates the developmental program during axonal regeneration: Induction of a specific β-tubulin isotype. Proc Nat Acad Sci, 85:4530-4533.

Hoffman, PN and Lasek, RJ (1980). Axonal transport of the cytoskeleton in regenerating motor neurons: constancy and change. Brain Res 202:317-333.

Hoffman, PN, Cleveland, DW, Griffin, JW, Landes, PW, Cowan, NJ and Price, DL (1987). Neurofilament gene expression: A major determinant of axonal caliber. Proc Natl Acad Sci 84:3472-3476.

Hoffman, PN, Koo, EH, Muma, NA, Griffin, JW, Price, DL (1988). Role of neurofilaments in the control of axonal caliber in myelinated nerve fibers. In Lasek, RJ and Black, MM (eds): "Intrinsic Determinants of Neuronal Form and Function," New York: Alan R Liss Inc, pp 389-402.

Julien, J-P, Meyer, D, Flavel, D, Hurst, J, and Grosveld, F (1986).Cloning and developmental expression of the murine neurofilament gene family. Mol Brain Res, 1:243-250.

Lasek, RJ (1986). Polymer sliding in axons. J Cell Sci (Suppl) 5:161-179.

Lasek, RJ (1988). Studying the intrinsic determinants of neuronal form and function. In Lasek, RJ and Black, MM (eds): "Intrinsic Determinants of Neuronal Form and Function," New York: Alan R Liss Inc, pp 3-58.

Lasek, RJ and Hoffman, PN (1976). The neuronal cytoskeleton, axonal transport and axonal growth. In Goldman, R, Pollard, T and Rosenbaum, J (eds): "Cell Motility, vol C: Microtubules and Related Proteins," Cold Spring Harbor Press, pp 1021-1051.

Lasek, RJ, Oblinger, MM and Drake, PF (1983). The molecular biology of neuronal geometry: The expression of neurofilament genes influences axonal diameter. Cold Spring Harbor Symp Quant Biol 48:731-744.

Lewis, SA and Cowan, NJ (1985). Genetics, evolution and expression of the 68,000-mol-wt neurofilament protein: isolation of a cloned cDNA probe. J Cell Biol 100:843-850

Leonard, DGB, Gorham, JD, Cole, P, Greene, LA, and Ziff, EB (1988). A nerve growth factor-regulated messenger RNA encodes a new intermediate filament protein. J Cell Biol 106:181-193.

Lieberman, AR (1971). The axon reaction: A review of the principal features of perikaryal responses to axon injury. Int Rev Neurobiol 14:49-124.

Liuzzi, FJ and Lasek, RJ (1987). Astrocytes block axonal regeneration in mammals by activating the physiological stop pathway. Science 237:642-645.

McQuarrie, IG (1983). Role of the axonal cytoskeleton in the regenerating nervous system. In Seil, FJ (ed): "Nerve, Organ and Tissue Regeneration: Research Perspectives" New York: Academic Press, pp 51-86.

McQuarrie, IG and Lasek, RJ (1988). Transport of cytoskeletal elements from parent axons into regenerating daughter axons. J Neurosci 9:436-446.

Miller, FD, Tetzlaff, W, Bisby, MA, Fawcett, JW and Milner, RJ (1989). Rapid induction of the major embryonic α-tubulin mRNA, Tα1, during nerve regeneration in adult rats. J Neurosci 9: 1452-1463.

Oblinger, MM and Lasek, RJ (1984). A conditioning lesion of the peripheral axons of dorsal ganglion cells accelerates regeneration of only their peripheral axons. J Neurosci 4:1736-1744.

Oblinger, MM and Lasek, RJ (1985). Selective regulations of two axonal cytoskeletal networks in dorsal root ganglion cells. In O'Lague, P (ed): "Neurobiology: Molecular Biological Approaches to Understanding Neuronal Function and Development", New York: Alan R Liss, pp 135-143.

Oblinger, MM and Lasek, RJ (1988). Axotomy-induced alterations in the synthesis and transport of neurofilaments and microtubules in dorsal root ganglion cells. J Neurosci 8:1747-1758.

Oblinger, MM, Szumlas, RA, Wong, J, and Liuzzi, FJ (1989a). Changes in neurofilament gene expression affect the composition of regenerating axonal sprouts elaborated by DRG neurons in vivo. J Neurosci 9: 2645-2653.

Oblinger, MM, Wong, J and Parysek, LM (1989b). Axotomy-induced changes in the expression of a type III neuronal intermediate filament gene. J Neurosci 9:3766-3775.

Parysek, LM and Goldman, RD (1988). Distribution of a novel 57kDa intermediate filament (IF) protein in the nervous system. J Neurosci 8:555-563.

Parysek, LM, Chisholm, RL, Ley, CA and Goldman, RD (1988). A Type III intermediate filament gene is expressed in mature neurons. Neuron 1:395-401.

Pearson, RCA, Taylor, N and Snyder, SH (1988). Tubulin messenger RNA: *in situ* hybridization reveals bilateral increases in hypoglossal and facial nuclei following nerve transection. Brain Res 463:245-249.

Portier, M-M, deNechaud, B, and Gros, F (1984). Peripherin, a new member of the intermediate filament protein family. Dev Neurosci 6:335-344.

Ring, G, Reichert, F and Rotshenker, S (1983). Sprouting in intact sartorius muscles of the frog following contralateral axotomy. Brain Res 260:313-316.

Robinson, PA, Wion, D and Anderton, BH (1986). Isolation of a cDNA for the rat heavy neurofilament polypeptide (NF-H). FEBS 209:203-205.

Smith, KA, Goodison, KL and Parhad, IM (1988). The effect of neurofilament accumulation in axonal terminals on neurofilament gene expression. J Cell Biol 107:463a.

Watson, WE (1968). Observations on the nucleolar and total cell body nuclei acid of injured nerve cells. J Physiol (Lond) 196: 655-676.

Willard, MB and Simon, C (1983). Modulations of neurofilament axonal transport during the development of rabbit retinal ganglion cells. Cell 35:551-559.

Wong, J and Oblinger, MM (1987). Changes in neurofilament gene expression occur after axotomy of dorsal root ganglion neurons: An *in situ* hybridization study. Metab Brain Dis 2:291-303.

Wong, J and Oblinger, MM (1989) Differential regulation of type III and type IV intermediate filament genes in regenerating DRG neurons. American Soc Neurochem 20:p122.

Wong, J and Oblinger, MM (1990). A comparison of peripheral and central axotomy effects on neurofilament and tubulin gene expression in rat dorsal root ganglion neurons. J Neurosci (in press).

**Advances in Neural Regeneration
Research, pages 277–289**
© 1990 Wiley-Liss, Inc.

PROTO-ONCOGENES, STRESS PROTEINS AND SIGNALLING MECHANISMS
IN NEURAL INJURY AND RECOVERY

Michael R. Hanley and Hilary P. Benton

MRC Molecular Neurobiology Unit,
MRC Centre
Hills Road
Cambridge, CB2 2QH, U.K.

INTRODUCTION

The study of nerve regeneration has been frequently
subdivided into two sequential processes: injury and
recovery. It is likely that specific, perhaps overlapping,
signalling mechanisms must be activated to induce the
injured state and to initiate the repair processes once
damage has been detected. The biochemical events underlying
these processes will undoubtedly use the highly conserved
gene products and small molecule messengers of surface
signal transduction pathways. Thus, the ubiquitous cellular
"stress response" (Young and Elliott, 1989) provides a
powerful intellectual structure to examine how neural cells,
especially neurones, may respond to injury and to examine
how normal function may be restored. Similarly, neural
recovery may be profitably modelled after other types of
growth-stimulatory processes, such as mitogen-induced
proliferation or hypertrophy. In this context, these cell-
specific processes, proliferation, hypertrophy, or neuronal
projection growth, may incorporate a common panel of genes
which underlie all forms of environmentally stimulated
growth, as is shown in Figure 1. These genes are likely to
include, if not be identical with, the proto-

Possible Receptor-driven Growth Processes

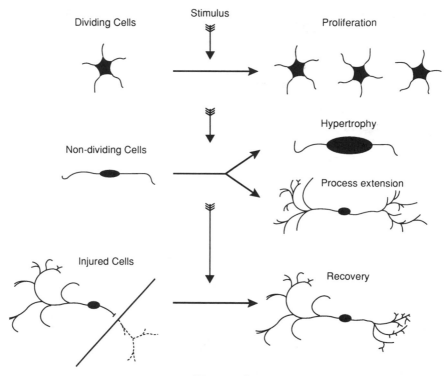

Figure 1.

oncogenes. In the transduction of both injury and repair
signalling, the stress response genes and proto-oncogenes
will have to coordinate disparate intracellular events by
co-opting constitutive communication networks. Here, we
discuss general issues of the involvement of three classes
of identified genes; stress proteins, proto-oncogenes, and
calcium signalling components, in the processes of neural
injury and recovery. Although much of the corroborative
evidence will be drawn from non-neural populations, emphasis
will be placed on explicit evidence for involvement of these
classes of response genes and their encoded paths of action
in neurones.

NEURAL INJURY

The stress response
The process which is commonly referred to as the "stress
response" involves the induction of a number of genes (Table
1) following any one of a variety of different cellular
perturbations.

Table 1
Stress-induced Proteins

Inductive stimuli	Responsive genes
Heat shock	Hsp70 family
Calcium overload	(BiP, GRP78)
Nutrient deprivation	Hsp90 family
Prolonged anoxia	(Endoplasmin, GRP94)
pH shock	

Induction of these genes by heat shock (Pelham, 1989) is the
most extensively studied mechanism of induction of these
proteins but probably not the most physiologically relevant
in many tissues, such as brain. It is now well established
that the heat shock proteins include the glucose-regulated
proteins (Lee, 1987), which are induced by a number of
adverse conditions, including oxygen or nutrient deprivation
and perturbations in cellular pH and calcium homeostasis
(Lee, 1987). The stress response does not only occur in
actively-growing permanent cell lines, which by definition
have an altered pattern of gene expression, but is a normal
part of the physiological response repertoire of every
eukaryotic cell. In, for example, differentiated primary
cultures of connective tissue cells, the stress response can
be dramatically elicited by addition of calcium perturbants
(Benton et al, 1988). Figure 2 shows the characteristic
pattern of protein synthesis changes in the induction of the
stress response; in this case following treatment of
differentiated primary chondrocytes with the calcium
ionophore, A23187. In this differentiated cell population
the stress protein induction is dramatic and comparable to
that seen under similar conditions in cells such as mouse
3T3 fibroblasts or HeLa cells (Watowich and Morimoto, 1988).
This inevitably raises the questions of what is the nature
and function of the diagnostic proteins whose synthesis is

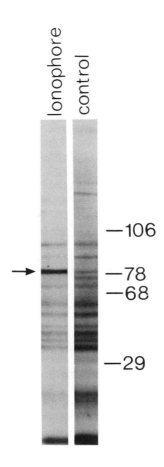

<u>Figure 2</u> Calcium perturbant-induced stress response, as monitored by effects on protein synthesis in porcine primary articular chondrocytes. Monolayer cultures were treated with the calcium ionophore A23187 (1µM) for 24 hours and ^{35}S-methionine-labelled proteins have been separated by SDS-gel electrophoresis and the labelled proteins have been exposed by fluorography. The arrow notes the position of the major calcium-induced stress protein.

induced under stressed conditions. Several classes of heat
shock or stress response proteins are recognized and they
are summarized in Table 1. They fall into distinctive
molecular weight categories, regardless of the responsive
cell population, suggesting a functional unity to the
phenomenon of cell stress. Much effort has been directed to
identifying possible functions for these proteins, and it
appears that each size class, although heterogeneous,
nevertheless includes several proteins with parallel
functions. The greatest attention has been directed to the
hsp70 family (Lindquist, 1986) and the array of activities
suggested for the class of hsp70 proteins is indicated in
Table 2.

Table 2
Proposed Functions for Hsp70 family

> Binding of malformed proteins
> Inhibition of movement through e.r.
>   of malformed proteins
> Cytoskeletal re-arrangement
> Uncoating of clathrin-coated vesicles
> Lysosomal degradation of intracellular
>   proteins

In most mammalian cell types, there are two principal forms
of hsp70: hsp73, an abundant constitutively-expressed
protein; and hsp72, a dramatically stress-responsive
protein. Following stress activation these proteins appear
transiently in the nucleus, and later, during recovery,
appear in close association with the ribosomal sites of
protein synthesis. The circumstantial evidence that these
proteins, and related stress proteins, comprise both
cellular defence and repair systems follows from the
frequent demonstration that a mild stress tolerises many
cells to a subsequent, more vigorous challenge. Indeed, in
fibroblasts, microinjection of neutralizing antibodies
eradicates this conditioning effect, so that mild stresses
become lethal (Riabowol et al, 1988). It is evident by
inspection of Table 2 that hsp70 proteins would be acting to
remove damaged proteins, maintain normal organelle function,
and minimize propagation of damage when the cell is in a
weakened state. For proliferating cells, the population can
restore normal behavior by replenishment, but for a

permanently non-dividing cell population, such as neurones, these proteins may provide the only protective pathways between restoration of function and irreversible decline.

Although coming under increasing scrutiny, the specific aspects of the stress response in neurones and glial cells have not been described in detail. However, hyperthermia has been shown to induce hsp70 gene expression in mammalian neurones (Sprang and Brown, 1987). Intriguingly, some neuronal populations, such as hippocampal neurones, appear to constitutively express high levels of hsp70 transcripts. Moreover, isolated cultured neurones are unable to survive mild thermal stress, much like the observations for fibroblasts, if they are microinjected with anti-hsp70 antibodies (Khan and Sotelo, 1989). In all neural cells, a universal early genetic response to any form of injury, including heat shock (Dragunow et al, 1989), is the induction of the c-fos proto-oncogene (Schwartz et al, 1989). Thus, the promiscuous response, c-fos, is a potential prerequisite to the more specific injury pattern of stress protein gene induction.

Reticuloplasmins

Many of the stress-induced proteins are now recognized to be major components of the lumen of the endoplasmic reticulum (Koch, 1987), such as GRP94 or GRP75. These proteins have a common panel of physical characteristics, being acidic glycoproteins with high calcium-binding capacities. These properties have led to the consideration that they function in maintaining the structural integrity of the endoplasmic reticulum, and are therefore subject to induction during stress as part of endoplasmic reticulum rearrangements (Booth and Koch 1989). These proteins are ubiquitous components of endoplasmic reticulum, and provide antigenic markers of the physical state and intracellular distribution of ER. For example, one such reticuloplasmin, endoplasmin, has been used to provide a spatial map of ER in a neuronal cell line (Hanley et al, 1988). The importance of the reticuloplasmins in the context of cell injury is that, being stress proteins, they simultaneously provide a monitor of the progression of the response, but also can be used immunocytochemically to follow the dynamics of the ER under these conditions. Unexpectedly, many cells show a morphological distortion and eventual vesiculation of the ER, as a common early event to stress conditions, but particularly to those involving perturbations in environmental or intracellular calcium (Koch et al, 1988; Booth and Koch, 1989). The events that have been described comprise a cycle of break-up and recovery, which is shown schematically in Figure 3.

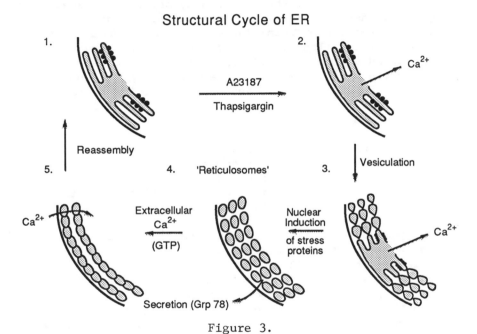

Figure 3.

In brief, the initial fragmentation of the ER appears in response to loss of calcium from the ER lumen. This loss can be triggered by calcium ionophore, or by calcium-pump arrest, using the novel tumor promotor, thapsigargin (Jackson et al 1987; Hanley et al, 1988). It is clear that the actual stress signal is loss of luminal calcium content, rather than cytosolic calcium elevation, because cytosolic calcium buffering does not alter the induction of the stress response (Drummond et al, 1988). Within several minutes of sustained calcium depletion from the ER, it begins to form vesicles, termed reticulosomes, which may be an underlying repeating ER substructure (Koch et al, 1988). In the time period during which the fragmentation of the ER is proceeding, the induction of stress genes in the nucleus is first detected. In the sustained presence of a stress, the luminal ER proteins appear to be secreted to the environment. It is at this point that the cells either initiate a restorative process or degenerate. The restoration event proceeds by a reassembly of the reticulosomes, only in the presence of extracellular calcium, into tubular ER structures. The appeal of this morphological cycle is that it clearly defines intracellular steps, and identifies explicit internal sites, at which injury progression or reinitiation of normal function can be followed. Thus, although many of these events have not been described in any neural cell population, it suggests several themes which have already attracted considerable support for their involvement in injury and repair; calcium homeostasis, alterations in genetic activity, and the role of ER and new protein synthesis in recovery.

More speculatively, one can suggest a unifying model based on these notions in which the common trigger event in induction of the stress state, which is the early warning of an impending cell crisis, is a catastrophic decline in ATP levels. When this occurs, ER pump activity will be arrested, and, as results from the use of thapsigargin have shown, pump arrest leads to rapid loss of ER calcium content. Put a different way, the presence of this rapid pump-leak system for ER acts to sample constantly the cytoplasmic ATP content, so that the leak process is immediately manifest upon reduction of ATP levels. The reason that calcium may need to be unloaded at the early stages of a stress response may not be to act as a signal, but rather to be depleted as a signal. Because calcium is a vital intracellular messenger, loss of its normal control following cellular damage could exacerbate the severity of the damage enormously (Scharfman and Schwartzkroin, 1989), by activating many identified calcium-regulated degradative enzymes. Thus, the cell may unload this potentially dangerous mediator while some homeostatic control persists. The fragmentation of the ER suggests the time frame in which protracted damage can be compensated for, or in which progressive deterioration begins. It seems likely that the secretion of some of the stress proteins, such as GRP70 in

Figure 2, may be the final protective strategies used by the
cell. Of course, this raises the very interesting
possibility that enhancing the extracellular levels of these
proteins may assist recovery (Pelham 1989); a proposition of
great importance in neuronal injury. The restoration of
normal ER morphology may be a good reporter for the overall
health of the cell, and it is interesting that its recovery
as an organelle requires external calcium. This echoes one
of the recurrent paradoxes of neuronal injury; that calcium
is simultaneously capable of inducing and repairing damage.

NEURAL REPAIR

Proto-Oncogenes

The image of the ER cycle poses the question of whether any
exogenous stimulants can productively intervene in these
events to bias the recovery pathways. In the nervous
system, a class of diffusible "trophic" factors have the
correct properties to act in this way. That is, they do not
only appear to function in developmental selection against
induced cell death (Barde, 1988), but they also act to
protect against damage and facilitate repair in the adult
state. Thus, it is of considerable interest that trophic
activity on target neurone populations has been observed
with oncogene-related growth factors (Hanley, 1989), which
stimulate cell division in cells with proliferative
potential. One common denominator in mitogen-stimulated
cell growth has been the obligate involvement of the ras p21
family (Mulcahy et al, 1984). When mutant tranforming ras
is injected into PC12 cells, however, it induces commitment
to differentiation (Hanley, 1989) which is very similar to
that induced by nerve growth factor. Indeed, neutralizing
antibodies to cellular ras species blocks the ability of
nerve growth factor to induce PC12 cell differentiation
(Hanley 1989). These early indications that ras might be an
essential signalling element in trophic factor receptor
pathways were explored systematically in several distinct
neuronal primary cultures (Borasio et al, 1989) sensitive to
different trophic factors, nerve growth factor, brain-
derived neurotrophic factor, and ciliary neurotrophic
factor. The striking conclusion has been that all trophic
factor actions can be mimicked by mutationally-activated ras

when introduced intracellularly. Thus, formal links between
the genetics of proliferative pathways, and trophic pathways
have been established. Casting the net more widely, how
many of the known neural proto-oncogenes may have normal
functions in the injury and recovery processes? Ras is now
recognized to be the archetype of a large superfamily of
related monomeric GTP-binding proteins (Santos and Nebreda,
1989), many of which are found in high levels in mammalian
neurones (Olofsson et al, 1988). Some of these are emerging
as very interesting candidates for transducers in trophic
factor mechanisms. For example, the rap1 protein (also
known as Krev) is able to reverse ras-induced cell
transformation (Kitayama et al, 1989). Thus, it would be
important to establish whether this antagonism of ras
pathways extends to the trophic factors. Another
interesting subfamily of relevance to neuronal regeneration
is the rab family. One specific member of the family, rab 3
(also known as smg25A) is induced in PC12 cells by nerve
growth factor (Sano et al, 1989). This has very recently
been shown to be selectively associated with synaptic
vesicles (Mollard et al, 1990). One striking point is that
the physical properties of rab, and its microdiversity,
recall descriptions of one of the "growth-associated
proteins" (GAPs) that is induced during nerve regeneration,
GAP-24 (Skene, 1984). Could GAP-24 be rab 3 or a closely-
related GTP-binding protein? This assignment of a GAP to a
species of GTP-binding protein would raise a number of
interesting issues about whether there is a requirement for
GTP turnover during robust nerve regrowth, particularly in
the light of evidence for involvement of GTP in
intracellular calcium regulation (Chueh et al, 1987).

The unifying hypothesis that these oncogene relationships
and interactions may suggest is the concept that trophic
factors recruit elements of proliferative response cascades
for a growth-related, but non-proliferative, function
(Figure 1). Thus the ultimate protective or restorative
mechanisms for trophic factor receptors may be the boosting
of levels of expression or patterns of activity of gene
products such as the ER calcium pump, heat shock proteins,
cytoskeletal elements, and free radical scavenger enzymes.
The objectives of these regulatory alterations would be to
enhance calcium buffering, remove denatured or degraded

macromolecules, erect protective intracellular barriers to preserve compartmentation, and limit the adventitious appearance of toxic products of neural trauma.

SUMMARY AND CONCLUSIONS

The understanding of the events in neural damage and regeneration have benefited greatly from genetic approaches which make no assumptions about the nature of the gene products. However, it is worth calling attention to three discrete but functionally overlapping categories of identified genes; stress response, proto-oncogenes, and calcium signalling; that may have central roles in these phenomena. The conspicuous virtue is that the molecular tools are already available. Moreover, exploring how these gene products may function in the nervous system context can benefit by analogy with what is known in other tissues or cells.

REFERENCES

Barde Y-A (1988). What, if anything, is a neurotrophic factor? Trends Neurosci. 11:343-346.

Benton HP, Jackson TR, Hanley MR (1989). Identification of a novel inflammatory stimulant of chondrocytes; early events in cell activation by bradykinin receptors on pig articular chondrocytes. Biochem. J. 258:861-867.

Booth C, Koch GLE (1989). Perturbation of cellular calcium induces secretion of luminal ER proteins. Cell 59:729-737.

Borasio GD, John J, Wittinghofer A, Barde Y-A, Sendtner M, Heumann R (1989). ras p21 protein promotes survival and fibre outgrowth of cultured embryonic neurons. Neuron 2:1087-1096.

Chueh S-H, Mullaney JM, Ghosh TK, Zachary AL, Gill DL (1987). GTP and inositol 1,4,5-trisphosphate-activated intracellular calcium movements in neuronal and smooth muscle cell lines. J. Biol. Chem. 262:13857-13864.

Dragunow M, Currie RW, Robertson HA, Faull RLM (1989). Heat shock induces c-fos protein-like immunoreactivity in glial cells in adult rat brain. Exp. Neurol. 106:105-109.

Drummond IAS, Livingston D, Steinhardt RA (1988). Heat shock
    protein synthesis and cytoskeletal rearrangements occur
    independently of intracellular free calcium increases in
    Drosophila cells and tissues. Rad. Res. 113:402-413.
Hanley MR (1989). Proto-oncogenes in the nervous system.
    Neuron 1:175-182.
Hanley MR, Jackson TR, Cheung WT, Dreher M, Gatti A, Hawkins
    P, Patterson SI, Vallejo M, Dawson AP, Thastrup O (1988).
    Molecular mechanisms of phospholipid signalling pathways
    in mammalian nerve cells. Cold Sping Harbor Symp. Quant.
    Biol. 53: 435-445.
Jackson TR, Patterson SI, Thastrup O, Hanley MR (1988). A
    novel tumour promoter, thapsigargin, transiently
    increases cytoplasmic free calcium without generation of
    inositol phosphates in NG115-401L neuronal cells,
    Biochem. J. 235:81-86.
Khan NA, Sotelo J (1989). Heat shock stress is deleterious
    to CNS cultured neurones microinjected with anti-HSP70
    antibodies. Biol.Cell. 65:199-202.
Kitayama H, Sugimoto Y, Matsuzaki T, Ikawa Y, Noda M (1989).
    A ras-related gene with transformation suppressor
    activity. Cell 56:77-84.
Koch GLE (1987). Reticuloplasmins: a novel group of proteins
    in the endoplasmic reticulum. J. Cell Sci. 87:491-492.
Koch GLE, Booth C, Wooding FBP (1988). Dissociation and
    reassembly of the endoplasmic reticulum in live cells. J.
    Cell Sci. 91:51-522.
Lee AS (1987). Co-ordinated regulation of a set of genes by
    glucose and calcium ionophores in mammalian cells.
    Trends Biochem. Sci. 12:20-23
Linquist S (1986). The heat shock response. Ann. Rev.
    Biochem. 55:1151-1191.
Mollard GFV, Mignery GA, Baumert M, Perin MS, Hanson TJ,
    Burger PM, Jahn R, Sudhof TC (1990). rab3 is a small GTP-
    binding protein exclusively localized to synaptic
    vesicles. Proc. Natl. Acad. Sci. USA 87:1988-1992.
Mulcahy LS, Smith MR, Stacey DW (1984). Requirement for ras
    proto-oncogene function during serum stimulated growth of
    NIH 3T3 cells. Nature 313:241-243.
Olofsson B, Chardin P, Touchot N, Zahraoui A, Tavitian A
    (1988). Expression of the ras-related ralA, rho12 and rab
    genes in adult mouse tissues. Oncogene 3:231-234.

Pelham HRB (1989). Heat shock and the sorting of luminal ER proteins. EMBO J. 8:3171-3176.

Riabowol KT, Mizzen L, Welch WJ (1988). Heat shock is lethal to fibroblasts microinjected with antibodies against hsp70. Science 242:433-436.

Sano K, Kikuchi A, Matsui Y, Teranishi Y, Takai Y (1989). Tissue-specific expression of a novel GTP-binding protein (smg p25A) mRNA and its increase by nerve growth factor and cyclic AMP in rat pheochromocytoma PC-12 cells. Biochem. Biophys. Res. Commun. 158:377-385.

Santos E, Nebreda AR (1989). Structural and functional properties of ras proteins. FASEB J. 3:2151-2163.

Scharfman HE, Schwartzkroin PA (1989). Protection of dentate hilar cells from prolonged stimulation by intracellular calcium chelation. Science 246:257-260.

Schwartz M, Cohen A, Stein-Izsak C, Belkin M (1989). Dichotomy of the glial cell response to axonal injury and regeneration. FASEB J. 3:2371-2378.

Skene JHP (1984). Growth-associated proteins and the curious dichotomies of nerve regeneration. Cell 37:697-700.

Sprang GK, Brown IR (1987). Selective induction of a heat shock gene in fibre tracts and cerebellar neurons of the rabbit brain detected by in situ hybridization. Mol. Brain Res. 3:89-93.

Watowich SS, Morimoto RI (1988). Complex regulation of heat shock-and glucose-responsive genes in human cells. Mol. Cel l. Biol. 8:393-405.

Young RA, Elliott TJ (1989). Stress proteins, infection, and immune surveillance. Cell 59:5-8.

**Advances in Neural Regeneration
Research, pages 291–307
© 1990 Wiley-Liss, Inc.**

HOX-2 HOMEOBOX GENES AND RETINOIC ACID: POTENTIAL
ROLES IN PATTERNING THE VERTEBRATE NERVOUS SYSTEM

Nancy   Papalopulu,   Paul   Hunt,   David
Wilkinson,   Anthony   Graham   and   Robb
Krumlauf

Lab of Eukaryotic Molecular Genetics
National Institute for Medical Research
The Ridgeway, Mill Hill, London NW7 1AA

INTRODUCTION

Classical genetics and experimental embryology
have generated a great deal of information on
nervous system anatomy and development. However
a new gene family, homeobox containing genes,
promises to provide insight into the molecular
basis of patterning in the vertebrate nervous
system. This hope is based on the discovery
that a set of genes, first discovered in
Drosophila, are involved in controlling
embryonic pattern formation and share a common
element, termed the homeobox. This motif
encodes a 60 amino acid domain that can bind to
DNA, and it is believed that homeodomain
proteins are nuclear proteins that exert
their biological functions by modulating
transcription. In *Drosophila,* a network of genes
is involved in pattern formation, and one
subset, the *Antennapedia*-like homeobox genes
(ANT-C and BX-C or HOM-C genes), specify
segment phenotype according to position along
the anteroposterior (A-P) axis (Akam, 1987, 1989;
Ingham, 1988;). An important aspect of the
process of specifying segment identity is that
the HOM-C genes are expressed in segment-
restricted patterns.

Many of the *Drosophila* segmentation and homeotic genes are also expressed in the embryonic nervous system. The segmentation genes *eve, en,* and *ftz* are expressed in a specific subset of neurons in every segment of the developing central nervous system and seem to be involved in neuronal determination (Doe et al., 1988a, 1988b). The homeotic genes are expressed at their highest levels in the embryonic nervous system (Doe and Scott, 1988). However, unlike the segmentation genes, they are not expressed in every segment of the CNS and are therefore not believed to be involved in the specification of segmentally reiterated features of the CNS. The homeotic genes tend to show peaks of expression in given parasegments and lower levels of expression in more posterior regions. Mutations in these genes affect those regions of the CNS that exhibit the highest levels of expression for each gene, suggesting that the *Drosophila* genes are involved in specifying the identity of segments once they have formed, and regulating their subsequent anteroposterior differentiation (Doe and Scott, 1988).

The homeodomain is highly conserved over a broad phylogentic spectrum, and the *Drosophila* motif has been used to isolate homeobox containing genes from many organisms, including mammals. By analogy to *Drosophila*, it is hoped that the vertebrate homeobox genes will provide clues to the processes of segmentation and positional information in these species. However, the processes of segmentation in arthropods and vertebrates are believed to have evolved independently, and it is not clear that the genes perform similar functions in these diverse groups. Initial studies on the mammalian homeobox genes have therefore centered on the nature of their organization and expression to gather support for their functional involvement in development. The murine genome contains at least 28 "*Antp*"-like homeobox genes that are organized into four clusters termed Hox-1, Hox-2, Hox-3, and Hox-5. The clustering of this class of homeobox genes (Hox) is a general phenomenon in most species, and the clusters within a vertebrate species appear to be related by duplication and divergence. In *Drosophila* there is a correlation between the physical order of the ANT-C and BX-C homeobox genes and their expression along the A-P axis (Harding et al., 1985; Akam, 1987). Recently it has been shown that the murine Hox clusters display a similar correlation between the position of a gene in the cluster and its domain of expression along the A-P axis, particularily in the central nervous system (CNS). Within a murine cluster starting at the 5' end, each adjacent 3' gene shows a successively more rostral limit of expression in the neural tube (Duboule and Dolle, 1989; Graham et al., 1989). This similarity between mouse and *Drosophila* is not limited only to patterns of expression, but also extends to the level of sequence identity and chromosomal organization. We argue that the conservation between the species in sequence identity, linear order of related genes in the cluster, and domains of expression along the A-P axis reflect a common evolutionary origin for these homeobox genes from an ancestral cluster that existed prior to the split between the deuterostome and protostome lineages (Akam, 1989; Duboule and Dolle, 1989; Graham et al., 1989). These studies support the idea that murine homeobox complexes may represent part of an evolutionarily conserved mechanism in positional signalling along the A-P axis of the embryo.

In this paper we examine the expression of Hox-2 homeobox genes in the developing neural tube, and show that the boundaries of expression of the genes have segment-specific patterns in the developing hindbrain. The data indicate that the Hox-2 genes may play a role in the specification of vertebrate segments in a manner analogous to that of their *Drosophila* homologues. We also examine the types of signalling molecules capable of activating Hox-2 expression, and show that the vitamin A derivative, retinoic acid (RA), can differentially regulate the Hox-2 complex. There is a correlation between the degree of induction by RA and the position of a gene in the Hox-2 cluster in both mouse F9 cells and *Xenopus* embryos. These findings suggest that RA could act as a potential morphogen in the embryo to help in establishing partially overlapping and graded domains of homeobox expression.

RESULTS AND DISCUSSION

Conservation and Segment-Specific Expression

In earlier studies we have shown that the Hox-2 cluster contains nine genes which are all arranged with the same 5'-3' direction with respect to transcription (Graham et al., 1988; Rubock et al., 1990). By sequence analysis and *in situ* hybridization we found that there were common features of structure and expression shared between the mouse Hox-2 complex and the *Drosophila* HOM-C complex (summarized in Fig.1B, bottom). Alignment of the most closely related mouse and *Drosophila* homeobox genes from their respective clusters shows that they are arranged in an identical order along the chromosome. The arrow above the clusters indicates that genes at the left are expressed in posterior regions of the embryo and that there is a trend towards successively more anterior domains of expression as one moves along the cluster in both species. In the mouse Hox-2 complex, Hox-2.5 has the most posterior boundary of expression in the neural tube and each 3' gene has progressively more anterior limits of expression in anterior nerve cord in the developing 12.5 day old embryo (Graham et al., 1989). At this stage the anterior boundaries of expression did not correlate with any clear morphological structure. In vertebrates the spinal cord is not believed to be intrinsically segmented and the regular array of ganglia in the PNS is a consequence of interactions with the segmented paraxial somitic mesoderm (Keynes and Stern, 1988). However, recent evidence suggests that repeated bulges (rhombomeres) which appear in the developing hindbrain are important segmental units in

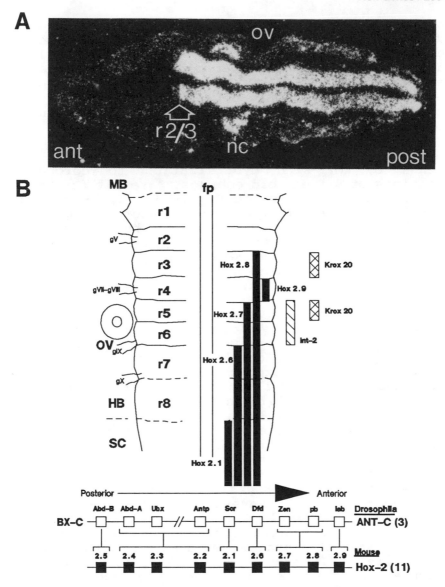

Figure 1. Homology between *Drosophila* and mouse homeobox clusters, and segmental expression in the hindbrain. (A) Hox-2.8 darkground *in situ* (arrow: rhombomere 2/3 boundary). (B) Summary of Hox-2 structure, evolutionary conservation and two-segment periodicity of expression in the hindbrain.

pattern specification in the vertebrate neural development (Lumsden and Keynes, 1989; Wilkinson et al., 1989a). The rhombomeres are anatomically detectable only at early embryonic stages (mouse embryonic day 9-10.5). The anterior boundaries of Hox-2 expression observed in 12.5 day old embryos could correlate with segment-specific patterns in earlier staged embryos.

We therefore analyzed the expression of Hox-2 genes by *in situ* hybridization to coronal sections of 9.5 day old embryos. A result for the Hox-2.8 gene is shown in Figure 1A. The Hox-2.8 gene is expressed from the most posterior regions (right of section) in the neural tube to a sharp anterior boundary. This boundary represents the junction between rhombomeres 2 and 3 (see arrow, Fig 1B.), based on position relative to the otic vesicle (OV). In addition to expression in the neural tube, Hox-2.8 is also expressed in two crescent shaped domains (nc) adjacent to rhombomere 4, which correspond to the developing VIIth/VIIIth sensory ganglia. These ganglia are derived from neural crest cells (nc) revealing that Hox genes are expressed in both neural tube and neural crest cells. When all of the Hox-2 genes are examined on near adjacent sections (Wilkinson et al., 1989b), a segmental pattern of expression is obsereved and the results are summarized in Figure 1B. Starting with the Hox-2.1 gene, each successive gene up to and including Hox-2.8 has an anterior boundary of expression which maps to a junction between rhombomeres. These expression limits occur at two-segment intervals, which is intriguing, as previous studies have indicated a two-segment periodicity in neuronal development within the hindbrain (Lumsden and Keynes, 1989). Furthermore, experiments on the expression pattern of the zinc-finger-encoding gene, *Krox-20,* showed that it was expressed in a rhombomere restricted manner, being detected only in rhombomeres 3 and 5 (Wilkinson et al., 1989a). Together these data, along with the Hox-2 patterns, suggest the existence of molecular mechanisms operating at two-segment intervals in the hindbrain. In experiments examining the timing of Hox-2 expression in the hindbrain (Wilkinson et al., 1989b), it was found that segment-restricted expression is already established in 8.5 day old embryos before the appearance of the rhombomeres, but not in 8.0 day old embryos, when the *Krox-20* gene is segmentally restricted. This suggests that the Hox-2 genes may act later in the process of segmentation than genes such as *Krox-20*.

Retinoic Acid and Induction of Hox-2 Expression

The colinear expression domains of Hox-2 genes along the embryonic A-P axis may be important for specifying positional information. One possibility is that a graded signal or morphogen is present in the embryo and that the Hox-2 patterns are established by a differential gene response to this signal. We were interested in examining possible molecular signals involved in establishing this pattern. Many homeobox genes are stimulated by the treatment of cultured cells by RA, and we were interested in determining if all Hox-2 genes respond to RA and if they displayed a differential response. In Figure 2A, four different mouse tissue culture cell lines have been treated with 5×10^{-7}M RA for 24 hrs and examined for Hox-2.1 RNA responsiveness; F9 is an embryonic teratocarcinoma line, EK-CCE and EK-HD14 are embryonic stem cells (ES) capable of contributing to the germline, and 3T3 cells are fibroblasts. Hox-2.1 levels are not detectable in the untreated stem cells (-lanes), but accumulate to very high levels in the RA treated cells (+lanes). The ES cells CCE and HD14 also show high levels of Hox-2.1 induction upon RA treatment; however, the gene is already dectable in the untreated stem cells and the degree of the response is different in these lines. The levels of Hox-2.1 do not appear to change in 3T3 cells in response to RA, although this may be due to lack of the appropriate receptors. Figure 2A therefore illustrates that Hox-2 genes can be stimulated by RA treatment and that the degree of the response varies between different cell lines.

A

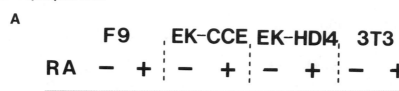

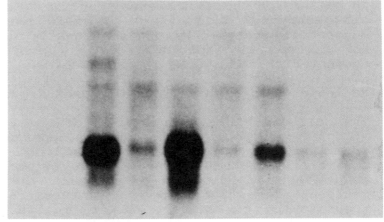

B

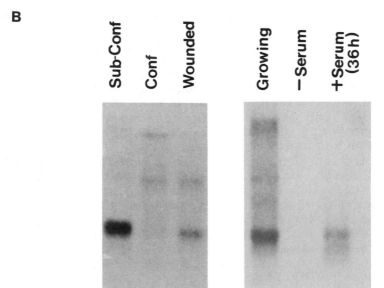

Figure 2. Induction of Hox-2.1 expression. (A) Response of Hox-2.1 to retinoic acid (RA) in embryonic stem (CCE & HD14), teratocarcinoma (F9) and fibroblast (3T3) cells. (B) Induction by serum stimulation and scrape wounding.

A recent study has suggested that growth factors, such as FGF, play an important role in patterning the embryo and regulating homeobox expression (Ruiz i Altaba and Melton, 1990). We therefore examined effects on Hox-2.1 gene expression resulting from variations in the culture conditions. Mouse 3T3 cells express the Hox-2.1 gene and, when grown to confluence or induced to enter the resting state by serum deprivation, the levels of Hox-2.1 are repressed (Figure 2B). If serum is reapplied to the culture, reappearance of Hox-2.1 expression is detected between 24-36 hrs after treatment. This is a very slow response and we tried a variety of purified growth factors in an attempt to identify the inducing signal. No significant induction was observed with enriched or purified preparations of beta-TGF, PDGF, FGF, ECDGF or NGF, but insulin did generate a weak response. Wounding cells is also known to induce cellular growth, and we scrape wounded a confluent population of 3T3 cells. The Hox-2.1 gene was induced 6 hrs after scraping (Figure 2B). These results show that Hox-2.1 is capable of responding to a variety of different signals, but that the growth factor response appears to be a very slow process and may not represent a direct stimulation by growth factors themselves. We have therefore not clearly identified the nature of the inducing signal.

In contrast, the high degree of sensitivity of Hox-2.1 to RA in Figure 2A suggests that the gene could be a direct target of RA. To further examine the nature of RA sensitivity we examined a detailed time course of the response. Figure 3A shows that the Hox-2.1 gene begins to accumulate RNA after only 15 min of treatment with RA in F9 teratocarcinoma cells. The levels increase steadily and peak around 15 hrs, remaining high for 3 days before declining to low levels 5 days after initial exposure to RA. The speed of this response supports the idea that Hox-2 genes could be direct targets of RA. But this response is not primarily at the transcriptional level, as there is only a slight

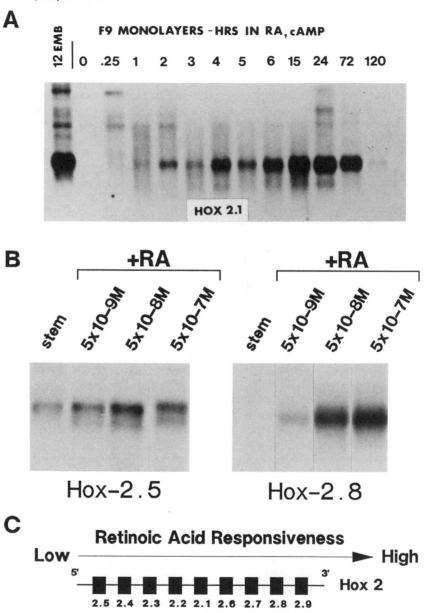

Figure 3. Responsiveness of Hox-2 genes to retinoic acid. (A) Time course of Hox-2.1 induction. (B) Variation of response with concentration. (C) Summary showing colinearity between RA response and gene order in cluster.

increase in the rates of transcription of Hox-2.1 in RA treated versus untreated F9 cells (data not shown).

To examine the relative sensitivity of Hox-2 genes to RA, we measured the degree of response of all nine genes with respect to variations in the concentration of RA. The comparative experiments were all performed in F9 cells to avoid variations in differential responsiveness between cell types, such as shown in Figure 2A. F9 stem cells were treated with three concentrations of RA ($5x10^{-9}$ -$5x10^{-7}$ M) and the levels of the Hox-2 genes before and after treatment measured by northern blotting. Examples of results for the Hox-2.5 and 2.8 genes are shown in Figure 3B. Expression of Hox-2.5 is detected in the untreated cells, and the increase in response to RA is very slight, even at the highest concentration. There is a gradual increase in the levels of Hox-2.5 as successively higher concentrations of RA are applied. In contrast, Hox-2.8 is not detected in the untreated cells and is induced to accumulate large amounts of RNA. There is clearly a dose response to RA for the Hox-2.8 gene in that levels significantly increase between $5x10^{-9}$ and $5x10^{-8}$ M RA and are highest at $5x10^{-7}$ M. The RA dose response for each gene is different, as shown here for Hox-2.5 and 2.8. However, there is a clear relationship between the position of a gene in the Hox-2 cluster and its level of response to RA. Hox-2.5 at the 5' end of the complex is the least sensitive gene, and successive genes in the cluster (moving towards Hox-2.9) show increasing responsiveness. These results are summarized in Figure 3C, and are remarkably analogous to the colinear patterns of expression we observed in the developing neural tube and hindbrain. The differential response of Hox-2 genes to a source of RA could both set up a gradient of homeobox expression and establish partially overlapping domains of expression. These data have been generated using cultured cells, and it would be useful to know whether a similar colinear RA response occurs in embryos.

RA Induction of Hox Genes in *Xenopus* Embryos

RA has received much attention as a potential embryonic morphogen, particularily in limb morphogenesis, where RA treatment alters the patterning of developing and regenerating limbs (for review see Brockes, 1989). In chick, RA-induced phenotypic alterations to the limb are identical to those generated by grafting a zone of polarizing activity (ZPA) to the anterior part of the limb bud, and support the idea that RA may play a role in normal embryonic patterning.

Homeobox genes from many species have been isolated, and there is a high degree of homology and conservation in sequence, organization and expression of the Hox clusters in all vertebrates, including *Xenopus*. Several members of the Hox-2 cluster in *Xenopus* have been cloned by De Robertis and colleagues (Wright et al., 1989), in particular Xlhbox 6 (Hox-2.5) and Xlhbox 4 (Hox-2.1). Figure 4A shows the relative position and organization of some of the members of the *Xenopus* related Hox-2 cluster, as compared to the mouse. Amphibian embryos have several advantages for examining early events during embryogenesis, and recently it was shown that RA can induce altered phenotypes in the developing *Xenopus* nervous system of the embryo (Durston et al., 1989). Since Hox-2 genes are normally expressed in the neural tube, we examined the degree to which endogenous *Xenopus* Hox-2 genes are induced by RA, to test whether the colinear and relative RA responsiveness of Hox-2 genes observed in mouse tissue culture cells occurs *in vivo* in *Xenopus* and might be related to the RA phenotype.

Figure 4B shows the results of a comparison between treated and untreated *Xenopus* embryos on the levels of expression of the Xlhbox 4 (Hox-2.1) and Xlhbox 6 (Hox-2.5) genes. The *Xenopus* probes were kindly provided by Dr. Eddy DeRobertis. The Xlhbox 6 RNA is detected by stage 24 in both treated and untreated embryos. However

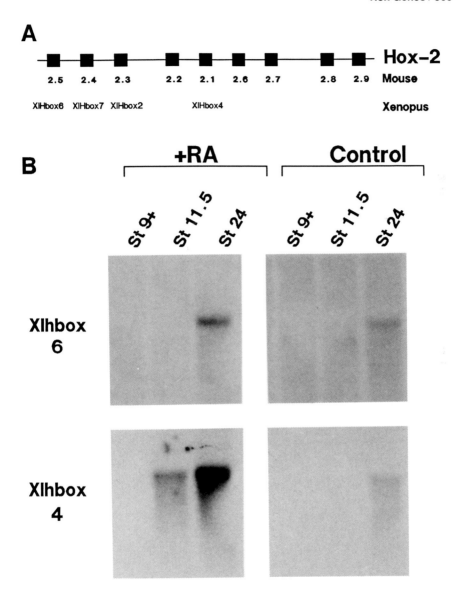

Figure 4. Induction of Hox-2 genes in retinoic acid (RA) treated *Xenopus* embryos. (A) Diagram of the mouse Hox-2 cluster with related *Xenopus* genes listed below. (B) Levels of Xlhbox 4 and 6 RNA in RA treated and control embryos at several stages.

the levels are slightly higher in embryos exposed to RA. There appears to be very little difference in Xlhbox 6 expression in RA treated embryos. In contrast, the Xlhbox 4 RNA accumulates to high levels at much earlier stages in treated embryos. The results show that the two *Xenopus* homeobox genes respond differently in the embryo to RA treatment, and that the degree of responsiveness is similar to the pattern we observed in F9 cells. The *Xenopus* related Hox-2.5 gene (Xlhbox 6) was very low in RA sensitivity and the Hox-2.1 related (Xlhbox 4) had a higher level of response. More members of the *Xenopus* cluster must be tested, but these data support the idea that homeobox genes could be direct targets of RA in the embryo, and that the colinear RA responsiveness of Hox-2 genes could be a feature of the Hox-2 complex itself, conserved during vertebrate evolution.

CONCLUSIONS

The findings in this paper demonstrate that homeobox genes have segmental patterns of gene expression in the developing vertebrate hindbrain. They lend strong support for the idea that rhombomeres are segmental units that play an important role in patterning the nervous system. The boundaries of Hox-2 expression occur at two-segment intervals, but are one rhombomere out of phase with the branchial motor system. This two-segment periodicity is potentially important, because many aspects of neural development and anatomy in the hindbrain suggest that mechanisms specifying pairs of segments are involved in organizing this region of the neural tube. While this study has focused on the patterning in the boundaries of expression, the relative levels of homeobox expression within a rhombomere may also be important in specifying segment identity. Some of the Hox-2 genes have very high levels of RNA in rhombomeres near their anterior boundary, and lower levels in more posterior rhombomeres. The effects of variable levels of expression on specification of the rhombomeres needs to be examined.

The Hox-2 genes are also expressed in neural crest derivatives in the hindbrain. This may be significant as it is believed that cranial neural crest is imprinted with positional information before it migrates from the neural plate. It is possible that the patterns of homeobox expression serve to provide positional cues to the neural crest for this imprinting process, by marking its initial A-P origin. The timing of the segment-restriced Hox-2 expression is consistent with a role not in establishing the segments themselves, but in specifying differences in the structures which may determine their individual phenotype. This is a role analogous to their *Drosophila* counterparts, which are involved in determining segment identity, and illustrates that the vertebrate Hox genes have an ancient conserved role in specifying regional variations in pattern along the body axis.

The colinear expression of Hox-2 genes in the neural tube, where the position of a gene in the cluster reflects its relative expression along the A-P axis, is an important evolutionary conserved feature of Hox genes. Retinoic acid has the ability to generate rapid graded homeobox responses in cultured cells and possibly embryos. The colinear differential sensitivity of Hox-2 genes to RA is a surprising finding, and suggests one molecular means the embryo could use to regulate homeobox expression. Many potential embryonic sources of RA have been identified (such as the notocord, early floorplate and Hensen's node); and in addition, RA receptors and cytoplasmic binding proteins have been found to have interesting expression patterns in the neural crest, CNS and PNS (Maden et al., 1990). This suggests that RA may have a normal role in neural development. It will be important to know whether RA modulates the levels of homeobox expression and/or the domains of expression. To test for the in vivo effects of RA, we are treating mouse and chicken embryos with RA and examining the level and domains of Hox-2 expression by *in situ* hybridization. In this way we hope to directly assay the embryonic responsiveness of homeobox genes to RA. The Hox-2 RA responsiveness, the ability of RA to induce neural tube (*Xenopus*) and craniofacial (mouse) abnormalities, and the effects of RA on the limb suggest that links between RA and homeobox genes will be an exciting area of future attention in the embryo.

REFERENCES

Akam ME (1987). The molecular basis for metameric pattern in the *Drosophila* embryo. **Development 101**: 1-22.

Akam M (1989). Hox and HOM: Homologous gene clusters in insects and vertebrates. **Cell 57**: 347-349.

Brockes J (1989). Retinoids, homeobox genes, and limb morphogenesis. **Neuron 2**: 1285-1294.

Doe CQ, Scott MP (1988). Segmentation and homeotic gene function in the developing nervous system of *Drosophila*. **T.I.N.S. 11**: 101-106.

Doe CQ, Hiromi Y, Gehring WJ, Goodman CS (1988a). Expression and function of the segmentation gene *fushi tarazu* during *Drosophila* neurogenesis. **Science 239**: 170-175.

Doe CQ, Smouse D, Goodman CS (1988b). Control of neuronal fate by the *Drosophila* segmentation gene *even-skipped*. **Nature 333**: 376-378.

Duboule D, Dolle P (1989). The murine Hox gene network: its structural and functional organisation resembles that of *Drosophila* homeotic genes. **EMBO J 8**: 1507-1508.

Graham A, Papalopulu N, Lorimer J, McVey JH, Tuddenham EGD, Krumlauf R (1988). Characterisation of a murine homeobox gene, Hox 2.6, related to the *Drosophila Deformed* gene. **Genes Dev 2**: 1424-1438.

Graham A, Papalopulu N, Krumlauf R (1989). The murine and *Drosophila* gene complexes have common features of organisation and expression. **Cell 57**:367-378.

Harding K, Weden C, McGinnis W, Levine M (1985). Spatially regulated expression of homeotic genes in *Drosophila*. **Science 229:** 1236-1242.

Keynes RJ, Stern CD (1988). Mechanisms of vertebrate segmentation. **Development 103:** 413-429.

Lumsden A , Keynes R (1989). Segmental patterns of neuronal development in the chick hindbrain. **Nature 337:** 424-428.

Maden M, Ong DE, and Chytil F (1989). Retinoid binding protein distribution in the developing mammalian nervous system. **Neuron,** in press.

Ruiz i Altaba A, Melton D (1990). Axial patterning and the establishment of polarity in the frog embryo. **T.I.G.S. 62:** 57-64.

Rubock MJ, Larin Z, Cook M, Papalopulu N, Krumlauf R, Lehrach H (1990). A yeast artificial chromosome containing the mouse homeobox cluster Hox-2. **Proc Natl Acad Sci USA,** in press.

Wilkinson DG, Bhatt S, Chavier P, Bravo R, Charnay P (1989). Segment-specific expression of a zinc-finger gene in the developing nervous system of the mouse. **Nature 337:** 461-464.

Wilkinson DG, Bhatt S, Cook M, Boncinelli E Krumlauf R (1989b). Segmental expression of Hox-2 homeobox-containing genes in the developing mouse hindbrain. **Nature 341:** 405-409.

Wright CVE, Cho KYW, Oliver G, DeRobertis EM (1989). Vertebrate homeodomain proteins: families of region-specific transcription factors. **T.I.B.S. 14:**52-56.

Advances in Neural Regeneration
Research, pages 309–323

NEURAL PATTERN FORMATION IN THE *DROSOPHILA* EYE

Ronald D. Rogge and Utpal Banerjee

Department of Biology and Molecular
Biology Insitute, Univ. of Calif. LA
Los Angeles, CA, 90024

It appears that insights into the mechanisms of neuronal regeneration will come only with an understanding of the basic processes that control the development of neurons. Unfortunately, the molecular mechanisms governing this developmental process are largely unknown, and only a very small number of key players have been identified.

The *Drosophila* eye has, in the past few years, gained recognition as an informative system in which one can ask questions about the molecular mechanisms of neuronal pattern formation. In principle, one of two modes of development could be envisioned. The first possibility is that cell fate is determined purely by lineage. This is often the case in early embryonic development where asymmetric cell divisions compartmentalize different components of the cytoplasm into the dividing daughter cells. In some organisms like the nematode *C.elegans*, the cell divisions are stereotypic and the lineage of every cell is known (Sulston and Horvitz, 1977). A second mode of development relies on interaction of a cell with its microenvironment. This could include interactions with membrane bound molecules on neighboring cells, secreted molecules like growth factors, or components of the extracellular matrix. As more examples become available, it is clear that a vast majority of neurons follow this second mode of development. Even in such organisms as

C.elegans, where cell lineage plays an important role in development, laser ablation and mutant studies show that the fate of any one cell is not invariant, but depends upon its environment and its developmental stage (Sulston and White, 1980).

Recent cell marking techniques in vertebrates have made it possible to determine cell lineage in the developing nervous system . It has been found in studies of the retina and the developing neural crest, that the fate of a cell is not determined by its lineage, but instead, by its environment (Turner and Cepko, 1987; Price and Thurlow, 1988; Holt et al., 1988 ; Wetts and Fraser, 1988). A cell in the right place at the right time takes on the specified fate, irrespective of its ancestry and birth date. This argues for interaction between the cell and its surround in determining neural fate. Over a decade ago, Ready et al. (1976), established that neurons in the *Drosophila* eye develop by an identical mechanism.

The eye develops as a single cell layered epithelium, called the eye disc. Development is marked by a dorso-ventral groove along the eye disc epithelium shown in Figure 1A. This groove, called the morphogenetic furrow, initiates at the posterior end of the disc and moves anteriorly. As shown in Figure 1B, cells ahead of the furrow are not patterned or differentiated. Immediately posterior to the furrow, these cells start forming clusters of neurons. Each cluster contains eight neurons (R1-R8), and gives rise to an ommatidium (facet) of the adult compound eye. Each of these eight neurons becomes an identified photoreceptor cell.

The general role of cell-cell interaction in the patterning of the photoreceptor neurons in the *Drosophlia* eye was first suggested by Ready et al.(1976) and Lawrence and Green (1979) , who showed by genetic mosaic analysis, that cells in the developing eye disc are not clonally related to each other. Some mechanism other than lineage must dictate which cell takes on the fate of an identified neuron. Tomlinson and Ready (1987),

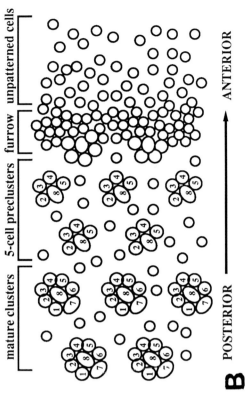

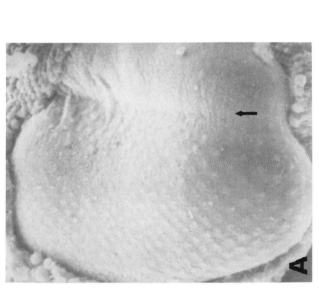

B POSTERIOR   ANTERIOR

Figure 1.

A. Scanning electron micrograph of a wild type eye disc. Anterior is to the right. The arrow marks the morphogenetic furrow.

B. Schematic representation of photoreceptor cluster formation in the eye disc. The morphogenetic furrow moves from posterior to anterior along the disc. Anterior to the furrow, cells are undifferentiated. Posterior to the furrow, initial clusters of five are formed, followed by the addition of cells R1, R6 and R7 to give rise to the mature eight cell clusters.

showed that cells in a developing photoreceptor
cluster differentiate in a specific order.
Immediately following the furrow, clusters of five
cells are visible. The central cell differentiates
first, becoming the R8 neuron. This is followed by
the pairwise differentiation of R2, R5; and R3, R4.
Three more cells join later,to complete the eight
cell cluster. Two of these cells differentiate to
become R1 and R6, followed by the final recruitment
of R7. This stereotypic differentiation pattern
led Tomlinson and Ready to propose that the fate of
a cell is determined by interactions along the
membranes of neighboring cells (1987).In this
model, a combination of cues are necessary to
specify each cell type.

Role of the *sevenless* and *bride of sevenless* Genes in Determination of R7 Fate

Much information about cell-cell interaction
has been derived from molecular analysis of the
sevenless (*sev*) gene (Banerjee et al., 1987a;Hafen
et al., 1987). In *sevenless* mutants, R7 fails to
differentiate in every ommatidium. Figure 2
compares electron microscope sections tangential to
the eye of wild type and *sevenless* flies. The
sevenless gene has been cloned and it codes for a
8.2 kb transcript that is expressed apically in the
eye disc epithelium, posterior to the morphogenetic
furrow. Sequence analysis has shown that the gene
product has an intracellular region that is highly
homologous to the tyrosine kinase domains of
oncogenes such as *ros* and *src;* and the EGF and
insulin receptors. The molecule is also predicted
to contain a large extracellular domain. The
sevenless molecule is likely to belong to the large
tyrosine receptor-kinase class (Bowtell et al.,
1988; Basler and Hafen, 1988).

Genetic mosaic studies show that the function
of the *sevenless*[+] product is essential only in
R7(Harris et al., 1976). The neighboring cells can
contain a mutant copy of this gene, and still
develop normally. Thus the function of *sevenless*
is cell autonomous. It was therefore surprising to
find that the *sevenless* protein is not limited to
the R7 cell. It is expressed, in other

photoreceptor cells and the non-neuronal cone cells
as well (Banerjee et al., 1987b; Tomlinson et al.,
1987). Perhaps this broader expression of the
sevenless protein represents the pluripotency of
the cells at the morphogenetic furrow. Any cell
could become R7, if it received the proper signals.

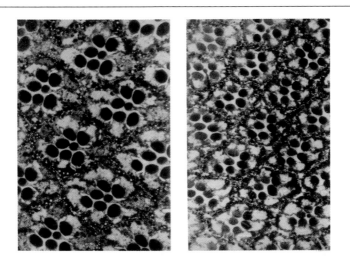

Figure 2.
Left panel: Section tangential to the adult eye of a wild
type fly. The typical trapezoidal pattern in each
ommatidium arises from the rhabdomeres of the six outer
cells R1-R6. The smaller, central rhabdomere belongs to R7.
R8 appears in a lower plane of section.
Right panel: A similar section for a *sevenless* mutant
shows that R7 is missing from every facet of the eye.

Within these cells, the localization of the
sevenless protein is limited to the apical-most
region of the epithelium. The protein is expressed
on the membranes of the microvilli extending into
the overlying extracellular matrix. This apical
localization, shown in Figure 3, underscores the
importance of the microvillar region, whose exact
role in cellular determination is as yet unclear.
If *sevenless* represents a receptor for a
developmental signal, what could one say about the
signal itself? A strong candidate for the signal

has been identified by Reinke and Zipursky (1988)
who have isolated a mutation called *bride of
sevenless* (*boss*), that has the same phenotype as
sevenless, i.e., cell R7 is missing from each facet
of the compound eye. The two mutations define
different genes that map to different chromosomes.
Genetic mosaic analysis has revealed another
important difference between the two genes. While
the function of *sevenless* is autonomous to R7, the
function of the *boss* gene is quite unnecessary in
R7 itself. Instead, the product of the *boss* gene
is required in R8 for the proper development of R7.
An R7 cell lacking *boss* product can develop
normally; but in a cluster, if the R8 lacks *boss*
product, the R7 will not develop. The *boss* gene
is being cloned, but the genetics strongly suggests
that it is likely to encode the developmental
signal that leads to the R7 cell fate.

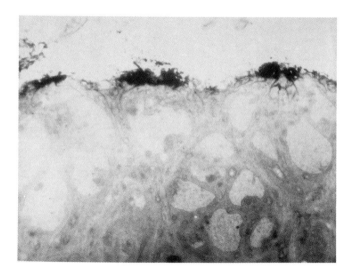

Figure 3.
Transmission EM of wild type eye disc stained with a
monoclonal antibody raised against the *sevenless*
protein. The *sevenless* protein is localized to the
apical tufts of microvilli overlying each cluster.

Role of Some Other Genes in Pattern Formation.

The *Drosophila* eye is put together by the well regulated functioning of over two hundred genes. Perturbations in any of these can lead to an abnormal eye phenotype. Some of these genes have been shown to have a direct role in the initial patterning of neurons in the eye disc. A few representative examples are presented here.

The mutation *rap* (*rhabdomeres abberant in pattern*) leads to an abnormal number of rhabdomeres in each ommatidium of the compound eye (Karpilow et al., 1989). Genetic mosaic studies for this mutation have shown that R8 must contain the *rap*$^+$ gene product for normal patterning of the cells in the ommatidium. This result points to the general importance of the central R8 cell in specifying the pattern of the rest of the neurons.

The *notch* gene codes for a transmembrane protein with EGF-like repeats in its extracellular domain (Wharton et al., 1985; Kidd et al., 1986). This gene was first identified for its role in the development of the embryonic nervous system, where it mediates the decision between neural and epidermal cell fate. In the absence of the *notch* gene product, cells canot choose the epidermal fate, but choose instead the default pathway to become neurons. The *notch* product seems to mediate inhibitory interactions between neurons, preventing neighboring cells from taking on identical fates. The role of *notch* in the development of the eye has been studied by Cagan and Ready (1989). Their studies show that the *notch* mutation can affect either the inhibitory or the inductive interactions between cells in the eye. Thus, unlike the *sevenless* gene which has an instructive role in cellular determination, the product of the *notch* gene seems to have a more general, permissive role.

The role of growth factor genes on eye development has been best established by the study of the *Ellipse* gene. In *Ellipse* mutants, there is a marked reduction in the number of ommatidia in the adult eye (Baker and Rubin, 1989). This dominant eye mutation is a gain of function allele of the *Drosophila* EGF receptor gene. Staining with antibodies demonstrates that clustering of neurons is abnormal at the morphogenetic furrow during development in the eye disc. Baker and Rubin suggest that increased levels of EGF receptor activity might correspond to regions where accessory cells, rather than neurons, are formed.

Finally, a new class of genes have been recently identified that seem to play an interesting role in the development of neurons in the eye. The genes within this class are cell specific transcription factors. The *rough* gene, for example, codes for a homeobox containing protein (Tomlinson et al., 1988; Saint et al., 1988), and its function is only needed in R2 and R5 for the proper development of R3 and R4. A second gene *seven up* codes for a product that is highly homologous to steroid receptors and participates in the determination of the fate of R3,R4,R1 and R6 (Mlodzik et al., 19ˆ). A lack of this gene product is proposed to transform each of these cells to R7. It is likely that intracellular transcription factors act in response to extracellular signals. It is hoped, that as more genes are analyzed in greater detail, we will know more about the various intervening steps.

The Enhancer Trap Method

The technique of enhancer trap or enhancer detector was first proposed in *Drosophila* by O'Kane and Gehring (1987). The method involves inserting the bacterial *lac* Z gene into the genome of the fly. Genetic crosses can be employed to mobilize this element to different parts of the genome. Many such independent insertions have been created and maintained as separate lines of flies. If in a particular line, the *lac* Z gene happens to insert close to a *Drosophila* enhancer sequence, flies from that line express β-galactosidase with the spatio-temporal specificity of the enhancer. This method can be used to identify genes that are expressed in an interesting pattern, irrespective of their mutant phenotype. The *lac* Z gene activity can be visualized in a fly that is heterozygous for the insertion. Thus even if the insertion was homozygous lethal, one could determine the specificity of the enhancer sequence in the developing eye. One such pattern is illustrated in Figure 4. In this case, the *lac* Z gene is expressed as a narrow band at the morphogenetic furrow. On screening 2,500 enhancer trap lines with separate and independent insertions, about twenty lines showed *lac* Z expression restricted to the furrow. Since important developmental decisions are made at the morphogenetic furrow, it is anticipated that some of the genes identified by this method will encode molecules of relevance to neuronal pattern formation. Other patterns that are currently being studied in our laboratory include ones in which expression of the *lac* Z gene in the eye disc is limited to R7 or R8. The only difference between the various neurons at this stage is their developmental history, and molecules that are exclusively expressed on one cell type are expected to be of developmental relevance.

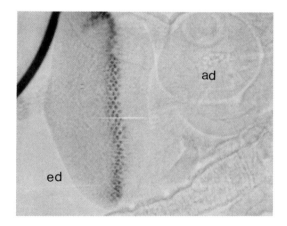

Figure 4.
An enhancer trap line that expresses the *lac* Z gene exclusively at the morphogenetic furrow.
This figure shows the eye-antenna disc stained with an antibody against β-galactosidase. The region of dark staining corresponds to the furrow. Anterior is to the right. **ed:** eye disc. **ad:** antenna disc. The eye disc gives rise to the adult eye and the antenna disc to the adult antenna.

Suppressor of sevenless

The *sevenless* gene is likely to be a receptor for a developmental signal that determines the fate of the R7 cell, and the *bride of sevenless* gene product is a good candidate for the signal that the receptor responds to. In an attempt to find other genes in this pathway, we have screened for second site dominant suppressors of the *sevenless* phenotype. This was prompted by the consideration that while the current search in several laboratories has been limited to those mutants that specifically lack R7 cells, other genes in this pathway might have functions elsewhere in the organism. For example, a molecule that is a substrate for the *sevenless* kinase, and initiates differentiation, might be required in many other tissues. A null mutation in such a gene will be difficult to isolate since it might have an unknown phenotype, including lethality. One way to generate mutations in the pathway would be to identify lesions in other genes that act as dominant, second site suppressors of *sevenless*. Since the effect is dominant, the genome has one normal copy of the "suppressor" gene, thus avoiding some of the possible adverse effects of mutating it in two copies. Several instances of such suppression have been discussed in the literature (examples: Lewis, 1945 ; Carlson et al., 1984 ; Jarvik and Botstein, 1975).

Dominant suppression due to the direct interaction of two gene products is expected only when both mutants make proteins, a slight defect in one being compensated by a defect either in structure or expression of the other. Thus, to identify a suppressor of the *sevenless* phenotype, mutagenesis was carried out using flies that make normal sized protein. A mutant that partially suppresses the *sevenless* phenotype was isolated on a *sevE4* background. We call this gene *Suppressor of sevenless (Sos)*, the allele name is JC2. Figure 5 shows a section tangential to the eye of a *sevE4;SosJC2* fly. In flies homozygous for the suppressor, about 36% of the ommatidia are wild type. The suppression can be mapped to a gene that is independent of *sevenless*.

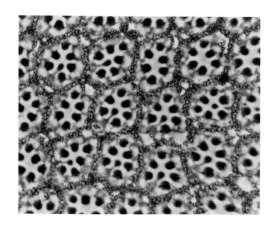

Figure 5.
Section tangential to the adult eye of a *sevE4;SosJC2* fly.
Some ommatidia are *sevenless*, others have a central R7 cell.

In color choice paradigms, the double mutant
sevE4;SosJC2 flies exhibit wild type behavior.
When given a choice between green and UV light,
wild-type flies overwhelmingly choose UV, but
sevenless flies, lacking the central UV sensitive
photoreceptor choose green. Double mutant
sevE4;SosJC2 flies overwhelmingly choose UV light
just like wild type. This implies that the central
cells not only have the morphology of R7 cells, but
they function as R7 cells as well.

Of the eighteen alleles of *sevenless* , *sevE4*
alone is suppressed by *SosJC2*. This allele
specificity further suggests that the product of
the *Sos+* gene interacts with that of *sevenless*.
If *SosJC2* was merely bypassing the *sevenless*
pathway (e.g., by spuriously phosphorylating the
sevenless substrate), one would then expect the
suppression to work even with the null alleles of
sevenless.

Genetic mosaic analysis was done to determine which cell must contain a mutant copy of the suppressor gene for R7 to develop in a *sevE4* background. The results showed that the suppression is autonomous to the R7 cell. A R7 cell is seen only when it carries the suppressor mutation. This suggests that the suppressor gene is acting intracellularly, perhaps downstream of the *sevenless* receptor.

The suppression of the *sevenless* phenotype by *Sos* follows a dosage effect. One copy of the mutant suppressor and one copy of the wild type gene gives rise to 17% suppression; two copies of the suppressor gives 36% suppression, and one mutant copy with no wild type component (achieved by using deletions) gives only 4% suppression. Thus the wild type and mutant genes seem to serve the same function. We therefore propose the hypothesis that the *Sos*JC2 mutation causes an overexpression of a gene downstream of the *sevenless* molecule. The defective kinase of *sevE4* could have residual activity that is able to rescue a R7 cell only when the *Sos*JC2 mutation causes this downstream gene to be overexpressed. This hypothesis can be tested once the *Sos* gene is analyzed at the molecular level.

Conclusions

Cells in the eye disc interact with each other, and also perhaps with their extra-cellular environment, to determine their fate. At the morphogenetic furrow, perhaps by random chance, a few of cells are determined to take on the fate of the R8 neuron. R8 is postulated to inhibit others from taking on the same neuronal fate, and is also responsible for the induction of other neuronal types. The example that is best established is the induction of the R7 cell. This induction is mediated by the interaction of the gene products of the *bride of sevenless* and the *sevenless* genes. The *Suppressor of sevenless* gene product also participates in the determination of the R7 cell, it remains to be seen if it also belongs to the same pathway.

REFERENCES

Baker N, Rubin GM (1989). Effect on eye development of dominant mutations in Drosophila homologue of the EGF receptor. Nature 340: 150–153.

Banerjee U, Renfranz PJ, Pollock JA, Benzer S (1987a). Molecular characterization and expression of *sevenless*, a gene involved in neuronal pattern formation in the Drosophila eye. Cell 49:281–291.

Banerjee U, Renfranz PJ, Hinton DR, Rabin BA, Benzer S (1987b). *The sevenless+* protein is expressed apically in cell membranes of developing *Drosophila* retina; it is not restricted to cell R7. Cell 51:151–158.

Basler K, Hafen E (1988). Control of photo-receptor cell fate by the *sevenless* protein requires a functional tyrosine kinase domain. Cell 54:299–311.

Bowtell DDL, Simon MA, Rubin GM (1988). Nucleotide sequence and structure of the *sevenless* gene of *Drosophila melanogster*. Genes and Development 2:620–634.

Cagan RL, Ready DF (1989). Notch is required for successive cell divisions in the developing Drosophila retina. Genes and Development 3:1099–1112.

Carlson M, Osmond BC, Neigeborn L, Botstein D (1984). A suppressor of SNF1 mutation causes constitutive high level invertase synthesis in yeast. Genetics 107:19–32.

Hafen E, Basler K, Edstroem JE, Rubin GM (1987). *Sevenless*, a cell-specific homeotic gene of Drosophila, encodes a putative transmembrane receptor. Science 236:55–63.

Harris WA, Stark WS, Walker JA (1976). Genetic dissection of the photoreceptor system in the compound eye of *Drosophila melanogaster*. J. Physiol. 256:415–439.

Holt CE, Bertsch TW, Ellis HM, Harris WA (1988). Cellular determination in the *Xenopus* retina is independent of lineage and birth date. Neuron 1:15–26.

Jarvik J, Botstein D (1975). Conditional lethal mutations that suppress genetic defects in morphogenesis by altering structural proteins. Proc Natl Acad Sci USA 72:2738-2742.

Karpilow J, Kolodkin A, Bork T, Venkatesh T (1989). Neuronal development in the Drosophila compound eye: rap gene function is required in photoreceptor cell R8 for ommatidial pattern formation. Genes and Development, in press.

Kidd S, Kelley MR, Young MW (1986). Sequence of the Notch locus of Drosophila: relationship of the encoded protein to mammalian clotting and growth factors. Mol Cell Biol 6:3094-3108.

Lawrence PA, Green SM (1979). Cell lineage in the developing retina of Drosophila. Dev Biol 71:142-152.

Lewis EB (1945). The relation of repeats to position effects in *Drosophila melanogaster*. Genetics 30:137-166.

Mlodzik M, Hiromi Y, Weber V, Goodman CS, Rubin GM (1990). The Drosophila seven-up gene controls neuroblast and photoreceptor cell fates. Cell 60:211-224.

O'Kane C, Gehring WJ (1987) Detection in situ of genomic regulatory elements in Drosophila. Proc Natl Acad Sci USA 84:9123-9127.

Price J, Thurlow L (1988). Cell lineage in the rat cerebral cortex: a study using retroviral-mediated gene transfer. Development 104: 473-482.

Ready DF, Hanson TE, Benzer S (1976). Development of the *Drosophila* retina, a neurocrystalline lattice. Develop Biol 53:217-240.

Reinke R, Zipursky SL (1988). Cell-cell interaction in the *Drosophila* retina: The bride of sevenless gene is required in cell R8 for R7 cell. Cell 55:321-330.

Saint R, Kalionis B, Lockett TJ, Elizur A (1988). Pattern formation in the developing eye of *Drosophila melanogaster* is regulated by the homeobox gene, rough. Nature 334:151-154.

Sulston JE, White JG (1980). Regulation and cell autonomy during postembryonic development of *C. elegans*. Devl Biol 78:577-597.

Sulston J, Horvitz R (1977). Post embryonic cell lineages of the nematode Caenorhabditis elegans. Dev Biol 56:110-156.

Tomlinson A, Bowtell DDL, Hafen E, Rubin GM (1987). Localization of the *sevenless* protein, a putative receptor for positional information, in the eye imaginal disc of Drosophila. Cell 51:143-150.

Tomlinson A, Kimmel BE, Rubin GM (1988). Rough, a Drosophila homeobox gene required in photoreceptors R2 and R5 for inductive interactions in the developing eye. Cell 55:771-784.

Tomlinson A, Ready DF (1987). Neuronal differentiation in the Drosophila ommatidium. Dev Biol 120:366-376.

Turner DL, Cepko CL (1987). A common progenitor for neurons and glia persists in rat retina late in development. Nature 328:131-136.

Wharton KA, Johansen KM, Xu T, Artavanis-Tsakonas S (1985). Nucleotide sequence from the neurogenic locus Notch implies a gene product that shares homology with proteins containing EGF-like repeats. Cell 43:567-581.

Wetts R, Fraser SE (1988). Multipotent precursors can give rise to all major cell types of the frog retina. Science 239: 1142-1145.

Advances in Neural Regeneration
Research, pages 325–327
© 1990 Wiley-Liss, Inc.

SPONTANEOUS RECOVERY OF FUNCTION AFTER SPINAL CORD INJURY

Inder Perkash

Department of Surgery, Stanford University and Spinal Cord Injury Service, VA Medical Center, Palo Alto, CA

There is ample evidence that neural regeneration and neural plasticity are attempts on the part of the nervous system to recover both anatomy and function following neurotrauma in human beings. The knowledge gained from clinical and animal studies of central nervous system regeneration and recovery of function is therefore important to develop therapeutic modalities and also to be able to prognosticate recovery in human beings following neurotrauma.

In our series of cases of clinical recovery we followed 178 newly spinal injured patients admitted during 1984-1989 to a regional spinal injury center. Of these, 31 patients had associated head injury. Of the total number, 82 were paraplegic and 96 were tetraplegic. The mean age of the patients was 56 years, with a range of 19 to 87 years.

On admission, there were 91 patients with Frankel A, 10 with Frankel B, 58 with Frankel C, 19 with Frankel D and none with Frankel E leisions. (Frankel A = Complete motor and sensory loss. Frankel B = Complete motor with incomplete sensory deficit. Frankel C = Useless motor function and intact sensations. Frankel D = Motor and sensory modalities intact but motor function not completely normal. Frankel E = Normal.) At follow-up 1 to 5 years later there were 80 with Frankel A, 4 with Frankel B, 53 with Frankel C, 39 with Frankel D and 2 with Frankel E lesions. There was significant recovery leading to 205% gain in Frankel D. No significant significant recovery was noticed in different age groups when compared with each other. Intra-Frankel classification change was evident in each group from A to E, with the highest number changing from C to D. Bowel and bladder recovery was subtle.

In the following chapters, both basic and clinical studies of spontaneous recovery of function are presented. Physiological correlates of spinal shock and recovery of function following partial spinal cord transection are described by Lillian Publos and co-workers. They show that following unilateral transection, chemical barriers are set up due to liberation of histamine or serotonin-like inhibitory substances which depress neural activity, rather than loss of descending facilitation of afferent input. They also demonstrate enhanced responsiveness to 'C' fiber stimulation when they use lidocaine to block dorsolateral funiculus transmission.

Harry Goshgarian has interesting data to show plastic morphological changes within 4 hours after an ipsilateral spinal cord hemisection at C-2. In his model, the conversion of ineffective to effective synapses only takes several hours and results in the functional recovery of a portion of the animal's diaphragm which had been paralyzed by spinal cord injury. A recent quantitative assessment of phrenic nerve activity indicates that there is a temporal correlation between the induction of the morphological alterations and the amount of functional recovery that can be measured in the paralyzed hemidiaphragm. Thus, the neuronal and glial alterations observed in the phrenic nucleus could represent the morphological substrate for the unmasking of functionally ineffective synapses in the spinal cord injury model.

Alterations of neural activity that accompany

deficits and recovery from restricted spinal lesions are presented by Charles Vierck and colleagues. They show that animals cannot discriminate between different train durations, suggesting that tactile sensations are not maintained by a repetitive stimulation. This does indicate that information supplied from caudal segments may necessarily not be adequately coded as a stimulus for recovery.

Trophic linkages between spinal motoneurons and muscles are examined by Eduardo Eidelberg. Cordotomy leads to irreversible transformation of slow to fast twitch muscle fibers in the rat. Many motoneurons show changes after cordotomy, but most eventually recover. Disuse per se does not induce significant loss of motoneurons.

David Burke discusses reflex patterns in spinal cord injured patients and doubts the existence of a disinhibited nociceptive flexion withdrawal reflex to explain flexor spasms in response to innocuous stimuli. He believes that the reflex patterns in spinal injured are not intrinsically abnormal phenomena.

The section concludes with a detailed description of characteristics and extent of recovery after human spinal cord injury by Milan Dimitrijevic and his cohorts. They discuss changes in neurocontrol of motor activity and possible mechanisms of the changes.

**Advances in Neural Regeneration
Research, pages 329–340**
© 1990 Wiley-Liss, Inc.

PHYSIOLOGICAL CORRELATES OF SPINAL SHOCK AND RECOVERY OF
FUNCTION FOLLOWING PARTIAL SPINAL CORD TRANSECTION

L.M. Pubols, D.A. Simone, J. Atkinson, H. Hirata[1],
and P.B. Brown

The Robert S. Dow Neurological Sciences Institute/
Department of Neurosurgery, Good Samaritan Hospi-
tal and Medical Center, Portland, Oregon 97210
(L.M.P., D.A.S., J.A., H.H.), Department of Physi-
ology, West Virginia University Health Sciences
Center, Morgantown, West Virginia 26506 (P.B.B.)

INTRODUCTION

While spontaneous recovery of function following
spinal cord injury has often been observed both clinically
and experimentally (e.g., Perkash, this volume; Murray and
Goldberger, 1974), the mechanisms that underlie this
recovery are poorly understood. In this laboratory we
have used the lumbar dorsal horn of the cat's spinal cord
as a model to study these mechanisms. Our standard lesion
has been unilateral transection of the dorsolateral
funiculus (DLF) at the level of T_{12}. This partial
transection interrupts much of the descending input to the
ipsilateral dorsal horn. It also axotomizes those dorsal
horn cells which project rostrally via the DLF. The most
obvious behavioral effect of this lesion immediately
postoperatively is hyperextension of the ipsilateral
hindlimb, with an inability to use the limb for standing
or walking. Over a period of several weeks, however, the
hyperextension abates, and there is recovery of the use of
the limb for posture and locomotion.

---

[1]Dr. Hirata's current address is: Department of
Anesthesiology, Yale University School of Medicine, 333
Cedar Street, New Haven, CT 06510

Our studies of the electrophysiology of L_6 and L_7 dorsal horn neurons have shown that these cells also show a temporary loss of function after T_{12} DLF lesions (Pubols et al., 1988). These neurons lose responsiveness to peripheral inputs during the first 24 hours following the lesion, and recover this responsiveness over a period of weeks. This chapter reviews these findings, and more recent work which provides clues to the physiological mechanisms that underlie these changes.

METHODS

For these studies we used adult cats, some of which had received a transection of the right dorsolateral funiculus at T_{12}. Dorsal horn cells in L_6 and L_7 were studied electrophysiologically in normal and lesioned animals anesthetized with sodium pentobarbital. The response properties of the neurons were evaluated using natural mechanical stimulation of the skin and electrical stimulation of hindlimb nerves. Cells were classed as low threshold (LT) if they responded maximally to innocuous forms of mechanical stimulation, such as movement of hairs or gentle skin pressure, high threshold (HT) if they required noxious levels of mechanical stimulation, e.g., pinching with blunt forceps, to reach threshold, and multireceptive (MR) if they responded in a graded fashion to both noxious and non-noxious mechanical stimuli.

In some experiments involving normal animals, individual dorsal horn cells were studied before and after injection of 2 μl of 2% lidocaine into the right T_{12} DLF. Fast Green dye was added to the lidocaine to mark the spread of the injection. Injections usually spread rostrocaudally for at least 1 cm, but were confined to the right lateral funiculus, and did not invade the dorsal columns or contralateral side.

RESULTS

Acute Transection of the Dorsolateral Funiculus Depresses Responsiveness to Peripheral Stimuli

During the first 24 hours following a dorsolateral funiculus lesion, responsiveness to peripheral stimulation was severely depressed. Table 1 shows that for a group of 5 animals studied during this period nearly half of the electrode penetrations contained no cells which responded to peripheral stimulation (mechanical stimulation of the skin or electrical stimulation of A fibers in the sural nerve). Normal animals had far fewer unresponsive penetrations (10.9%), a difference which was highly significant when the percentage for each animal was calculated separately and used as the basis for group comparisons (t = 5.27, d.f. = 7, p < 0.01). Responsiveness recovered over a 4 week period, and the percentage for animals studied at 28-30 days is similar to that for normals.

Table 1. Percent of Electrode Penetrations Lacking Cells Responsive to Peripheral Stimuli (% Nil Penetrations)

	# of Animals	Nil Penetrations/ Total Penetrations	%
Normal	4	5/46	10.9
DLF Lesion			
<24 hr.	5	29/61	47.5
3 days	2	9/32	28.1
14 days	3	6/40	15.0
28-30 days	5	5/48	10.4

An examination of the time course of response depression suggested that this occurs fairly rapidly. Elevated percentages of penetrations without responses to peripheral stimuli were observed from the earliest post-

lesion time studied, approximately 90 minutes after making
the lesion.

Lidocaine Blockade of the DLF Fails to Mimic the Effects of Acute DLF Transection

To account for the acute depression in responsiveness
to peripheral stimuli, we proposed that a DLF lesion might
lead to a loss of descending inhibition acting on interneurons that mediate primary afferent inhibition (Pubols
et al., 1988). Alternatively, it was proposed that other
effects of the injury such as blood flow changes,
diffusion of agents from the injury site, or release of
transmitters or other substances from degenerating nerve
terminals, might be responsible for depressed responding.
To test the first hypothesis, experiments were performed
using lidocaine injection, rather than traumatic injury,
to block transmission in the dorsolateral funiculus. If
interruption of descending inhibition is the mechanism
that causes depressed responsiveness, it was reasoned that
lidocaine blockade should mimic the effects of an acute
DLF lesion. If not, then some mechanisms other than
release of local inhibitory circuits from descending
inhibition are implicated.

Preliminary studies of 3 LT, 3 MR, and 3 HT cells
studied both before and after lidocaine blockade of the
ipsilateral T_{12} DLF have revealed that this procedure does
not result in depressed responsiveness to afferent
stimulation (natural stimulation of the skin and graded
electrical stimulation of A and C fibers in the tibial
nerve). In fact, in all cells with nociceptive inputs (MR
and HT), responsiveness to A-delta and/or C-fiber
stimulation was enhanced, while their responses to
stimulation of A-beta fibers were unaffected. Sensitivity
to natural stimulation was also enhanced for some MR and
HT cells. The 3 LT cells had no C-fiber responses, and
little, or no, A-delta response, and their responses to
electrical and natural stimuli were unaffected by
lidocaine injection into the DLF.

The responses of one MR cell to tibial nerve
stimulation before and after lidocaine injection are
illustrated in Figure 1. C-fiber responses were only

elicited by the strongest stimuli employed (50X threshold, 1 msec pulse duration), and had latencies greater than 100 msec. Therefore, responses occurring during the first 100 msec were considered to be a reflection of A-fiber activity, and responses with latencies of 101-500 msec were attributed to C-fiber activation. Figure 1 shows that C-fiber responses in this unit were greatly enhanced by lidocaine injection.

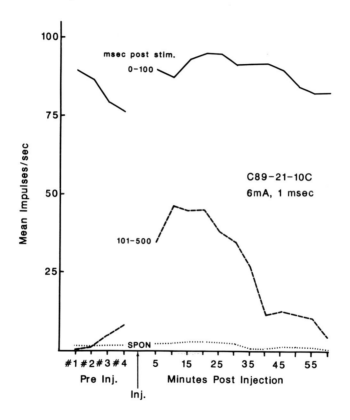

Figure 1. Response to tibial nerve stimulation at C-fiber strength in one MR cell before and after lidocaine injection of the DLF. Response rate is the mean for 25 consecutive trials at 1 trial/sec. The response to C-fiber activation occurs with a latency greater than 100 msec. Impulses occurring within the first 100 msec following the stimulus are due to A-fiber activation. SPON - rate of spontaneous activity.

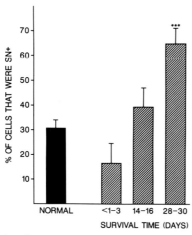

Figure 2. Mean percent of cells that responded to sural nerve stimulation in a group of normal (n = 10), <1-3 day lesion (n = 4), 14-16 day lesion (n = 3), and 28-30 day lesion (n = 5) animals. Error flags: standard error of the mean. Asterisks: mean that differed significantly from normal (p < 0.001). (From Pubols et al., 1988; reprinted with permission.)

Table 2. Increase in SN Response as a Function of Submodality and RF Locus

	% of cells giving impulses to SN stim.		
	Normal	Chronic DLF lesion	
LT< RF on toes	16.7< 2.8	39.1< 5.92	
RF off toes	13.9	33.2	
			(p<.01)
HT	45.0	55.2	(ns)
MR	35.2	55.2	(ns)

Figure 3. Receptive field locus as a function of response to sural nerve stimulation for all cells having a cutaneous receptive field. Each symbol represents one cell. Numbers refer to the hindlimb regions illustrated in the figurine at the lower left. Symbols have been placed in the box which corresponds to the hindlimb region, or regions, in which the receptive fields were located. Boxes proceeding from left to right go from more distal to more proximal hindlimb regions. Boxes proceeding from top to bottom encompass successively greater numbers of hindlimb regions, i.e., have successively larger receptive fields. LT - low threshold cell, HT - high threshold cell, MR - multireceptive cell. (From Pubols, in press; reprinted with permission.)

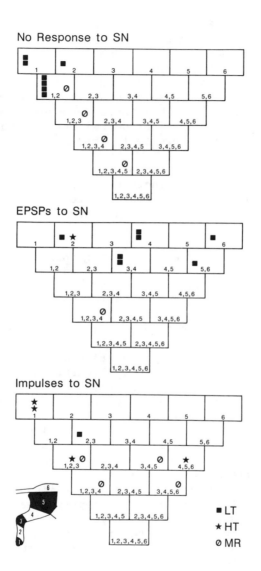

Figure 3.

Chronic DLF Lesions Strengthen Responses to Afferent Input

   While acute DLF lesions lead to temporary depression
in responsiveness, chronic DLF lesions result in enhanced
response to peripheral stimuli (Pubols et al., 1988).
While about 1/3 of the L_6 and L_7 dorsal horn cells in the
normal animal respond with impulses to sural nerve
stimulation, about 2/3 do so at 4 weeks following DLF
transection (Figure 2). This increase occurs primarily
within the subpopulation of LT dorsal horn neurons with
receptive fields on the proximal hindlimb (Table 2).

Cell Types Most Likely to Increase Responding to Sural
Nerve Stimulation After DLF Lesions Are Also Likely to
Have Subliminal Responses to Sural Nerve Stimulation in
Normal Animals.

   Studies of the dorsal horn using intracellular
methods suggest that strengthening of weak synaptic inputs
from the sural nerve is likely to be the mechanism by
which the increased efficacy of sural nerve stimulation is
achieved following chronic DLF lesions (Pubols, in press).
In addition to the cells that give impulses to sural nerve
stimulation in normal animals, a further 26% respond with
EPSPs, but not impulses, to this stimulus. As shown in
Figure 3, these are predominantly low threshold cells with
proximal receptive fields. High threshold and
multireceptive neurons tended either to give impulses or
no response to sural nerve stimulation, rather than EPSPs,
while low threshold cells tended to give either EPSPs or
no response. Within the low threshold class, all of the
cells without detectable EPSPs to sural nerve stimulation
had receptive fields on the toes and/or foot, while all of
those that displayed EPSPs had receptive fields proximal
to the toes, including some with receptive fields on the
hip or back. Thus, the subpopulation of cells that made
the greatest contribution to the increase in
responsiveness to sural nerve stimulation with chronic DLF
lesions is also the subpopulation with subliminal
responses to this stimulus in normal animals.

DISCUSSION

Our results using lidocaine are consistent with other evidence that the DLF contains descending pathways that mediate tonic inhibition of nociceptive inputs (e.g., Sandkuhler et al., 1987a), and do not support the hypothesis that depressed responsiveness with acute DLF lesions might be due to disinhibition of primary afferent depolarization. This assumes that lidocaine is equivalent to acute transection in blocking all descending activity. Experiments of Sandkuhler et al. (1987b), strongly suggest that this is the case, but one further control might be to study the same cell before and immediately after DLF transection.

Mechanisms proposed to cause the depressed responsiveness must be ones which are consistent with its fairly rapid onset and with the distance between the lesion and recording sites, which was approximately 9 cm. Depressed responsiveness was seen as early as 90 min post lesion, but the development of this phenomenon within the first 90 min has not yet been studied. Such data would obviously be of interest in suggesting, or ruling out, various potential mechanisms.

In view of the immediately enhanced responding to peripheral stimulation seen with lidocaine blockade, one might hypothesize that the increased responding to sural nerve stimulation in chronic DLF lesion animals was simply a reflection of release of descending inhibition, which was masked at earlier survival times by injury-induced depression in responsiveness. However, lidocaine injection into the DLF selectively disinhibited the high threshold (A-delta and C-fiber) input to nociceptive neurons, and had no effect upon the response properties of non-nociceptive neurons. Chronic DLF lesions, on the other hand, increased the A-fiber responses of non-nociceptive neurons. The possibility exists that some LT cells have a weak input from A-delta afferents, and that this A-delta input is under descending inhibitory control. However, we have not observed any A-delta responses in the 3 LT cells studied with lidocaine injection. Therefore, it appears that additional factors are involved in strengthening the responses of LT neurons to their afferent inputs.

One of the factors that lead to strengthening of weak projections after spinal cord injury may be the formation of new synapses, as suggested by the work of Goshgarian et al. (1989) and Murray and Goldberger (1974). Another potential mechanism is receptor up-regulation in response to partial denervation. Peptidergic receptors are of particular interest in this regard, since both primary afferents and descending pathways contain neuropeptides, such as substance P (LaMotte, 1986). Wright and Roberts (1978) observed a supersensitivity to substance P in dorsal horn neurons after dorsal root section. Further investigation is required to determine whether removal of descending substance P innervation also results in supersensitivity to substance P. Serotonin receptors might also show changes after DLF lesions, since much of the descending serotonergic input to the dorsal horn derives from raphe-spinal projections in the dorsolateral funiculus (Bowker et al., 1981; Bullitt and Light, 1989). While serotonin is usually thought to inhibit dorsal horn neurons, Randic and Yu (1976) found that iontophoretically applied serotonin excited non-nociceptive cells in the dorsal horn. Previous work (Seybold, 1985; Pubols et al., unpublished observations) has shown that serotonin receptors are found in laminae II - IV of the dorsal horn. Further work is needed to establish whether these are affected by acute and chronic DLF transection.

SUMMARY

1. Unilateral transection of the dorsolateral funiculus causes acute depression of evoked activity in dorsal horn neurons caudal to the lesion.

2. This effect appears to be due to factors unrelated to blockade of descending neural activity, since lidocaine blockade of the DLF does not depress evoked activity, and enhances the responsiveness of nociceptive neurons.

3. Responsiveness recovers within 4 weeks following DLF lesions, and weak inputs to non-nociceptive neurons become strengthened. This does not appear to be due to release of descending inhibition, since non-nociceptive neurons were unaffected by lidocaine blockade of the DLF. Other mechanisms which might cause an increased efficacy of weak

projections include collateral sprouting and receptor upregulation.

ACKNOWLEDGMENT

The authors wish to acknowledge the expert technical
assistance of S. Dawson, L. Kane, D. Fear, and J. Gregory.
This work was supported by research grant NS19523 from the
National Institutes of Health and by the Spinal Cord
Laboratory Development Fund of the Good Samaritan Hospital
and Medical Center Foundation.

REFERENCES

Bowker, RM, Westlund, KN and Coulter, JD (1981).
  Serotonergic projections to the spinal cord from the
  midbrain in the rat: An immunocytochemical and
  retrograde transport study. Neurosci Lett 24: 221-226.
Bullitt, E and Light, AR (1989). Intraspinal course of
  descending serotonergic pathways innervating the rodent
  dorsal horn and lamina X. J Comp Neurol 286: 231-242.
Goshgarian, HG, Yu, X-J, and Rafols, JA (1989). Neuronal
  and glial changes in the rat phrenic nucleus occurring
  within hours after spinal cord injury. J Comp Neurol
  284: 519-533.
LaMotte, CC (1986). Organization of dorsal horn neurotransmitter systems. In Spinal Afferent Processing,
  edited by TL Yaksh, New York Plenum, pp 97-139.
Murray, M and Goldberger, ME (1974). Restitution of
  function and collateral sprouting in the cat spinal
  cord: The partially hemisected animal. J Comp Neurol
  158: 19-36.
Pubols, LM, Hirata, H, and Brown, PB (1988). Temporally
  dependent changes in response properties of dorsal horn
  neurons after dorsolateral funiculus lesions.
  J Neurophysiol 60: 1253-1267.
Pubols, LM. Characteristics of dorsal horn neurons
  expressing subliminal responses to sural nerve
  stimulation. Somatosensory and Motor Research
  (in press).
Randic, M and Yu, HH (1976). Effects of 5-hydroxytryp-
  tamine and bradykinin in cat dorsal horn neurones
  activated by noxious stimuli. Brain Res 111: 197-203.

Sandkuhler, J, Fu, QG, and Zimmermann, M (1987a). Spinal pathways mediating tonic or stimulation-produced descending inhibition from the periaqueductal gray or nucleus raphe magnus are separate in the cat. J Neurophysiol 58: 327-341.

Sandkuhler, J, Maisch, B, and Zimmermann, M (1987b). The use of local anesthetic microinjections to identify central pathways: A quantitative evaluation of the time course and extent of the neuronal block. Brain Res 68: 168-178.

Seybold, V (1985). Distribution of histaminergic, muscarinic and serotonergic binding sites in cat spinal cord with emphasis on the region surrounding the central canal. Brain Res 342: 291-296.

Wright, DM and Roberts, MHT (1978). Supersensitivity to a substance P analogue following dorsal root section. Life Sciences 22: 19-24.

**Advances in Neural Regeneration
Research, pages 341–353
© 1990 Wiley-Liss, Inc.**

POSSIBLE MORPHOLOGICAL AND PHYSIOLOGICAL CORRELATES TO
THE UNMASKING OF A LATENT MOTOR PATHWAY AFTER SPINAL
CORD INJURY

Harry G. Goshgarian

Department of Anatomy and Cell Biology
Wayne State University, School of
Medicine, Detroit, Michigan 48201

INTRODUCTION

As we have discussed in this symposium, there are
numerous instances in which spontaneous recovery of
function occurs after spinal cord injury. Many of these
examples of functional restitution do not involve
regeneration in the injured spinal cord at all (Basbaum
and Wall, 1976; Guth, 1976; Goshgarian and Guth, 1977;
Devor and Wall, 1981a,b; Devor, 1983; Seltzer and Devor,
1984). Rather, it has been suggested that functional
recovery could be achieved through the activation of
normally latent pathways found in the non-damaged
regions of the spinal cord (Goshgarian et al., 1989).
Little is known about the mechanisms involved in the
unmasking of these pathways (Cragg and McLachlan, 1978;
Devor et al., 1986). Why are they normally latent and
what are the sequelae of spinal cord injury which govern
their unmasking and ultimate functional expression?
Electrophysiological studies conducted primarily on
sensory pathways not only in the spinal cord, but also
in many other regions of the CNS have suggested that the
pathways are latent because their synaptic connections
are initially functionally ineffective in firing the
postsynaptic target neuron (see Goshgarian et al., 1989
for literature review). Shortly after injury to the
nervous system or other various manipulations, however,
the functionally ineffective synapses are converted to
ones which can initiate activity in the postsynaptic
cell. The result is spontaneous functional restitution.

Early studies from our laboratory have related functionally ineffective synapses to a latent motor pathway in the injured spinal cord (Goshgarian and Guth, 1977; Goshgarian, 1979, 1981). In these studies, we employed a well known respiratory reflex known as the "crossed phrenic phenomenon" (CPP) to demonstrate injury-induced neural plasticity in the mammalian spinal cord. Briefly, the CPP can be described as follows (Fig. 1). Cervical spinal cord hemisection rostral to the level of the phrenic nucleus will paralyze the ipsilateral hemidiaphragm. If the phrenic nerve to the opposite, functioning side of the diaphragm is then cut (i.e., if the animal is subjected to severe respiratory stress), functional recovery is achieved in the hemidiaphragm paralyzed by spinal cord hemisection. This example of spontaneous functional restitution of muscle paralyzed by spinal cord injury has been referred to as the crossed phrenic phenomenon (Chatfield and Mead, 1948).

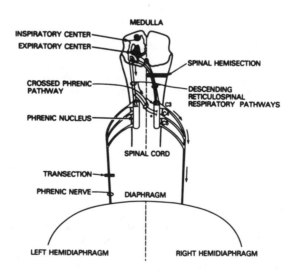

Fig. 1   Diagram of the descending respiratory pathways and the surgical procedures required to induce the crossed phrenic phenomenon (see text).

Our previous studies have shown that there is a delayed expression of the CPP in guinea pigs (Goshgarian and Guth, 1977) and young adult rats (Goshgarian, 1979). That is, if these animals are subjected to spinal hemisection followed immediately by contralateral phrenicotomy, the CPP is either not expressed at all or it is relatively weak and the animals usually die of asphyxia shortly after surgery. However, if several hours are allowed to pass after spinal hemisection before the contralateral phrenicotomy is carried out, the animals display a prominent CPP (Goshgarian and Guth, 1977; Goshgarian, 1979; O'Hara and Goshgarian, 1988).

The above results imply that there are rapid, lesion-induced changes that occur in the spinal cord within hours after injury which unmask functionally ineffective synapses and allow the animal to more fully express the CPP. Although the unmasking of functionally ineffective synapses has been demonstrated physiologically throughout the CNS, and several physiological mechanisms for their unmasking have been hypothesized over the years (Cragg and McLachlan, 1978; Devor et al., 1986), a morphological basis underlying the unmasking of the connections has only recently been suggested (Goshgarian et al., 1989).

The purpose of this chapter is to briefly describe specific morphological alterations of the normal ultrastructure of the rat phrenic nucleus which can be detected as early as 4 hours after an ipsilateral spinal cord hemisection and to suggest that these alterations could represent the morphological basis for the unmasking of functionally ineffective synapses in our spinal cord injury model. Furthermore, data from a quantitative electrophysiological analysis of phrenic nerve activity during the CPP will be presented to show that there is a temporal correlation between the enhanced expression of the CPP and the induction of the injury-induced morphological alterations in the phrenic nucleus. The morphological results summarized in this chapter have been described in detail in a previous publication (Goshgarian et al., 1989), but the physiological results thus far have only been described in abstract form (O'Hara and Goshgarian, 1988).

MATERIALS AND METHODS

Young adult (6-14 weeks old) male and female
Sprague Dawley rats were used in both the morphological
and electrophysiological experiments of this
investigation. All animals were anesthetized with 4%
chloral hydrate (400 mg/kg, i.p.) prior to surgery,
perfusion, and physiological monitoring of phrenic nerve
activity during the CPP.

Morphological Studies

The CPP was not induced in the animals for
morphological study. The sole purpose of the study was
to describe the rapid changes that occur in the phrenic
nucleus following a rostral, ipsilateral spinal cord
hemisection. Horseradish peroxidase (HRP) was applied
to the transected left phrenic nerve two days before
sacrifice in all animals to retrogradely label phrenic
motoneurons for identification under the electron
microscope. At 4 hours, 1 day, 2 days, and 4 days prior
to sacrifice, 4 rats at each time interval were
subjected to a left cervical spinal cord hemisection at
C_2. Four control animals were sacrificed without
hemisection.

Following surgery, the animals were perfused by a
mixture of 2.5% glutaraldehyde and 0.5% paraformaldehyde
in 0.1M phosphate buffer. The cervical spinal cord was
removed and HRP-labeled neurons in the phrenic nucleus
were processed for EM examination as previously
described (Goshgarian et al., 1989). The morphological
features of the phrenic neuropil were analyzed
qualitatively and then quantitated by a Bioquant IV
morphometric analysis system. Significant differences
in morphological features of the phrenic neuropil
between groups were determined by a two-tailed Student's
t-test. Significance was established at $p < 0.05$.

Physiological Studies

Following a left C_2 hemisection, both phrenic
nerves were exposed in the neck where they pass ventral
to the roots of the brachial plexus. The left phrenic

nerve was placed on recording electrodes while the right
phrenic nerve was blocked with a 2% xylocaine solution
to induce the CPP. CPP activity was recorded between 12
and 15 minutes after the spinal hemisection. After the
initial recording was completed, the xylocaine was
washed from the right phrenic nerve with saline, and the
animal's wounds were closed. A second recording of
crossed phrenic activity was made in each animal after
an interval of 1,2,4,12, or 24 hours post hemisection.
Four animals were used at each interval. The recording
conditions were standardized at each recording session.

Crossed phrenic activity was amplified with a
Tecktronix AM502 differential amplifier (gain, 100K)
using a bandpass of $0.1\text{-}1\text{KH}_2$ for all of the recordings.
The signals were electronically rectified, integrated,
and recorded on a Gould/Brush 2400 Series Analog
Recorder. The area beneath the integrated compound
nerve potentials, representing our quantitative
assessment of phrenic nerve activity, was measured with
a Bioquant system. The average integrated area of 15
consecutive crossed phrenic bursts was obtained for each
recording session. After subtracting out EKG activity,
the average area obtained at the first recording session
was subtracted from the average area obtained at the
second recording session. The difference between the
initial and second recording was expressed as a ratio of
the initial recording multiplied by 100% for each
animal.

For statistical analysis, an average percent
increase and standard error of the mean were calculated
for the group of 4 animals at each time interval.
Significant increases for each of the group means was
assessed using 95% confidence intervals. One-way
analysis of variance was used to test for a significant
difference between groups. Significant differences
between individual pairs of groups were determined using
Duncan's multiple range test.

RESULTS

Morphological Studies

The normal ultrastructure of the rat phrenic nucleus has already been described in detail by our laboratory (Goshgarian and Rafols, 1984; Goshgarian et al., 1989) and is summarized in figure 2, top drawing. The majority of the dendrites of phrenic motoneurons are oriented rostrocaudally in the spinal cord and surround phrenic motoneuron cell bodies in transverse sections through the phrenic nucleus. Normally, the longitudinally oriented dendrites (D1-D6) are isolated from each other by thin, intervening astroglial processes (dotted areas). Occasionally, short dendrodendritic membrane appositions (e.g., between D1 and D2; and between D5 and D6) with punctum adhaerens (open block arrow) are seen. Synaptic terminals in the phrenic nucleus usually form single synapses with a postsynaptic profile (e.g., T_1-T_4), but an occasional double synapse (between T_5 and D5 and D6) is also observed. We have defined double synapses as presynaptic boutons establishing active synaptic zones with more than one postsynaptic profile in the same plane of section.

Both qualitative and quantitative morphometric analysis indicated that by 4 hours post hemisection (Fig. 2, center drawing), the mean length of the dendrodendritic appositions increased significantly (p<0.01) from 1.42 ± 0.09 to 1.89 ± 0.12 um. The mean dendrodendritic apposition length further increased to 2.20 ± 0.20 um by 1 day post hemisection. The increase in dendrodendritic apposition length is most likely due to an active withdrawal of astroglial processes away from their normal position in between adjacent dendrites (exemplified by the directions indicated by the solid block arrows). In addition, by 4 hours post hemisection, the number of double synapses (between T_1 and D1,D2, and between T_4 and D5,D6) increased significantly (p<0.01) from the normal value of 71 ± 8 to 110 ± 8 synapses.

At 4 days post hemisection (Fig. 2, bottom drawing), the mean percentage of appositions per total

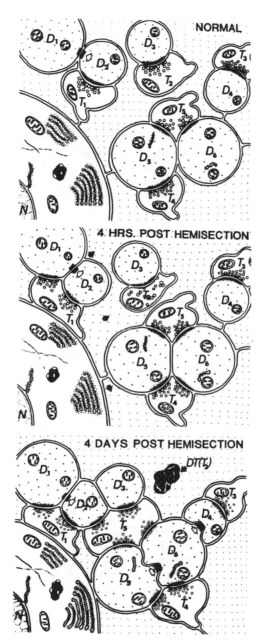

Fig. 2 Diagram of the rapid morphological alterations
that occur in the rat phrenic nucleus (see text).

dendrite number increased significantly (p<0.01) from
the normal value of 4.68 $\pm$ 0.69% to 7.46 $\pm$ 0.79%.
Several of these new appositions were relatively short,
and thus the mean length of the dendrodendritic
appositions reverted back to normal levels at this time.
Several dendrites displayed irregular contours (D4-D6)
with finger-like processes and puncta adhaerentia (e.g.,
open block arrows between D5 and D6). In addition, a
slight decrease in the number of double synapses was
accompanied by a corresponding increase in the number of
triple and quadruple synapses (e.g., T_5 in Fig. 2,
bottom drawing). Degenerated terminals (Fig. 2, DT
which represented T_2 in top and middle drawings) were
usually incorporated into glial processes.

Physiological Studies

In the rat, crossed phrenic activity can be induced
within minutes after spinal hemisection, but this
activity is very weak. At one hour post hemisection,
there was no significant increase in crossed phrenic
activity as compared to the initial control recording
(Fig. 3). The mean for the one hour post hemisection
group was 13.15 $\pm$ 19.58% increase over the initial
recording. Two hours post hemisection, however, there
was a statistically significant increase in crossed
phrenic activity with the mean for this group being
73.56 $\pm$ 18.81% increase over the initial recording.
Four hours post hemisection a marked enhancement of
crossed phrenic activity was found with the mean for
this group being 237.10 $\pm$ 70.25%. Twelve hours post
hemisection the increase in crossed phrenic activity
over the control recordings maintained its relatively
elevated value with the mean for this group being 217.77
$\pm$ 40.26%. A similar situation was observed in the 24
hour post hemisection group (211.91 $\pm$ 48.53%). Thus,
crossed phrenic activity is markedly enhanced by 4 hours
post hemisection and this enhancement in activity
persists out to 24 hours post hemisection (the longest
survival time studied).

DISCUSSION

Investigators have maintained that there should be

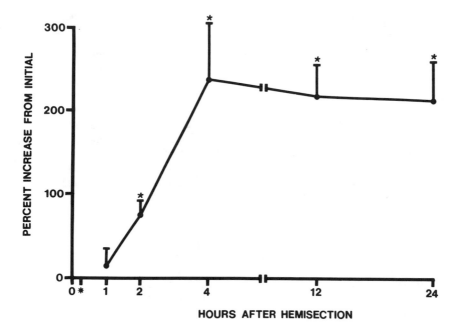

Fig. 3. The percent increase in crossed phrenic
activity at various post-hemisection
intervals. Asterisk on horizontal axis
denotes the initial recording at 15 min
post hemisection. First significant
increase over initial recording is at 2
hours (see text).

no morphological substrate underlying the rapid
unmasking of functionally ineffective synapses after CNS
injury presumably because of the consensus that
injury-induced morphological changes are relatively slow
(Devor et al. 1986). Furthermore, it has been suggested
that there is no need to propose a morphological basis
for the unmasking of functionally ineffective synapses
since their expression after CNS injury can be explained
by well known physiological principles such as the
release of the target cell from chronic post-synaptic
inhibition or the development of denervation-induced
hypersensitivity (Cragg and McLachlan, 1978).

It is possible, however, that the rapid morphological alterations which occur in the phrenic nucleus may be related to the unmasking of functionally ineffective synapses in our spinal cord injury model involving the crossed phrenic phenomenon. It has been suggested that glial process retraction from in between adjacent neural membranes would result in a rise in the extracellular potassium concentration because the glial processes would no longer be available to absorb the potassium which is released from the physiologically active cells (Halton et. al., 1984; Hatton, 1985, 1986). Elevated extracellular potassium would increase neuronal membrane excitability by partial depolarization (Hatton, 1985, 1986). In addition, the increase in neural membrane apposition resulting from glial retraction may create the development of electrical field effects around groups of neurons. The result of these field effects would be to synchronize the firing of cells, especially if electrical excitability were already elevated by depolarizing extracellular ion concentrations (Hatton, 1985).

Thus, in our model, there is no need to propose the presence of individual abnormal or immature synapses which are rapidly coverted after CNS injury to ones capable of initiating activity in the postsynaptic target neuron. It is possible that functionally ineffective synaptic terminations from the crossed phrenic pathway (Fig. 1) may be both physiologically and morphologically normal, but quantitatively insufficient to fully depolarize phrenic motoneurons in spinal hemisected young adult rats. Thus, when the animals are subjected to respiratory stress immediately after spinal hemisection, the summated action potentials of the crossed phrenic input may not be able to fire many cells. Within hours after spinal cord injury, however, glial retraction and increases in phrenic membrane apposition could result in enhanced excitability of phrenic motoneurons. This enhanced excitability coupled with the rapid presynaptic augmentation of input mediated by double synapse formation, could be the mechanism enabling previously ineffective synapses of the crossed phrenic pathway to activate many more phrenic motoneurons and thus bring about meaningful functional restitution.

A major problem in physiologically assessing an injury-induced increase in crossed phrenic activity in rats is the inter-animal variation in the amount of activity that can be generated immediately after spinal cord hemisection. This variation is due to spinal cord circuitry which is established during the normal development of the animal. The present physiological experiments were designed to differentiate between crossed phrenic activity that can be generated by developmentally acquired circuitry and the enhanced activity that is generated from injury-induced modifications to this circuitry. This was accomplished by subtracting the mean integrated area under the 15 minute waveforms from the mean area under the waveforms generated at a later post hemisection interval and expressing the difference as a ratio of the initial activity. The result of this procedure is an assessment of hemisection induced enhancement of activity with each animal serving as its own control.

The present physiological study has shown that there is a significant augmentation of crossed phrenic activity in young adult rats as early as 2 hours after a C_2 spinal cord hemisection. By 4 hours post hemisection, however, the increase in activity reaches a maximum as compared to the initial activity seen immediately after spinal cord hemisection. The augmented activity is then maintained through the 24 hour duration of the study. The above physiological results correlate temporally with the morphological changes observed in the phrenic nucleus within 4 hours after C_2 hemisection and suggest that glial retraction and synaptogenesis may be related to the increased activity (Goshgarian et al., 1989). Additional experiments are being conducted in our laboratory to establish causality between the herein described morphological and physiological events.

ACKNOWLEDGEMENT

This work was supported by U.S. Public Health Service grant NS-14705.

REFERENCES

Basbaum AI, Wall PD (1976). Chronic changes in the
response of cells in the adult cat dorsal horn
following partial deafferentation. The appearance of
responding cells in a previously non-responsive
region. Brain Res 116:181-204.
Chatfield PO, Mead S (1948). Role of the vagi in the
crossed phrenic phenomenon. Am J Physiol 54:417-422.
Cragg B, McLachlan E (1978). A mechanism for the
observed recovery from ineffectiveness of synapses in
the central nervous system. J Theor Biol 71:433-440.
Devor M (1983). Plasticity of spinal cord somatotopy
in adult mammals: Involvement of relatively
ineffective synapses. Birth Defects: Orig Art
Series 19:287-314.
Devor M, Basbaum AI, Seltzer Z (1986). Spinal
somatotopic plasticity: Possible anatomical basis
for somatotopically inappropriate connections. In
Goldberger ME, Gorio A, Murray M (eds):
"Development and Plasticity of the Mammalian Spinal
Cord," Padova, Italy:Liviana, pp 211-227.
Devor M, Wall PD (1981a). Effect of peripheral nerve
injury on receptive fields of cells in the cat spinal
cord. J Comp Neurol 199:277-291.
Devor M, Wall PD (1981b). Plasticity in the spinal
cord sensory map following peripheral nerve injury in
rats. J Neurosci 1:679-684.
Goshgarian HG (1979). Developmental plasticity in the
respiratory pathway of the adult rat. Exp Neurol
66:547-555.
Goshgarian HG (1981). The role of cervical afferent
nerve fiber inhibition of the crossed phrenic
phenomenon. Exp Neurol 72:211-225.
Goshgarian HG, Guth L (1977). Demonstration of
functionally ineffective synapses in the guinea pig
spinal cord. Exp Neurol 57:613-621.
Goshgarian HG, Rafols JA (1984). The ultrastructure
and synaptic architecture of phrenic motor neurons in
the spinal cord of the adult rat. J Neurocytol
13:85-109.
Goshgarian HG, Yu X-J, Rafols JA (1989). Neuronal
and glial changes in the rat phrenic nucleus
occurring within hours after spinal cord injury. J
Comp Neurol 284-519-533.

Guth L (1976). Functional plasticity in the
  respiratory pathway of the mammalian spinal cord.
  Exp Neurol 51:414-420.
Hatton GI (1985). Reversible synapse formation and
  modulation of cellular relationships in the adult
  hypothalamus under physiological conditions. In
  Cotman, CW (ed): "Synaptic Plasticity", New York:
  Guilford Press, pp 373-404.
Hatton GI (1986). Plasticity in the hypothalamic
  magnocellular neurosecretory system. Fed Proc
  45:2328-2333.
Hatton GI, Perlmutter LS, Salm AK, Tweedle CD
  (1984). Dynamic neuronal-glial interactions in
  hypothalamus and pituitary: Implications for control
  of hormone synthesis and release. Peptides 5 (suppl.
  1):121-138.
O'Hara TE, Goshgarian HG (1988). Increased phrenic
  nerve activity occurring within hours of an
  ipsilateral C_2 spinal cord hemisection in adult rats.
  Soc Neurosci Abst 14(1):606.
Seltzer Z, Devor M (1984). Effect of nerve section on
  the spinal distribution of neighboring nerves. Brain
  Res 306:31-37.

Advances in Neural Regeneration
Research, pages 355–368
© 1990 Wiley-Liss, Inc.

ALTERATIONS OF A CORTICAL NETWORK OF NEURONS
FOLLOWING INTERRUPTION OF THE DORSAL SPINAL COLUMNS

Charles J. Vierck, Jr.[1], Barry L. Whitsel[2],
Albert T. Kulics[3] and Brian Y. Cooper[1]

[1]Department of Neuroscience and Center for
Neurobiological Sciences, University of
Florida College of Medicine, Gainesville, FL
32610
[2]Department of Physiology, School of Medicine,
University of North Carolina, Chapel Hill, NC
27514
[3]Department of Physiology and Neurobiology,
Northeastern Ohio Universities' College of
Medicine, Rootstown, OH 44272

In anticipation of techniques that might
restore sensory capacities following "repair" of a
spinal transection (e.g., by implantation of fetal
tissue), an optimistic view is that new connections
could be supplied from caudal segments to
projection neurons in the dorsal horn rostral to
the transection. However, it is unlikely that
functions of the dorsal columns (containing primary
afferent projections to the medulla) could be
restored. Thus, the maximal functional recovery
that might be attained following repair of a
transection can be modeled by restricting
somatosensory transmission to pathways originating
in the dorsal horn. Such a model is provided by
testing capacities for discrimination of
somatosensory stimuli applied to regions innervated
by spinal segments caudal to a lesion of the dorsal
columns.

Previous investigations of the pathway from
the dorsal columns (DCs) to the brainstem (gracile
and cuneate nuclei), ventrobasal thalamus and
primary somatosensory cortex (S-I) have generally

emphasized and revealed substrates for spatial resolution. For example, a high degree of topographic order and detail, and predominant representations of the distal extremities have been demonstrated by recordings within this system (e.g., Dreyer et al., 1974; Ferrington et al., 1988). Therefore, textbook descriptions of spinal pathways have asserted that spatial discriminations are lost following interruption of the dorsal columns. However, a series of psychophysical investigations of monkeys have shown that a variety of spatial and intensive discriminations are not deteriorated (or are disrupted only temporarily) by lesions of the dorsal columns (reviewed by Vierck and Cooper, 1990).

Monkeys have been trained on paradigms which provided threshold estimates for the following discriminations: a) touch detection and pressure discrimination (Vierck, 1977), b) absolute localization (Vierck et al., 1988), c) the presence of a gap between two simultaneous contacts (the two-point threshold; Vierck and Cooper, 1990), d) the relative positions of two points applied sequentially (Vierck et al., 1983), e) the relative size of objects impressed on the skin (Vierck, 1973), and limb position sense (Vierck, 1984). In each case, the stimuli were applied to either hindlimb, and rostral (thoracic) lesions of the dorsal column on the ipsilateral side did not produce enduring deficits. Thus, ascending pathways originating in the dorsal horn can support many spatial capacities that have been regarded as hallmarks of discriminative somesthesis. However, consideration of the ascending connections that might be reestablished by repair of a spinal transection demands attention to other aspects of somatosensory resolution as well.

As shown in figure 1, long projections from segment A (below a transection) would no longer terminate in the dorsal column nuclei or the thalamus, leaving a zone of the thalamocortical projection system severely deafferented (A: cells symbolized by open circles). However, a portion of the deafferented zone would receive inputs from

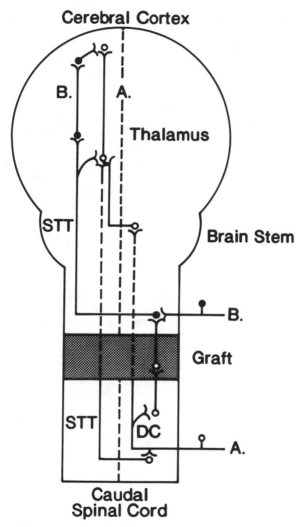

Figure 1. A diagram of hypothetical ascending connections after repair of a spinal transection. Long dorsal column (DC) and spinothalamic (STT) axons from below the lesion (A) will degenerate (dashed lines on either side of the midline). However, a graft might relay information from caudal segments to rostral STT cells (B). At thalamic and cortical levels, the intact projection systems (B) provide some input to the deafferented neurons (A).

nearby regions that are fully innervated by intact pathways (B: closed circles). Evidence to support the driving of deafferented cortex from inputs to adjacent, innervated regions is provided by experiments involving section of peripheral nerves (Merzenich et al., 1984) and by many demonstrations of a wide representation within the S-I cortical map of a small spot on the skin surface (e.g., Woolsey et al., 1942; Juliano and Whitsel, 1987). Thus, if inputs from caudal segments could be provided to some of the rostral projection neurons supplying these collateral inputs, as shown in Fig. 1, it is conceivable that the deafferented zone of cortex would respond to stimulation within dermatomes caudal to the lesion.

If the connections diagrammed in Fig. 1 could be established by repair of a spinal transection, somatotopic representation of the segments caudal to the lesion would be impoverished. Even if information were transmitted through grafted tissue at the lesion site, all inputs from caudal segments would be to one or a few rostral segments containing long projection neurons (Jakeman and Reier, 1990). Therefore, tests of spatial resolution may be of less relevance to the questions under consideration than are evaluations of capacities to resolve the temporal features of somatosensory input. For example, if stimulation of the ventral surfaces of the feet could be detected and timed, any capacity for ambulation would be aided.

When temporal features of tactile stimulation have been varied in tests of discrimination, the importance of dorsal column input to rostral projection targets has been revealed. The first hint of this came from a study of spatiotemporal resolution in which monkeys learned to respond differentially to brushing across a small patch of skin in proximal-distal or distal-proximal sequences. Interruption of the dorsal columns produced enduring deficits on this test of spatiotemporal resolution (Vierck, 1974). For a more pure test of temporal resolution, monkeys have been trained to discriminate different frequencies of tactile stimulation. Normally, the animals distinguished between 10 Hz and 12-14 Hz, but after section of the ipsilateral dorsal column the animals could not differentiate 10 from 35 Hz (Vierck et al., 1985). Also, several monkeys have been trained to discriminate different intervals between two pulses of electrical stimulation. Preoperatively, an interval of 100 msec was discernable from 120 msec, but after a dorsal column lesion, one of these monkeys has not produced comparable performance at intervals of 70 vs. 120 msec (A. Kulics and C. Vierck, unpublished observations).

In order to determine whether the deficits in temporal discriminations were restricted to a difficulty in resolution of intervals between pulses, we have subsequently trained monkeys to discriminate between different durations of stimulation at 10 Hz. Much to our surprise, section of the dorsal column produces a severe deficit on this task (C. Vierck and B. Cooper, unpublished observations). Preoperatively, 3 animals could reliably distinguish 3 pulses (over a train duration of 200 msec) from 5, 6 or 7 pulses, but after the lesion they could not respond appropriately to trains containing as many as 30 tactile stimuli (train durations of 1.5 to 3 sec).

The severe deficit in discriminating the duration of tactile stimulation indicates that interruption of the dorsal column deprives rostral projection targets of a type of input that is required for maintenance of responsivity to repetitive stimulation. The tests of temporal discrimination required that the subjects receive a series of stimuli on each trial and then report on differences in intervals or durations. In contrast, the earlier tests of spatial and intensive capacities presented the critical cue at the first contact on each trial (following intertrial intervals of 10 seconds or longer). That is, lesioned animals could detect and locate stimuli that were presented separately, but even gross differences in duration were not discriminable when the stimuli were presented in rapid succession.

The inability of CNS neurons to support a discrimination of stimulus duration could result from a variety of deficiencies in activation of the partially deafferented neurons by intact pathways. The worst of these possibilities - a lack of driving by the stimulus - is unlikely. If this were the case, animals with dorsal column lesions would not be capable of detecting and localizing tactile stimuli. Also, neurophysiological investigations have demonstrated activation of cortical neurons within regions of the S-I cortex that are partially deafferented by interruption of the dorsal columns (Dreyer et al., 1974; Eidelberg and Woodbury, 1972). Other possible disruptions of these neural networks could result from relative imbalances of excitation and inhibition. For example, inhibition could build up, so that the neurons become progressively unresponsive to high rates of repetition. Alternatively, the network could be inadequately inhibited following activation by a stimulus, leading to prolonged afterdischarge.

For an evaluation of the effects of a spinal lesion on rostral networks that contribute to sensory experiences, it is important to sample comprehensively the activity of neurons within the appropriate regions. For this purpose, cortical evoked potentials have been recorded in animals with dorsal column lesions (Anderson et al., 1972). Relative to preoperative recordings, only subtle increases in latency and decreases in amplitude were noted for single traces. However, when pairs of electrical stimuli are presented, and S-I evoked potentials are averaged over repetitions of the pairs to awake monkeys, the response to the first stimulus is greatly attenuated, and little or no activity follows the second stimulus (Figs. 2 and 3; A. Kulics and C. Vierck, unpublished observations). Thus, the behavioral deficit in responsiveness to iterations is revealed by averaged recordings which accumulate only salient and consistent responses.

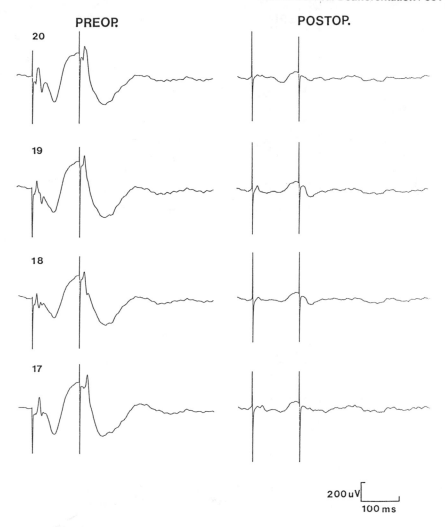

PREOP.   POSTOP.

20

19

18

17

200 uV
100 ms

Figure 2. Averaged evoked responses for 25 pairs
of pulses (100 msec ISI; 10 sec between pairs),
delivered to the hands of an awake monkey. Four
electrodes (#17-#20) were spaced 5 mm apart at
locations spanning the S-I hand representation.
Positivity is up. Preoperatively, fully developed
potentials were elicited at each location by each
pulse. Postoperatively, potentials could be
observed for individual stimuli (not shown), but
the averaged potentials were markedly attenuated.

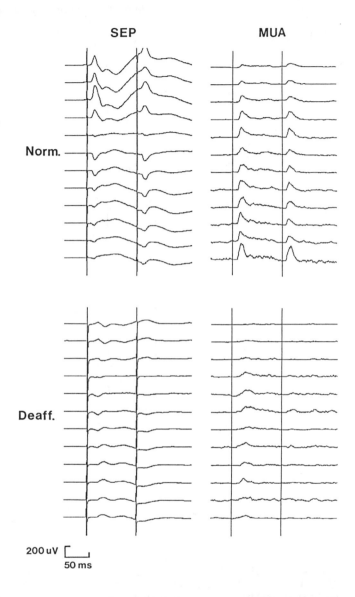

SEP　　**MUA**

Norm.

Deaff.

200 uV

50 ms

Figure 3. Averaged evoked responses (SEPs) and
multiple unit activity (MUA; integrated and half
wave rectified) for series of 10 paired stimuli to
the hands. Surface-to-depth recordings from S-I
(top-to-bottom of each panel) by an electrode
containing 12 tips, spaced at 400 um intervals.
The SEPs and MUA are attenuated throughout the
deafferented cortex, particularlly for the second
stimulus. Voltage calibration refers to SEPs only.

Evoked potentials are quite useful for sampling large areas of cortical tissue and evaluating whether any part of a somatosensory representation responds to stimulation at a given point on the skin. However, the need for averaging makes this technique marginally useful for assessing responses to individual stimuli. For this purpose, multiple unit recordings have been obtained from S-I cortex of monkeys (B. Whitsel, A Kulics and C. Vierck, unpublished observations). In one of these experiments, responses to brushing 3.0 x 1.0 cm areas of skin on the left forelimb or hindlimb were recorded 6 months following a left dorsal column lesion at an upper thoracic level. Stimulation of the left arm activated normally innervated cortex, and the hindlimb region of the right S-I cortex was deprived of input from the dorsal columns. In order to thoroughly test responsivity to repetitive stimulation, series of 100 stimuli were delivered at interstimulus intervals of 0.44 to 10 sec.

An example of clear differences in responsivity of normal and DC-deafferented cortex is shown in Fig. 4. The panels on the left present the activity of a cluster of fully afferented neurons in the forelimb region of S-I to 100 repetitions of the brushing stimulus. The difference between levels of activity during the interstimulus intervals (ISIs: top left panel) and during the stimulus (middle panel) is shown in the bottom left panel. Each stimulus produced a response, and the rate of driven activity was approximately 5 times the spike rate during the ISIs. In contrast, the panels on the right side of Fig. 4 demonstrate weak and inconsistent activation of a cluster of neurons in the DC-deafferented hindlimb region of S-I. A striking feature of this record is an extreme variability in activity along the series of ISIs (top panel) and stimuli (middle panel). Clearly this group of neurons was not consistently activated by the repetitions, as shown in the bottom right panel; the difference between driven and interstimulus activity is often miniscule or negative.

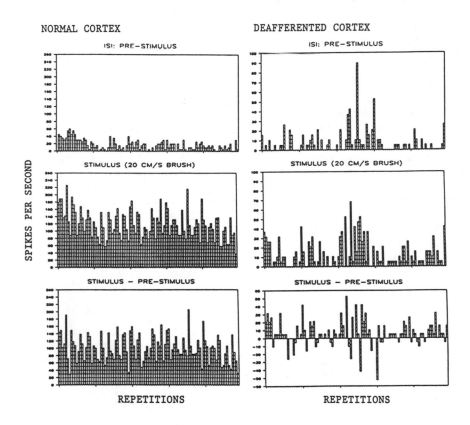

Figure 4. Responses of clusters of S-I neurons in a normally innervated region responding to forelimb stimulation (**left panels**) and in a DC-deafferented region responding to hindlimb stimulation (**right panels**). One hundred repetitions of the brushing stimulus were delivered to each site at a rate of 1.45 Hz (250 msec duration, 440 msec ISI). **Top panels:** rate of action potentials in the 250 msec preceding the 2nd to the 100th stimulus. **Middle panels:** rate of activity during the 2nd to the 100th stimulus. **Bottom panels:** subtractions of pre-stimulus (ISI) from driven activity for stimuli 2–100.

The activity patterns of DC-deafferented neurons during repetitive stimulation do not support the hypothesis that temporal discriminations of lesioned animals are disrupted by the presence of afterdischarge. Activity in the ISI for DC-deafferented neurons was generally lower than observed in recordings from normal cortex, and responses to stimulation were also less than normal. The lower levels of resting and driven activity within the DC-deafferented network appear to result from several different sources of suppression. As shown in Fig. 4 (right panels), for a series of stimulations at a rate of 2.3 Hz, both the spontaneous and driven activity waxed and waned in a pattern that was not reliably determined by the stimulus. In addition, the signal to noise ratio for driven / ISI activity was clearly influenced by the rate of stimulation, as demonstrated in the top panels of Fig. 5.

A cluster of neurons was activated by brushing within the peripheral receptive field at 10 cm/sec. In successive series of identical stimuli, the ISIs were either 10.44 sec (top left panel of Fig. 5) or 0.70 sec (top right panel). The histograms of average discharge rates during and after brushing show a greater responsivity when there were long pauses between stimuli. The rates of discharge in the ISIs were comparable in the two series, but stimulation at short ISIs did not increase the level of discharge over spontaneous rates.

In summary, interruption of the dorsal columns spares a variety of spatiotactile capacities but produces deficits in appreciation of the timing and duration of tactile stimuli. Recordings from the cortical termination of this projection reveal effects that can account for the psychophysical results: 1) responses of deafferented neurons to tactile stimuli are weak and variable (right panels of Fig. 4 and lower panels of Fig. 5); and 2) the signal to noise ratio is decreased abnormally by repetitive stimulation (upper panels of Fig. 5) at short ISIs. The responsivity of normal cortex is maintained over long periods of fast-paced stimulation (left side of Fig. 4).

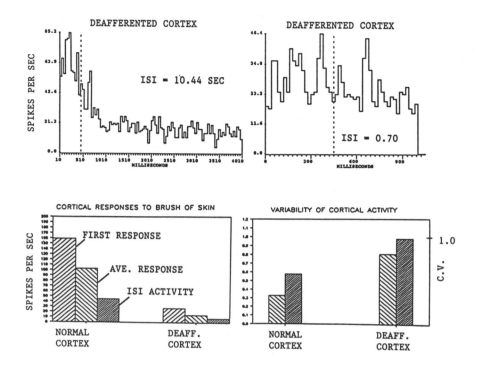

Figure 5. **Upper panels:** Histograms of the average
firing rate of a cluster of neurons within DC-
deafferented S-I cortex, when the brushing stimulus
is presented at 0.09 Hz (**left panel**; 440 msec
duration, 10 sec ISI) or 0.9 Hz (**right panel**; 440
msec duration, 0.7 sec ISI). The vertical dashed
lines denote stimulus offset. The rates of
activity were comparable in the interstimulus
intervals (the Y axes are autoscaled). **Lower
panels:** Averaged data are shown for 7 multiunit
recordings from normal (forelimb) cortex and for 5
multiunit recordings from deafferented (hindlimb)
cortex. **Left panel:** The first response of each
series of stimuli is compared with the average of
responses 2-100 and with the average rate of firing
during the ISIs. **Right panel:** Averaged
coefficients of variation (C.V.) for responses to
stimulation and for activity in the ISIs for normal
and deafferented cortex. Hatching on the right as
indicated on the left.

These results reveal an impediment to recovery from spinal cord injury that might not have been detected by experiments concerned with repair of more extensive lesions (e.g., transection). That is, a persistence of sensory and motor deficits would likely be attributed to inadequacies of repair techniques, but interruption of the dorsal columns produces impairments that would not be expected to ameliorate with establishment of a relay through a graft. In the absence of this direct projection of primary afferents to the brain stem, even intact pathways from the spinal cord do not reliably activate the primary somatosensory cortex, despite abundant projections to this network of neurons (Berkley, 1980). The DC-deafferented model facilitates examinations of techniques that might increase the afferent driving of rostral projections of somatosensory pathways originating in the dorsal horn.

ACKNOWLEDGEMENTS

The research in this report was supported by NINDS grant NS07261 and by NIDR grant DE07509. The technical support of James Murphy, Mark Tommerdahl and Jean Kaufman is gratefully acknowledged.

REFERENCES

Andersson SA, Norrsell K, Norrsell U (1972). Spinal pathways projecting to the cerebral first somatosensory area in the monkey. J Physiol 225:589-597.
Berkley KJ (1980). Spatial relationships between the terminations of somatic sensory and motor pathways in the rostral brainstem of cats and monkeys. I. Ascending somatic sensory inputs to lateral diencephalon. J comp Neurol 193:283-317.
Dreyer DA, Schneider RF, Metz CV, Whitsel BL (1974). Differential contribution of spinal pathways to body representation in postcentral gyrus of <u>Macaca mullata</u>. J Neurophysiol 37:119-145.
Eidelberg E, Woodbury CM (1972). Apparent redundancy in the somatosensory system in monkeys. Exper Neurol 37:573-581.

Ferrington DG, Downie JW, Willis WD (1988). Primate nucleus gracilis neurons: responses to innocuous and noxious stimuli. J Neurophysiol 59:886-907.

Jakeman LB, Reier PJ (1990). Axonal projections between fetal spinal cord transplants and the adult rat spinal cord: A Neuroanatomical tracing study of segmental interactions. J comp Neurol (In press).

Juliano SL, Whitsel BL (1987). A combined 2-deoxyglucose and neurophysiological study of primate somatosensory cortex. J comp Neurol 263:514-525.

Merzenich MM, Nelson RJ, Stryker MP, Cynader MS, Schoppmann A, Zook JM (1984). Somatosensory cortical map changes following digit amputation in adult monkeys. J Comp Neurol 224:591-605.

Vierck CJ (1973). Alterations of spatio-tactile discrimination after lesions of primate spinal cord. Brain Research 58:69-79.

Vierck CJ (1974). Tactile movement detection and discrimination following dorsal column lesions in monkeys. Exp Brain Res 20:311-346.

Vierck CJ (1977). Absolute and differential sensitivities to touch stimuli after spinal cord lesions in monkeys. Brain Res 134:529-539.

Vierck CJ (1984). The spinal lemniscal pathways. In Davidoff R (ed): "Handbook of the Spinal Cord," New York: Marcel Dekker, pp 673-750.

Vierck CJ, Cohen RH, Cooper BY (1983). Effects of spinal tractotomy on spatial sequence recognition in Macaques. J Neuroscience 3:280-290.

Vierck CJ, Cohen RH, Cooper BY (1985). Effects of spinal lesions on temporal resolution of cutaneous sensations. Somatosensory Res 3:45-56.

Vierck CJ, Cooper BY (1990). Epicritic sensations of primates. In Berkley MA, Stebbins WC (eds): "Comparative Perception," New York: John Wiley, pp 29-66.

Vierck CJ, Favorov O, Whitsel BL (1988). Neural mechanisms of absolute tactile localization in monkeys. Somatosensory Res 6:41-62.

Woolsey CN, Marshall WH, Bard P (1942). Representation of cutaneous tactile sensibility in the cerebral cortex of the monkey as indicated by evoked potentials. Bull Johns Hopk Hosp 70:399-441.

Advances in Neural Regeneration
Research, pages 369–377
© 1990 Wiley-Liss, Inc.

TROPHIC LINKAGES BETWEEN SPINAL MOTONEURONES
AND MUSCLES

Eduardo Eidelberg

Division of Neurosurgery, Audie L.
Murphy Memorial Veteran's Hospital,
and the University of Texas Health
Sciences Center at San Antonio
San Antonio, Texas   78284

There is a great deal of evidence, based upon studies
of development and of the consequences of lesions, that
motoneurones and muscles are linked by "trophic"
mechanisms in addition to the classical electrical
pathways. Some trophic effects seem to be mediated by
regulation of gene expression, others by
post-translational events. The trophic relationships
among neurons are generally less clear than are those
involving neuromuscular junctions, due to the difficulties
in accessibility of neuronal structures in situ, compared
to skeletal muscles. The classical example of trophic
interactions between motoneurones and their targets is the
study by Buller et al (1960) on the effects of
cross-innervation of slow and fast-twitch muscles (see
also Gordon et al., 1986).

Several years ago we became interested in the
development of muscle atrophy following lesions of the
"upper" motoneurons. This phenomenon is well known to
clinicians, but has rarely been explained by hypotheses
other than disuse. We started from a paper by Solandt and
Magladery (1942), in which it was shown that transection
of the spinal cord in adult rats, at T6, caused
substantial atrophy of the hindlimb muscles as well as
increased responsiveness of the same muscles to
intraarterial acetylcholine. Both phenomena became
apparent within a few days after cordotomy,   and both
regressed partially in the succeding weeks. These early
findings may be related to the demonstration by Nelson et
al (1979), and Nelson and Mendell (1979) that the unitary

Ia EPSP's of extensor motoneurones become larger with a
faster rise time after cordotomy, and remain enlarged for
days to months. We extended the observations of Solandt
and Magladery (1942) by defining the kind of motoneurones
and muscle fibers affected by cordotomy. In this we were
guided by previous reports by Midrio et al.(1988), Lieber
et al.(1986), and West et al.(1986) where it was shown
that cordotomy in the rat leads to extensive
transformation of slow twitch (S) to fast twitch (FR)
muscle fibers in the course of 4-6 weeks post-cordotomy.
This transformation was irreversible, and was demonstrated
by histochemistry, by SDS gel separation of myosin light
chains, and by measurement of the contraction properties
of the muscles in vitro (Eidelberg et al, 1989). We found
no changes in the properties of originally fast-twitch
muscles, such as EDL (extensor digitorum longus), except
for transient reduction in the crossectional area of their
muscle fibers.

Many investigators in this field have attributed the
effects of cordotomy upon skeletal muscles to disuse, and
there are many observations that partially support this
hypothesis. For example, immobilization of joints, or
suspension of the entire body, or of the hindquarters,
does lead to atrophy, but not to transformation of muscle
fiber   types (Spector, 1985). One alternative to disuse
was proposed by McComas et al (1973), who suggested that
lesions of the upper motoneurones affect the lower
motoneurones by transsynaptic orthograde degeneration
(Cowan, 1970). We addressed this hypothesis by looking
for morphological changes in the segmental motoneurones of
L4 through L6, where most of the sciatic motor pool is
found in rats. We transected the spinal cord, and
perfused the rats at varying intervals post-cordotomy.
The alpha motoneurones are counted in serial transversal
sections, stained with cresyl-violet, using the criteria
of Koningsmark (1970). The data showed a consistent and
statistically significant reduction in the number of
cells counted in rats operated 2-8 days before perfusion
(Eidelberg et al. 1989). The magnitude of the cell loss
was close to 20% of the counts from intact control rats.
When the ventral horn cells were studied by TEM in rats
prepared up to 8 days after cordotomy, most of the
motoneurones exhibited alterations such as nuclear
swelling, clumping of mitochondria, and disintegration of

the Nissl substance. These changes are non-specific, and
are observed also after axotomy, chemical poisoning,
ischemia, etc. The tissues obtained 16 days or longer
after cordotomy showed no apparent abnormalities. These
findings suggest that many motoneurones are affected by
cordotomy initially, but most recover eventually. Local
injection of colchicine into the spinal cord mimicked the
effects of cord transection (Karlsson and Sjostrand, 1969;
Pilar and Landmesser 1972). This suggests the likelihood
that the trophic system involves axonal transport.

We attempted to find out whether the fiber type
transformation (from slow to fast twitch) following
cordotomy would be paralleled by enlargement of the soma
of the motoneurones, in accordance with the "size
principle" (Henneman et al 1965). We transected the cord
in adult rats, and later injected WGA-HRP into two
muscles: SOL on the right and EDL on the left (see Fig. 1
and 2). The subjects were perfused and later, the
retrogradely labeled motoneurones were identified in
serial frozen sections of the lumbar cord treated by the
TMB method. The crossectional area of the soma of these
cells was measured with a Bioquant image analyzer. The
motoneurones in EDL and SOL pools became smaller, not
larger, for 1-2 weeks and then returned to control size.
There was no significant difference in the size of SOL
(slow) and EDL (fast) motoneurones (see Ishihara et al,
1988. and Ulfhake and Kellerth, 1982).

Currently we are investigating the use of six day old
rats prepared by unilateral sciatic nerve section or by
cervical hemisection, as an in vivo test for putative
neurotrophic factors. In this study, 6 day old rats
undergo right sciatic nerve section with simultaneous in
situ application of "cell growth" candidates, the left
sciatic remaining intact and untreated. In other 6 day
postnatal rats, a right side cervical (C2) spinal cord
hemisection and concurrent application of cell growth
factors is performed. In all cases the animals are
allowed to mature to 6 weeks of age. Those animals with
sciatic nerve cuts are perfused, lumbar spinal cord tissue
stained with cresyl violet and stained motoneurones
tabulated. Hemisected rats are injected at C6
(bilaterally) with WGA-HRP two days prior to perfusion,
frozen brain sections are reacted (using the TMB method),

Fig. 1. Changes in crossectional area of soleus motoneurones at different times following thoracic spinal cord transection.

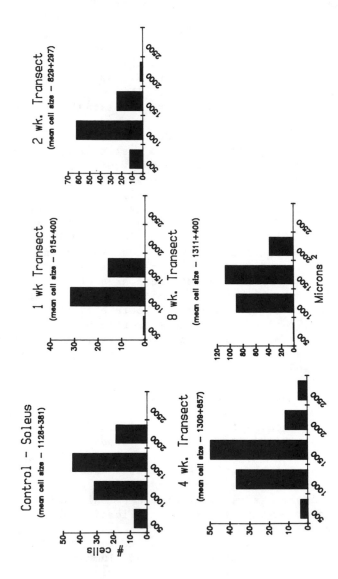

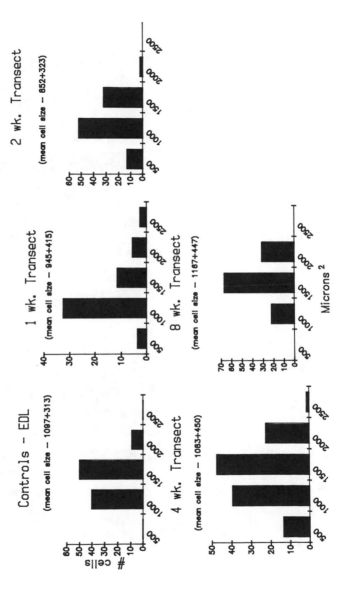

Fig. 2. Changes in crossectional area of EDL motoneurones as a function of time after cordotomy.

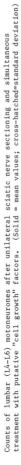

Fig. 3.   Counts of lumbar (L4-L6) motoneurones after unilateral sciatic nerve sectioning and simultaneous treatment with putative "cell growth" factors. (Solid = mean values; cross-hatched=standard deviation)

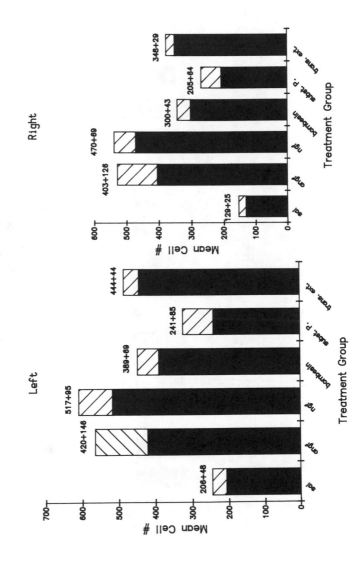

Fig. 4. Counts of **rubrospinal** neurons following cervical spinal cord (C2) hemisection and simultaneous treatment with various "cell growth" factors. (Solid = mean values; cross-hatched= standard deviation.)

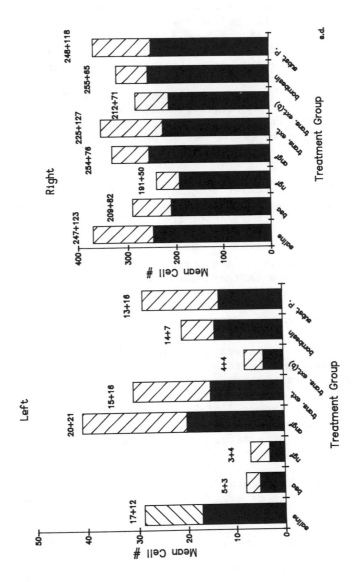

and labelled neurons in the area of the red nucleus
tabulated. The preliminary data of the sciatic nerve
section (Fig. 3) series suggests a protective effect
acting upon the motoneurones. Treatment of the lesion
site with substance P, NGF, or Anti-NGF reduced retrograde
mortality of motoneurones significantly. Treatment with
saline, bombesin, or an isolated muscle extract resulted
in an approximate 50% cell mortality on the lesioned side.
Data from the cervical hemisected rats (Fig. 4) indicates
that of all the putative "cell growth" factors tested thus
far, NGF appeared to have the least protective influence.
Other substances are yet to be tested.

REFERENCES

Buller A J, Eccles J C, Eccles R M (1960) Interactions
between motoneurones and muscles in respect of the
characteristic speed of their responses. J. Physiol.
(Lond) 150: 417-439

Cowan W M (1970) Anterograde and retrograde transneuronal
degeneration in the central and peripheral nervous system.
In: Contemporary Research Methods in Neuroanatomy, W.J.H.
Nauta and S.O.E. Ebbeson Eds. Springer Verlag, N.Y.
217-250

Eidelberg E, Nguyen L H, Polich R and Walden J G (1989)
Transsynaptic degeneration of motoneurones caudal to
spinal cord lesions. Brain Res Bull. 22: 39-45

Gordon T, Thomas C K, Stein R B, Erdebil S (1986)
Comparison of physiological and histochemical properties
of motor units after cross-reinnervation of antagonistic
muscles in the cat hindlimb. J. Neurophysiol 60: 365-373

Henneman E, Somjen G, Carpenter D O (1965) Functional
significance of cell size in spinal motoneurones J.
Neurophys 28:560-580

Ishihara A, Naithoh H, Araki H, Nishihira Y (1988) Soma
size and oxidative enzyme activity of motoneurones
supplying the fast twitch and slow twitch muscles in the
rat. Brain Res. 446: 195-198

Karlsson J-O, Sjostrand J (1969) The effect of colchicine
on the axonal transport of protein in the optic nerve and
tract of the rabbit. Brain Res. 13: 617-619

Koningsmark B W (1970) Methods for the counting of neurons. In Contemporary Research Methods in Neuroanatomy, W.J.H. Nauta and S.O.E. Ebbeson Eds., Springer Verlag N.Y. 341-380

Lieber R L, Johansson C B, Vahlsing H L, Hargens A R, Feringa E R (1986) Long-Term effects of spinal cord transection on fast and slow rat skeletal muscle. Exper. Neurol. 91: 423-434

McComas A F, Sica R E P, Upton A R M, Aguilar N (1973) Functional changes in motoneurones of hemiparetic patients. J. Neurol. Neurosurg. Psychiat. 36: 183-193

Midrio M, Betto D D, Betto R, Noventa D, Antico F (1988) Cordotomy-denervation interaction on contractile and myofibrillar properties of fast and slow muscles in the rat. Exper Neurol 100: 216-236

Nelson S G, Mendell L M, (1979) Enhancement in Ia-Motoneuron synaptic transmission caudal to chronic spinal cord transection J. Neurophys 42: 642-646

Nelson S G, Collatos T C, Niechaj A, Mendell L M (1979) Immediate increase in Ia-Motoneurone synaptic transmission caudal to spinal cord transection. J. Neurophys 42: 655-657

Pilar G, Landmesser L (1972) Axotomy mimicked by localized colchicine application. Science 177: 1116-1118

Solandt D Y, Magladery J W (1942) A comparison of effects of upper and lower motor neurone lesions on skeletal muscle. J. Neurophys. 5: 373-389

Spector S A (1985) Effects of elimination of activity on contractile and histochemical properties of rat soleus muscle. J. Neurosci. 5: 2189-2196

Ulfhake B, Kellerth J O (1982) Does a motoneurone size correlate with motor unit type in cat triceps surae? Br Res. 251: 201-209

West S P, Roy R R, Edgerton V R (1986) Fiber type and fiber size of cat and ankle knee, and hip extensors and flexors following low thoracic spinal cord transection at an early age. Exper. Neurol. 91: 174-182

Advances in Neural Regeneration
Research, pages 379–389
© 1990 Wiley-Liss, Inc.

EXTEROCEPTIVE REFLEXES AND FLEXOR SPASMS

David Burke

Department of Neurology, The Prince Henry Hospital
and School of Medicine, University of New South
Wales, Sydney 2036, Australia

INTRODUCTION

Spinal cord lesions can impair the supraspinal control
of spinal reflexes, both proprioceptive and exteroceptive,
and result in, for example, spasticity and clonus on the one
hand and flexor spasms on the other. The flexor spasm is
generally seen as an exaggeration of the nociceptive flexion
withdrawal reflex (Hagbarth, 1960; Kugelberg et al., 1960;
Dimitrijevic and Nathan, 1967, 1968), something to be
dampened down if not completely eliminated. However, there
may be no immediately identifiable trigger for flexor spasms
or they may be triggered by normally innocuous stimuli. For
flexor spasms to be manifestations of a nociceptive flexion
withdrawal reflex would require considerable change in
synaptic circuitry to allow volleys from mechanoreceptors
access to the reflex pathway, and this implies that
extensive remodelling (plasticity) occurs caudal to a spinal
cord lesion. There are two therapeutic implications of this
view of flexor spasms: first, that the flexor spasm is
intrinsically abnormal and should be suppressed and,
secondly, that physical and/or pharmacological therapies
could modify the pattern of synaptic plasticity.

An alternative view with radically different
therapeutic implications is that the flexor spasm is a
fragmentary expression of activity of the spinal locomotion
generator and represents merely the initiation of spinal
stepping or the flexion phase of walking (Sherrington,
1910). In cat and many other animal species, the locomotion

rhythm is generated by intrinsic spinal cord circuits which coordinate activity between limbs, even in the isolated spinal cord (Grillner and Dubuc, 1988). Peripheral inputs can modify this rhythm but are not essential for its generation, provided that the relevant spinal circuits are sufficiently excitable. The evidence for a spinal locomotion generator in human subjects is scant but, in the spinal patient, excitability is high and, as noted above, normally innocuous stimuli may provoke reflex activity. Therapeutic measures that suppressed a locomotion rhythm generator may have undesirable effects: for example, impaired mobility when on drugs such as baclofen might be due not to abolition of the "spastic splint" (as is often said) but to interference with the locomotion generator in a patient who is struggling to locomote.

Exteroceptive reflexes acting on alpha motoneurons (and therefore detectable in EMG recordings) have been reported to be different in normal subjects and spinal patients (for example, Shahani and Young, 1971; Meinck et al., 1983) but the reflex pattern has not been studied under functionally useful conditions: as a rule subjects have reclined on a couch, either at rest (Shahani and Young, 1971) or contracting the target muscle voluntarily (Meinck et al., 1983). If supraspinal inputs normally select from a number of possible reflex responses the one appropriate to a particular circumstance, the pattern seen in the spinal patient could be any one of those alternatives - abnormal not because of its pattern but because it is obligatory and can be manifest under inappropriate circumstances. The studies to be summarized below were predicated on the view that the variability of the reflex pattern in normal subjects must be fully appreciated before the reflex pattern in the spinal patient is considered "abnormal". The hypotheses were that considerable task-dependent variability would be demonstrable in normal subjects and that the abnormalities seen in the patients are primarily of intensity and inappropriate expression, rather than reflections of radically altered patterns of reflex connectivity.

GENERAL METHODOLOGY AND RATIONALE

Reflex changes in EMG activity and in muscle spindle discharge were sought in response to electrical stimulation

of the sural nerve at the ankle, using trains of five
non-painful stimuli delivered at 300 or 330 Hz. EMG of the
target muscles in the ipsi- and contralateral legs was
recorded using surface electrodes and, sometimes,
intramuscular wires. The activity was amplified, filtered,
rectified and averaged, using the sural stimulus as trigger.
The discharge of single muscle spindle afferents innervating
the pretibial flexor muscles was recorded from the peroneal
nerve using tungsten microelectrodes, and peristimulus time
histograms constructed using the sural stimulus as trigger.
The subjects reclined on a couch or stood in various
postures, as described below.

The rationale for choosing the sural nerve was that it
and the posterior tibial nerve supply all mechanoreceptors
in the sole of the foot. However, the posterior tibial
nerve is a mixed nerve innervating skin and muscle, while
the sural nerve is purely cutaneous. The feedback from
cutaneous mechanoreceptors is being increasingly recognized
as important in normal motor control, and the acts of
standing and walking are powerful stimuli to the sole of the
foot. Such inputs might reasonably be expected to modulate
the activity of motoneurons innervating particularly the
muscles that operate on the ankle (pretibial flexors and
triceps surae) and perhaps also proximal muscles of the same
limb and even muscles in the opposite limb. Widespread
effects would support the view that such reflexes normally
play a role during stance and locomotion.

TASK-DEPENDENT MODULATION OF EXTEROCEPTIVE REFLEXES OPERATING ON FUSIMOTOR NEURONS

When subjects reclined on a couch, stimuli to the sural
nerve failed to affect the discharge of spindle afferents
innervating the pretibial flexor muscles, whether those
muscles were relaxed (Gandevia et al., 1986) or contracting
voluntarily (Aniss et al., 1988). The voluntary contraction
was used to ensure that the receptor-bearing muscle was in
receipt of a functionally significant level of fusimotor
drive, so that any weak reflex effect on fusimotor neurons
would be more likely to be detected as a change in muscle
spindle discharge. Precisely the same stimuli had clear
effects on alpha motoneurons, as revealed by peristimulus
averages of rectified EMG.

When subjects stand quietly without support and with
eyes shut, there is normally little background EMG activity
in the pretibial flexors unless the body sways sufficiently
to provoke a reflex correction. Under these circumstances,
stimulation of the sural nerve induced changes in spindle
discharge that could not be explained by muscle stretch and
presumably resulted from reflex activation of fusimotor
neurons (Aniss et al., 1989). In a few instances, the
increase in spindle discharge occurred in muscles that had
little or no EMG and the stimuli failed to produce reflex
EMG activity. These findings suggest that the cutaneous
afferent volleys activated gamma motoneurons, and that in
this posture they had a lower threshold for such inputs than
alpha motoneurons. The appearance of a gamma motoneuron
reflex in the standing posture and the reversal of the
relative thresholds for alpha and gamma motoneurons indicate
that whether or not these reflexes are detectable may depend
on the task given to the subject: for the gamma motoneuron,
a reflex input from the sole of the foot might be of little
biological importance in a subject who is reclining on his
back.

Partly because of technical difficulties, comparable
studies have not been carried out yet for other muscle
groups; nor has this paradigm been investigated in spinal
patients. If, as might be expected, inputs from cutaneous
mechanoreceptors have an exaggerated reflex effect on gamma
motoneurons much as they have on alpha motoneurons, the
existence of this reflex would not be pathological per se.
The reflex pathway exists in reclining human subjects even
if activity in it is then normally minimal.

PATTERN OF EXTEROCEPTIVE REFLEXES OPERATING ON ALPHA MOTONEURONS

In standing human subjects, stimulation of the sural
nerve induced a reflex modulation of on-going EMG activity
of the tested muscles (tibialis anterior, triceps surae,
biceps femoris and vastus lateralis) in the ipsilateral leg.
Reflex modulation of EMG could also be detected in muscles
of the leg contralateral to the stimulus, but the strength
of the modulation was much less (D. Burke, H.G. Dickson and
N.F. Skuse, unpublished findings). For functional
antagonists, the earliest changes, within the first 50-100
ms, tended to be reciprocal or, at least, out of phase, but

the later activity (>150 ms) tended to be in phase. On
latency grounds, the earliest reflex changes must be spinal,
for the following reasons. First, the duration of the
stimulus train was 12 ms. Secondly, the conduction time for
the afferent side of the reflex arc is probably about 25 ms,
based on the latency of the spinal somatosensory evoked
potential to stimulation of the sural nerve at the ankle.
Thirdly, the conduction time in the fastest alpha
motoneurons is approximately 20 ms from cord to tibialis
anterior or triceps surae. (Note that the reflexes
demonstrated in the present experiments probably involved
low-threshold motoneurons with relatively slow motor
conduction.)

These findings confirm previous reports on
exteroceptive reflexes (e.g., Delwaide and Crenna, 1984;
Meinck et al., 1983) that inputs from mechanoreceptors (in
the present case, cutaneous mechanoreceptors) have reflex
actions on multiple muscles in both limbs. It can be
concluded that it is not intrinsically abnormal for
innocuous tactile stimuli to excite motoneurons innervating
multiple muscles of the lower limb, even muscles of the
opposite limb, as can occur in the spasms of a spinal
patient.

TASK-DEPENDENT MODULATION OF EXTEROCEPTIVE REFLEXES OPERATING ON ALPHA MOTONEURONS

In subjects who were standing, these reflexes had a
predictable variability that took two forms dependent
(i) on which muscles were active in the particular task, and
(ii) on the nature of the particular task (D. Burke, H.G.
Dickson and N.F. Skuse, unpublished findings).

Different Reflex Synergies

Trains of non-painful stimuli to the sural nerve
produced reflex changes only in those muscles that were
active, and the reflex effect consisted of modulation of the
on-going EMG envelope detectable only in stimulus-locked
averages. If subjects stood on a surface tilted
toe-upwards, vertical stance required activity in tibialis
anterior but not triceps surae, and in vastus lateralis more
than biceps femoris (Fig. 1A). Conversely, stance on a

surface tilted toe-down reinforced the need for activity of
triceps surae and biceps femoris at the expense of,
particularly, tibialis anterior (Fig. 1B). Hence different
muscle synergies were required to stand upright with the two
forms of surface tilt, and these synergies involved a
mixture of flexor and extensor activity at different
joints.

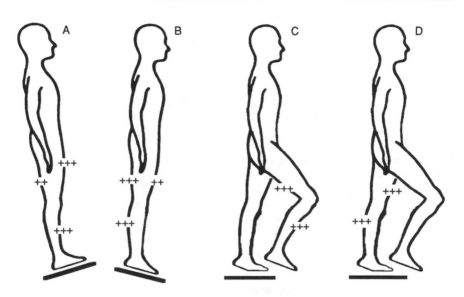

Figure 1. Muscle synergies adopted by subjects in different
postures, namely toe-up stance (A), toe-down stance (B),
flexion of ipsilateral leg (C) and stance on the ipsilateral
leg (D). The intensity of the background contraction and of
the reflex action in the sampled muscles is indicated by the
"+" symbol.

Standing on one leg with the other flexed as in the
flexion phase of walking resulted in reflex modulation of
the active flexor muscles in the flexed leg (tibialis
anterior and biceps femoris) when the ipsilateral sural
nerve was stimulated (Fig. 1C). Conversely, when the
extensors (triceps surae and vastus lateralis) were active
as in the extension phase of walking, the reflex changes
occurred in those muscles (Fig. 1D).

It is notable that the reflex pattern in these
different maneuvers involved a mixed flexor and extensor
synergy, a purely flexor synergy or a purely extensor
synergy, dependent on task. All that was required for
reflex activity to become manifest in a muscle was activity
in the relevant motoneuron pool. Given the high level of
motoneuron excitability in spinal patients even when at
rest, the appearance of comparable reflex activity in a
non-contracting muscle, be it flexor or extensor, would not
require extensive remodelling of spinal reflex circuits: the
reflex activity could result merely from the heightened
excitability.

Different Reflex Patterns

Evidence that the pattern of reflex activity of a
single muscle might differ in different tasks was sought for
tibialis anterior, a muscle involved when flexor spasms
occur in patients and when nociceptive flexion withdrawal
reflexes are elicited in normal subjects. The general
format of the reflex modulation of tibialis anterior EMG was
consistent across trials in the same subject and in
different subjects (Fig. 2), with an initial facilitation at
about 50-60 ms followed by more profound inhibition that was
usually interrupted by a second phase of facilitation (or
lessened inhibition) at about 80 ms.

The relative sizes of the initial and second phases of
facilitation varied in different maneuvers performed by the
same subjects. Because the contractions were functional,
their intensity was that required for the specific task and
the contraction level for different tasks could not be
matched perfectly (although they appeared to be comparable
from on-line audio and oscilloscope monitoring). To
determine whether these changes could be attributed to
different contraction levels, subjects performed a series of
voluntary contractions against increasing resistance (Fig.
2A). There was little change in the relative intensities of
the different components of the reflex pattern.

The greatest differences in reflex pattern in different
tasks were seen when balancing on an unstable surface was
compared with limb flexion (as in the flexion phase of
walking) and with stance on a surface tilted toe-up (Fig.
2B-D). With balancing, the initial facilitation was

prominent and the second merely a transient inflection on the subsequent inhibition. With the limb in flexion, the initial phase of facilitation was small or absent, and the second clearly exceeded any inhibition, producing a clear peak above the baseline level of activity.

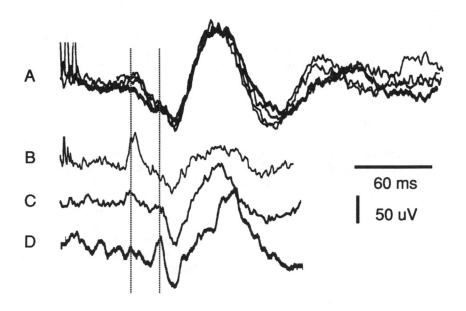

Figure 2. The pattern of reflex modulation of EMG of tibialis anterior. The upper panel (A) contains the responses recorded during four voluntary contractions performed against increasing resistance (0 Nm, 6 Nm, 25 Nm and 35 Nm), with the amplification of the averages adjusted to demonstrate the similarity of the responses. Panels B, C and D show, for the same subject, the reflex patterns when balancing on an unstable surface with the ipsilateral foot forward (B), during stance on a surface tilted toe-up (C), and during limb flexion (D). The vertical calibration applies only to B-D.

These results indicate that there are a number of different reflex pathways to the one motoneuron pool from the same afferent species (cutaneous mechanoreceptors). On

latency grounds, the short latency pathways (initial
facilitation, subsequent inhibition) can only be spinal and
it is possible that the second phase of facilitation is also
spinal (however, see Choa and Stephens, 1982; Jenner and
Stephens, 1982; Delwaide and Crenna, 1984). The intact
nervous system can choose between different reflex pathways
even when the tasks to be undertaken require activity in the
same muscle.

There are clear implications for the reflex pattern
seen in the initially quiescent muscles of spinal patients.
In an initially quiescent muscle, an inhibitory reflex will
go undetected, but facilitatory reflexes may produce a burst
of EMG. The latency of the reflex response will, of
necessity, be measured to that burst, even if it is not the
earliest reflex action on the motoneurone pool. If both
phases of facilitation result from activity in spinal reflex
circuits, the latencies seen in patients will depend on
which pathway is "open". It has been shown that the latency
of the exteroceptive reflex may vary in spinal patients, but
it can also appear to do so in normal subjects in different
tasks, as described above.

COMMENT

Within limits, exteroceptive reflexes acting on gamma
and alpha motoneurons of normal human subjects can vary,
dependent on the task in which the subject is involved.
Presumably, the source of the "variability" is the
supraspinal control of the reflex pathway and, presumably,
the rationale for the "variability" is optimal feedback for
that task. The view that exteroceptive reflexes act to
promote contraction of flexor muscles at different joints
and so promote the flexion phase of walking is overly
simple: they may do that, but they are also active during
different forms of stance.

In patients with spinal cord injury, the reflex
repertoire is more limited, and the relevant afferent
volleys enter a spinal cord that has heightened
excitability. There is, as yet, no conclusive evidence that
the afferent volley evokes a reflex pattern that is
intrinsically abnormal. Rather than studying initially
quiescent muscles, attention should be directed to the
pattern seen in patients whose muscles have background

activity, be that produced by a voluntary contraction of a paretic muscle or by sustained reflex activity, such as tendon vibration. It is conceivable that exteroceptive reflexes of spinal patients are abnormal in only two respects: heightened excitability of spinal cord circuitry in the resting state, and deficient supraspinal control of that circuitry.

ACKNOWLEDGEMENTS

This work was supported by the National Health & Medical Research Council of Australia. The author is grateful to his colleagues, named above and co-authors of published work.

REFERENCES

Aniss AM, Gandevia SC, Burke D (1988). Reflex changes in muscle spindle discharge during a voluntary contraction. J Neurophysiol 59:908-921.

Aniss AM, Diener, Hore, Burke & Gandevia (1989). Reflex activation of muscle spindles in human pretibial muscles during standing. J Neurophysiol submitted.

Choa BHG, Stephens JA (1982). Cutaneous reflex responses and central nervous lesions studied in the lower limb in man. J Physiol (London) 328:23P-24P.

Delwaide PJ, Crenna P (1984). Cutaneous nerve stimulation and motoneuronal excitability. II: Evidence for non-segmental influences. J Neurol Neurosurg Psychiatry 47:190-196.

Dimitrijevic MR, Nathan PW (1967). Studies of spasticity in man. 1. Some features of spasticity. Brain 90:1-30.

Dimitrijevic MR, Nathan PW (1968). Studies of spasticity in man. 3. Analysis of reflex activity evoked by noxious cutaneous stimulation. Brain 91:349-368.

Gandevia SC, Miller S, Aniss AM, Burke D (1986). Reflex influences on muscle spindle activity in relaxed human leg muscles. J Neurophysiol 56:159-170.

Grillner S, Dubuc R (1988). Control of locomotion in vertebrates: spinal and supraspinal mechanisms. In Waxman SG (ed) "Functional Recovery in Neurological Disease", Advances in Neurology, Vol. 47, New York: Raven Press, pp 425-453.

Hagbarth K-E (1960). Spinal withdrawal reflexes in the
human lower limb. J Neurol Neurosurg Psychiatry
23:222-227.

Jenner JR, Stephens JA (1982). Cutaneous reflex responses
and their central nervous pathways studied in man.
J Physiol (London) 333:405-419.

Kugelberg E, Eklund K, Grimby L (1960). An electro-
myographic study of the nociceptive reflexes of the lower
limb. Mechanism of the plantar responses.
Brain 83:394-410.

Meinck HM, Benecke R, Kuster S, Conrad B (1983). Cutaneo-
muscular (flexor) reflex organisation in normal man and
in patients with motor disorders. In Desmedt JE (ed):
"Motor Control Mechanisms in Health and Disease",
Advances in Neurology, vol. 44, New York: Raven Press,
pp 787-796.

Shahani BT, Young RR (1971). Human flexor reflexes.
J Neurol Neurosurg Psychiatry 34:616-627.

Sherrington CS (1910). Flexion-reflex of the limb, crossed
extension-reflex, and reflex stepping and standing.
J Physiol (London) 40:28-121.

**Advances in Neural Regeneration
Research, pages 391–405**
© **1990 Wiley-Liss, Inc.**

CHARACTERISTICS AND EXTENT OF MOTOR ACTIVITY RECOVERY AFTER SPINAL CORD INJURY

Milan R. Dimitrijevic, Mark A. Lissens and W. Barry McKay

Division of Restorative Neurology and Human Neurobiology, Baylor College of Medicine, Houston, Texas

INTRODUCTION

Reported clinical observations in humans with acute traumatic spinal cord injury (SCI) indicate that the loss of spinal cord functions can be spontaneously restored (Bracken et al., 1984). Actually, about 10% to 20% of traumatic, complete SCI subjects will regain some useful functions (Ducker et al., 1983; Young, 1989). When motor recovery occurs, the impaired functions begin to improve after a period of weeks and/or months (Dimitrijevic, 1988).

There are several factors that influence the characteristics and extent of recovery of spinal cord functions impaired by trauma: 1. Severity of axonal lesions, their number and distribution within the long ascending and descending tracts (Blight et al., 1987); 2. Severity and extent of injury to the spinal gray matter and the short, intermediate and long propriospinal axons of the fasciculus propriospinalis (Kakulas, 1985); 3. Presence of more than one spinal cord lesion, in particular one situated at a lower spinal level than the clinical lesion and is, therefore, not recognized (Dimitrijevic, 1987); 4. The presence of brainstem or brain lesions not clinically obvious; 5. The extent and number of established neurobiological recovery mechanisms; 6. The level of expertise of immediate and long-term medical care, such as transportation from the site of the accident to the medical institution, and whether the patient is treated in a regional spinal cord injury care unit or in a hospital that seldom admits patients with spinal cord injury (Donovan et al., 1984).

Throughout the years (1971 - 1989), we had an opportunity to work closely with specialists in spinal cord injury management in a regional spinal cord injury center, The Institute for Rehabilitation and Research, Houston, Texas, where we clinically and neurophysiologically examined and followed-up a large number of SCI subjects. In this chapter we shall summarize our observations on the characteristics and extent of motor activity recovery following SCI. We shall also describe the clinical and subclinical characteristics of SCI subjects, the outcome of different neurological motor activity and neurocontrol in groups of subjects who were initially clinically complete and discuss the preliminary observation that it is possible to modify established neurocontrol even in chronic ambulatory SCI subjects. Finally, we shall discuss the role of neurobiological mechanisms involved in motor activity recovery processes.

MATERIAL

We have seen 642 SCI subjects and of these 581 had spinal cord lesions above the T10 spinal cord segment. Of these 581 subjects from the Houston Data Base (HDB), 118 were seen the first time between the onset of injury and the first 6 months, 70 between 7 to 12 months, 111 between 1 and 2 years, 63 between 2 and 3 years and 219 after 3 or more years following injury. A large number of patients, years after injury, were referred to our group because of our expertise in assessing and controlling spasticity, altered sensation and/or pain. Many of these subjects came from regional rehabilitation centers from which they had graduated after optimizing their functional status and degree of independence.

The age of this group of 581 SCI subjects ranged from 2 to 64 years and consisted of 116 women and 465 men. The level of spinal cord injury was from C1 to T10 and the majority of the injuries were closed spinal cord injuries.

METHOD

All subjects were assessed clinically and neurophysiologically. We used the SPINAL CORD INJURY ASSESSMENT PROTOCOL routinely as well as the EXTENDED PROTOCOL FOR THE ASSESSMENT OF NEUROMUSCULAR FUNCTIONS AND NEUROCONTROL OF POSTURE AND GAIT. The first protocol for the assessment of spinal cord injuries consists of the clinical neurological evaluation by neurologists. The neurological criteria for complete spinal cord injury or transected spinal cord are very straightforward: there must be no brain motor control or perception of any sensory modality below the level of the lesion. Whenever any motor and/or sensory functions are partially present below the level of intact spinal cord functions, spinal cord injury is then recognized as being incomplete. All these findings, whenever possible, are summarized in terms of the functional anatomy of the spinal cord by recognizing diffuse or patchy incomplete spinal cord lesions or lesions of the anterior, posterior or hemistructures of the spinal cord. Following neurological evaluation, functional assessments by a physiatrist and a physical therapist were performed according to a protocol similar to Barthel's Index but adapted to SCI subjects (Mahoney et al., 1965; Fugl-Meyer et al., 1975).

When the clinical assessments are completed, a series of neurophysiological procedures are initiated. Multichannel, simultaneous recording of motor unit activity by surface electrodes from 12 to 16 muscle groups was applied to record motor unit activity even when movements were absent and the subjects paralyzed. During phasic and tonic stretch reflexes we also used polyelectromyographic recordings of motor unit activity to measure local and generalized responses (Dimitrijevic et al., 1983a; Sherwood, 1989).

Furthermore, this Brain Motor Control Assessment (BMCA) was used in paretic subjects to record neurocontrol of motor unit activity during movements. Unlike subjects whose nervous system functions are intact, different features of neurocontrol can be developed in SCI subjects for the same motor task, such as multi-joint flexion-extension of the lower limb or ankle dorsal-plantar flexion. The neurocontrol pattern recorded from an individual SCI subject will remain consistent for specific motor tasks but will differ from that of another SCI subject. Simultaneous recording from 12 to 16 muscle groups above and below the spinal cord lesion of motor evoked potentials elicited by magnetic transcranial stimulation of the motor cortex was performed in paralyzed and paretic subjects at the end of the BMCA protocol.

Sensory functions were examined by conventional neurological evaluation for touch, pin-prick, 2 point discrimination, vibration, heat and cold. When necessary, a quantitative method for cold, heat and vibration was also used (Beric, 1989; Lindblom, 1981). In addition, we carried out somatosensory evoked potentials by stimulating the median nerve at the wrist and the tibial nerve at the popliteal fossa while recording from surface leads over the cervical spinal cord (median nerve), lumbosacral spinal cord (tibial nerve) and scalp (Dimitrijevic et al., 1978, and 1983b; Beric et al., 1987a; Beric, 1989).

The extended protocol for the assessment of neuromuscular functions and neurocontrol of posture and gait was applied when the subjects' condition allowed it. This protocol consists of: 1. Lower motor neuron electromyography, qualitative and quantitative; 2. Tendon jerks, H-reflex, cutaneo-muscular reflex recording; 3. Muscle fatigue resistance - peripheral fatigue; 4. Muscle fatigue resistance - central fatigue; 5. Isokinetic dynamometry to measure muscle tone and force during concentric and eccentric muscle contraction; 6. Stabilometry (posturography); 7. Posturography with neurocontrol study of postural control mechanisms; 8. Gait neurocontrol study on a treadmill; 9. Gait neurocontrol study on a walking path; 10. Contingent negative variation (CNV) - touchometry; 11. Pain questionnaire and assessment of pain condition; 12. Movement related evoked potentials.

OBSERVATIONS

Characteristics and Extent of Recovery: Clinical Observations
Of the 58 SCI subjects, in whom the onset condition was well documented, we studied 35 subjects within the first year after the onset of injury, 5 subjects within 2 years and 18 subjects within 3 or more years. Initially, 48 of these 58 subjects, regardless of the observation period, manifested complete lesions; 7 of them were motor complete and sensory incomplete, while 3 were motor and sensory incomplete. Thus, the great majority of subjects suffered from complete spinal cord lesions. Of the 55 subjects who initially showed evidence of motor complete spinal cord lesion, 13 partially recovered and became motor incomplete after an observation period of 1, 2, 3 or more years.

Another group of 18 subjects was selected from our HDB of 581 subjects because they initially suffered from complete lesion and were studied in our program 2 or 3 years after injury. Their neurological deficits had not changed but they had developed muscle hypertonia and spasms. As you can see in Figure 1, spasticity developed in 4 of 18 subjects in a period of 5 months after injury. Spasticity can appear within the first 6 months after injury, between 8 and 12 months and even 17 months after injury. Thus, there is no specific time window when spasticity can appear in an initially clinically complete condition.

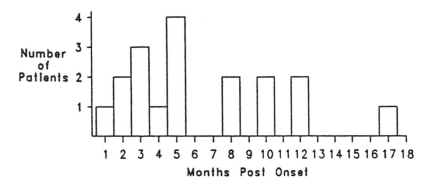

Figure 1. Onset of spasticity in 18 paralyzed SCI subjects.

<u>Characteristics and Extent of Recovery: Subclinical Observations</u>
The characteristics and extent of recovery were studied neurophysiologically in 3 different clinical categories of subjects: motor complete, motor incomplete (wheelchair-bound), motor incomplete (ambulatory). In the first group of 20 initially motor complete subjects, 12 of them showed evidence of subclinical motor incompleteness (Fig. 2). This discomplete finding was documented months and years after injury and when followed-up 5 to 7 years after the onset. Some changes in the neurophysiological findings were present in follow-up studies for only 2 of 12 subjects and consisted of fluctuations in amplitude and duration of motor unit activity but not in the features of neurocontrol. Thus, in the category of clinically complete SCI subjects there is a large proportion of neurophysiologically discomplete spinal cord injuries that do not change their characteristics and extent of recovery throughout the years. But we can also run into a rare exception when the subject changes from complete to discomplete, and from discomplete to incomplete but wheelchair-bound. In one of these 12 subjects in whom we documented discomplete lesion 5 years after injury, we recorded clinically and neurophysiologically an incomplete but wheelchair-bound condition 3 years later.

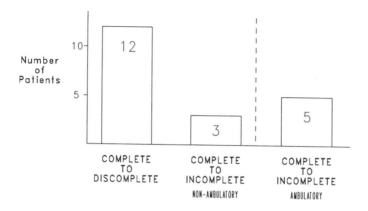

Figure 2. Extent of recovery in 3 subgroups of 20 SCI subjects who were initially motor complete.

In the second group of 3 subjects (Fig. 2), clinically incomplete and wheelchair-bound, we documented a more extensive recovery of motor activity, even though insufficient for locomotion. One of the 3 subjects studied did not reveal changes in neurocontrol 6 months and 2 years after spinal cord injury. Two other subjects studied 3 months and 1.5 year respectively after the onset of injury were followed-up on a yearly basis. They revealed changes in neurocontrol but never recovered enough to stand or walk.

When neurocontrol has a different feature, then such a difference is striking and can be easily recognized. Figure 3 illustrates different features of neurocontrol in 6 SCI subjects with different degrees of failure in performing an identical motor task. These subjects can be divided into 2 subgroups according to their neurocontrol features and ability to implement a motor task: 3 subjects fail to accomplish the same motor task and reveal corresponding altered neurocontrol while the other 3 are able to implement the same motor task but with different neurocontrol strategy.

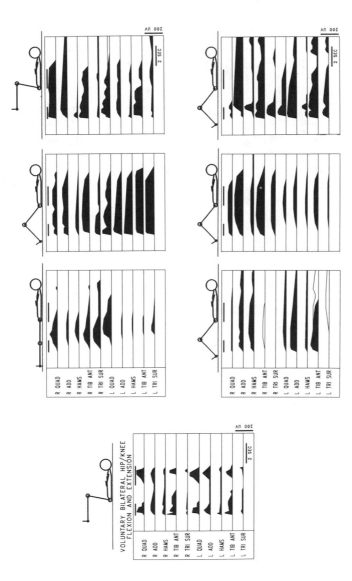

Figure 3. Performance of voluntary multi-joint motor task with EMG pattern in a healthy subject (left). Above, 3 different SCI subjects (T8, C3, T7) attempt to perform the same task with different degrees of clinical movement. Below, 3 other SCI subjects (T5, C6, C4) accomplish the same clinical movement with very different neurocontrol strategies.

Another example of 2 distinct features of neurocontrol in SCI subjects during an identical motor task is shown in Figure 4. In the wheelchair-bound subject there is a large amount of motor unit activity (above), while the ambulatory SCI subject generated less and more organized motor unit activity (beneath). Transcranial stimulation reveals just the opposite finding: only motor evoked potentials to the left and to the right dorsal ankle flexors in the wheelchair-bound SCI subject, and motor evoked potentials in all the recorded muscle groups in the ambulatory SCI subject. Thus, when suprasegmental control is significantly reduced and symmetrically organized, motor control can be triggered, revealing characteristic features of gross motor activity. However, when suprasegmental control is more extensive, it is possible to generate more localized motor unit activity: the so-called "local" response then becomes manifest. In other words, also "poorly" organized activity has its own definite organization and neurocontrol.

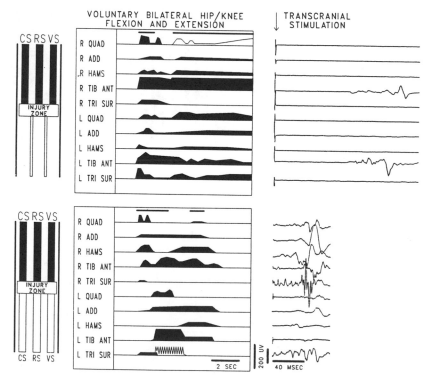

Figure 4.

Figure 4. BMCA (left) and transcranial stimulation (right) results from two SCI subjects. Above, a subject with clinically incomplete C7 lesion (wheelchair-bound) attempted voluntary multi-joint movement showing widespread activation and long latency motor evoked responses to transcranial stimulation present only in both tibialis anterior muscles. Below, a SCI subject with incomplete C5 lesion (ambulatory) shows more specific activation during voluntary movement and shorter latency responses to transcranial stimulation with more muscles responding. Motor evoked potentials are of larger amplitude and shorter latency time on the right side and lower amplitude, longer latency on the left.

In the third group of 5 subjects drawn from HDB, who initially suffered from complete motor lesion but recovered motor activity to such an extent that they could stand and walk (Fig. 2), we provided neurophysiological evidence that the neurocontrol of such gait is very different when compared to that of subjects with intact nervous systems. This finding suggests that the injured spinal cord can generate locomotion by means of strategies different from those of the healthy nervous system. Follow-up studies of neurocontrol features in these 5 subjects were carried out on a yearly basis and revealed no other changes than in the amplitude and duration of motor unit activity.

Modification of Neurocontrol in the Established Spinal Cord Lesion: Preliminary Results

On 2 occasions, we had an opportunity to include 2 SCI subjects, wheelchair users and non-functional ambulators, in a program of neuromuscular and functional electrical stimulation. The first subject, injured 25 years previously, participated for two years in a functional electrical stimulation (FES) program that was tailored to his particular condition. The second subject, injured 5 years before, participated in a functional electrical stimulation program only for two months. Both responded to FES with a significant change in the neurocontrol of volitional activity and gait and also with obvious changes in the clinical appearance of their gait. This new neurocontrol was retained without electrical stimulation. It is interesting to note that the first subject, who needed two years of daily FES, had predominantly tonic neurocontrol characteristics during volitional activity and gait, whereas the second subject, who had responded to months of FES, had predominantly phasic features in neurocontrol of volitional activity and gait. At present there are 2 more patients under treatment who also support the very preliminary observation that established spinal cord injury which does not show any so-called "spontaneous" alteration in neurocontrol, when exposed to externally controlled afferent input and facilitation of the existing motor function through FES, can after a varying period of time regain new neurocontrol of volitional activity and gait (Fig. 5).

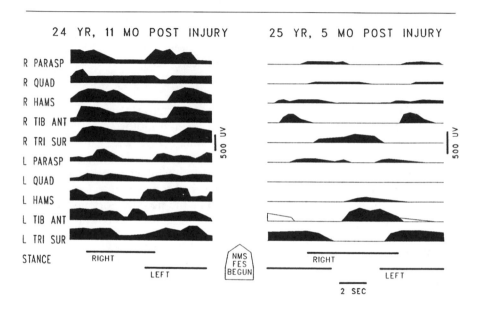

Figure 5. BMCA recording in an incomplete ambulatory post-traumatic T7 paraparetic during gait carried out 24, 25 years after the onset of injury, illustrating a significant change in the neurocontrol pattern between years 24 - 25 when NMS and FES programs were initiated.

DISCUSSION

According to these observations, it is obvious that the majority of subjects with clinically complete spinal cord lesion will in time regain at least some of their nervous system functions even in the absence of clinical evidence.   Others will reveal clinical signs of trace or gross but not functionally useful movement, while there are also some who can even recover the ability to stand and walk.   Thus, in the majority of initially clinically complete SCI subjects, the process for recovery of impaired functions can occur spontaneously but the extent of recovery can vary a great deal. It has been reported that approximately 10% to 20% of the subjects with initially complete spinal cord lesions will regain some functions (Young, 1989; Ducker et al., 1983). We have observed that this percentage is even larger when subclinical criteria are applied. This means that there is a wider range of partial recovery, covering subclinical and a variety of clinical aspects.

Let us discuss the possible underlying mechanisms in the 18 complete SCI subjects in whom spasticity developed within 1 to 17 months after injury. Is spasticity the result of "sprouting" of the uninjured primary sensory neurons and other spinal interneuronal axons and dendrites, or does spasticity result from improved conduction through long descending axons and the partially restored brain influence on segmental network? Excitatory residual brain influence, after spinal conduction is partially restored, will facilitate the spinal central excitatory state, and spinal reflexes will become excessive in amplitude and duration. Another explanation for the delayed appearance of spasticity can be that inhibitory brain influence on the spinal neuronal network is first restored and then followed by stronger excitatory input which will overcome inhibitory brain influence. Finally, a subclinical lesion of the cauda equina can suppress the manifestation of spasticity until lower motor neuron functions recover (Dimitrijevic, 1988; Dimitrijevic, 1987; Beric et al., 1987b).

In our previous studies on the clinically complete spinal cord lesion, we were able to demonstrate the presence of excitatory and inhibitory residual brain influence (Dimitrijevic et al., 1984; Cioni et al., 1987). Therefore, in order to explain the different delays in the onset of spasticity in subjects with initially complete spinal cord lesion, it is necessary to propose the existence of more than one underlying spinal and supraspinal mechanism. Our previous studies also support the suggestion that severe spasticity in complete SCI subjects is the expression of residual excitatory brain influence through impaired segments of the spinal cord (Dimitrijevic, 1988; Dimitrijevic, 1987).

Moreover, the neurophysiological analysis of 20 initially complete SCI subjects revealed that 12 of them had reached the stage of discomplete lesion, meaning that they revealed the presence of subclinical but definite brain excitatory influence on the segmental neuronal network. Spasticity was recorded clinically in all of these 12 subjects. This influence can also be demonstrated by means of the reproducible character of repeatedly elicited phasic, proprioceptive and exteroceptive reflexes which are otherwise unreproducible when elicited repetitively and deprived of additional external or suprasegmental excitation (Dimitrijevic et al., 1970; Dimitrijevic et al., 1973). This residual influence can be revealed by the tonic stretch reflex, whose presence depends upon brain influence (Dimitrijevic et al., 1977). When the influence of residual brain descending axons is more pronounced, Jendrassik-like reinforcement maneuvers will elicit motor unit excitation (Dimitrijevic et al., 1984). Further improvement in brain influence can even make it possible for the subject to initiate and stop flexor/extensor spasms or, in the absence of any movement, to elicit single motor unit activity in the muscles appropriate for the specific motor task which is otherwise clinically absent (Dimitrijevic et al., 1989).

Therefore, from the discomplete spinal cord lesion we can learn that steadily increasing residual brain influence can trigger and at first modify activity that is otherwise generated at the spinal network level, and that it will then incorporate into the spinal network simple, more restricted excitation and inhibition of different parts of spinal generators of activity. When brain influence is further improved by the next, larger population of conducting axons, the subject becomes motor incomplete by demonstrating the ability to initiate gross, multi-joint, patterned flexor/extensor slow and fatigable movements without gaining the ability to stand or walk. In this case, the brain utilizes a modest number of functioning descending axons to control spinal flexor generators, supraspinally dependent extensor generators and sometimes also to achieve the separation between each pair of spinal generators. With larger numbers of descending functioning axons, it becomes possible to carry out single- and multi-joint movements and to control equilibrium by integrating the activity of segmental and suprasegmental structures, such as brainstem, cerebellar and brain communication in generating automatic and skilful volitional motor activity. There is experimental evidence that axonal plasticity and remyelination can restore the functions of injured axons (Waxman, 1988 and 1989). Moreover, there are neurobiological evidences also for the activation of unused synapses to replace the activity of the injured ones as well as the utilization of the uninjured portion of the spinal tracts, residual brain influence or the utilization of alternate unaffected pathways (Easter et al., 1985; Marshall, 1985). Thus, there are several neurobiological processes that can contribute to the restoration or compensation for impaired spinal cord functions. While we are developing molecular biological restorative procedures for chronic and acute SCI this new information coming from human neurobiology might influence our present research strategy. We can either choose to rebuild the impaired anatomy or partially restore the anatomy and enhance the residual functions available.

In summary, residual brain influence can develop different neurocontrol features suggesting that recovery from spinal cord injury depends on the presence of conductiong axons and the locations of their endings within the spinal gray matter.

REFERENCES

Beric A, Dimitrijevic MR, Lindblom U (1987a). Cortical evoked potentials and somatosensory perception in chronic spinal cord injury patients. J Neurol Sciences 80:333-342.

Beric A, Dimitrijevic MR, Light JK (1987b). A clinical syndrome of rostral and caudal spinal injury: neurological, neurophysiological and urodynamic evidence for occult sacral lesion. J Neurol Neurosurg Psychiat 50:600-606.

Beric A (1989). Quantitative techniques in assessment of sensory abnormalities in patients with spinal cord injury. In Davis R, Kondraske GV, Tourtellotte WW, Syndulko K (eds): "Quantifying Neurologic Performance", Philadelphia: Hanley & Belfus, Inc, pp 84-95.

Bracken MB, Collins WF, Freeman DF, Shephard MJ, Wagner FW, Silken RM, Hellenbrand KG, Ramsohoff I, Hunt WE, Perot PL (1984). Efficacy of methylprednisolone in acute spinal cord injury. JAMA 251:45-52.

Blight AR, DeCrescito V (1987). Morphometric analysis of experimental spinal cord injury in the cat: the relationship of injury intensity to survival of myelinated axons. Neuroscience 19:321-341.

Cioni B, Dimitrijevic MR, McKay WB, Sherwood AM (1987). Voluntary supraspinal suppression of spinal reflex activity in paralyzed muscles of spinal cord injury patients. Exp Neurol 93:574-583.

Dimitrijevic MR, Nathan PW (1970). Studies of spasticity in man. 4. Changes in flexion reflex with repetitive cutaneous stimulation in spinal man. Brain 93:743-768.

Dimitrijevic MR, Nathan PW (1973). Studies of spasticity in man. 6. Habituation, dishabituation and sensitization of tendon reflexes in spinal man. Brain 96:337-354.

Dimitrijevic MR, Spencer WA, Trontelj JV, Dimitrijevic M (1977). Reflex effects of vibration in patients with spinal cord lesions. Neurol 27:1078-1086.

Dimitrijevic MR, Larsson LE, Lehmkuhl LD, Sherwood AM (1978). Evoked spinal cord and nerve root potentials in humans using a non-invasive recording technique. Electroencephalogr Clin Neurophysiol 45:331-340.

Dimitrijevic MR, Faganel J, Lehmkuhl LD, Sherwood AM (1983a). Motor control in man after partial or complete spinal cord injury. In Desmedt JE (ed): "Motor Control Mechanisms in Health and Disease", New York: Raven Press, pp 915-926.

Dimitrijevic MR, Prevec TS, Sherwood AM (1983b). Somatosensory perception and cortical evoked potentials in established paraplegia. J Neurol Sci 60:253-265.

Dimitrijevic MR, Dimitrijevic M, Faganel J, Sherwood AM (1984). Suprasegmentally induced motor unit activity in paralyzed muscles of patients with established spinal cord injury. Ann Neurol 16:216-221.

Dimitrijevic MR (1985). Residual motor functions in spinal cord injury. In Waxman SG (ed): "Advances in Neurology: Functional Recovery in Neurological Disease", New York: Raven Press, pp 139-155.

Dimitrijevic MR (1987). Neurophysiology in spinal cord injury. Paraplegia 25:205-208.

Dimitrijevic MR, Nix W, McKay WB, Sherwood AM (1989). Volitional motor control of motor units in paralyzed muscles in man with established spinal cord injury. Presented at the International Conference on "The Motor Unit, Physiology, Diseases, Regeneration and Rehabilitation", Munich, W Germany, July 14-16.

Donovan WH, Carter RE, Bedbrook G, Young JS, Griffith ER (1984). Incidence of medical complications in spinal cord injury: patients in specialized compared with nonspecialized centers. Paraplegia 22:282-290.

Ducker TB, Lucas JT, Wallace CA (1983). Recovery from spinal cord injury. Clin Neurosurg 30:495-513.

Easter SS, Purves D, Rakic P, Spitzer NC (1985). The changing view of neural specificity. Science 230:507-511.

Fugl-Meyer AR, Jaasko L, Leyman I, Olsson S, Steglind S (1975). The post-stroke hemiplegic patient: A method of evaluation of physical performance. Scand J Rehab Med 7:13-31.

Kakulas BA (1985). Pathology of spinal injuries. CNS Trauma 1:117-129.

Lindblom U (1981). Quantitative testing of sensibility including pain. In Stalberg E, Young RR (eds.): "Clinical Neurophysiology, Neurology I", London: Butterworths, pp 168-190.

Mahoney FL, Barthel DW (1965). Functional evaluation: The Barthel index. State Med I 14:61-65.

Marshall JF (1985). Neural plasticity and recovery of funtion after brain injury. In Smythies JR, Bradley RJ (eds): "International Review of Neurobiology", New York: Academic Press, pp 201-247.

Sherwood AM, Dimitrijevic MR (1989). Brain motor control assessment. Proc. of the Annual International Conference of the IEEE Engineering in Medicine and Biology Society 11:943-944.

Waxman SG (1988). Clinical course and electrophysiology of multiple sclerosis. In Waxman SG: "Advances in Neurology: Functional Recovery in Neurological Disease", New York: Raven Press, pp 157-183.

Waxman SG (1989). Demyelination in spinal cord injury. J Neurol Sci 91:1-14.

Young W (1989). Recovery mechanisms in spinal cord injury: Implications for regenerative therapy. In Seil FJ (ed): "Neural Regeneration and Transplantation", New York: Alan R. Liss, pp 157-169.

Index

A23187, 279
Acetylated tubulin, antibody to, growth cone
    guidance, 13
Acetylcholine
    neuromuscular junctions, synaptic competi-
        tion at, living mice, 39
    neurotransmitter phenotype regulation, de-
        veloping SCG sympathetic neurons,
        rat, 25, 26
    and spinal cord transection, motor neuron
        linkages with muscles, rats, 369
Acetylcholine receptors, 97
    axonal growth and synaptic plasticity, 2
    neuromuscular junctions, synaptic competi-
        tion at, living mice, 34, 35, 39
    postsynaptic loss of, 37
Acetylcholinesterase, 21, 22, 24, 25, 95, 97
β-Actin, gene expression in lesion-induced syn-
    aptogenesis, rats, 72, 73, 79–82, 84
Afferent fibers, group I, 220
Afferent input, increased response to, chronic
    spinal cord transection, partial recov-
    ery of function, cat, 336, 337
A fibers, 332, 333, 337
Alzheimer's disease, 4, 95
Amino acid sequence, fibroblast growth factor,
    basic, 116
4-Aminopyridine, 245–247
β-Amyloid precursor proteins, 112
Angiotensin, 112
ANT-C homeobox gene, 291, 293
Antenna disc, *Drosophila*, 317
Antennapedia-like homeobox genes, 291, 292
Anteroposterior axis and differentiation, verte-
    brate neural tube patterning,
    homeobox genes, 291–293, 305
Anti-NGF, spinal cord transection, motor neuron
    linkages with muscles, rats, 376
AP-1 transcription complex, NGF synthesis in-
    crease after sciatic nerve lesion, 126,

128, 130–132
APV, NMDA antagonist, 51
Aspartate, astroctyes, swelling-induced mem-
    brane transport changes, EAA release,
    207, 209–211
4-di-2-ASP, mitochondria stained in nerve ter-
    minals, 38
Astrocytes/astroglia
    cellular composition, 161
    CNS-PNS interface, 162, 188, 189
    cytokine responses, 163–164
    density in white vs. gray matter, 162
    fetal, transplants, and axonal growth in-
        crease, 172
    fibroblast growth factor, basic, 110, 116
    functions, 162–165
        blood-brain barrier, 162, 164
        potassium buffer, 163
    GFAP-positive, voltage-gated ion channels,
        satellite cells, 239–240, 245, 249, 250
    in injury and regeneration, 162, 165
        development, 162
    interaction with neuron growth cone, axonal
        regeneration, dorsal root transitional
        zone, adult mammals, 227–234
    -leptomeningeal interface, 191
    mediation of axon/neurite outgrowth,
        171–181
        axon growth inhibtion, lesioned CNS,
            174–175
        cell-cell interaction role, 175–177
        changes during development, 177–180
        channels, 176–177
        immature vs. mature, in vitro, 173–174
    neuritogenic factor secretion, 147, 148–153
        factor depletion effect, 148–149
    neurotrophic proteins supporting long-term
        brain neuron survival, 147, 153–154,
        156
        hippocampal neurons, 153, 154